Dandy
(1886-1946)

Grashey
(1876-1950)

Sweet
(1860-1926)

Law
(1875-1947)

Caldwell
(1870-1918)

Béclère, A.
(1856-1939)

Graham
(1883-1957)

MERRILL'S ATLAS OF
RADIOGRAPHIC POSITIONING & PROCEDURES

FIFTEENTH EDITION | VOLUME TWO

MERRILL'S ATLAS OF
RADIOGRAPHIC
POSITIONING
& PROCEDURES

Jeannean Hall Rollins, MRC, BSRT(R)(CV)(M)
Associate Professor
Medical Imaging and Radiation Sciences Department
Arkansas State University
Jonesboro, Arkansas

Bruce W. Long, MS, RT(R)(CV), FASRT, FAEIRS
Associate Professor, Emeritus
Radiologic and Imaging Sciences Programs
Indiana University School of Medicine
Indianapolis, Indiana

Tammy Curtis, PhD, RT(R)(CT)(CHES)
Professor and Program Director
Radiologic Sciences and School of Allied Health
Northwestern State University
Shreveport, Louisiana

ELSEVIER

Elsevier
3251 Riverport Lane
St. Louis, Missouri 63043

MERRILL'S ATLAS OF RADIOGRAPHIC POSITIONING
AND PROCEDURES, EDITION 15

ISBN: 978-0-323-83280-9 (vol 1)
ISBN: 978-0-323-83281-6 (vol 2)
ISBN: 978-0-323-83282-3 (vol 3)
ISBN: 978-0-323-83279-3 (set)

Notice

Practitioners and researchers must always rely on their own experience and knowledge in evaluating
and using any information, methods, compounds or experiments described herein. Because of rapid
advances in the medical sciences, in particular, independent verification of diagnoses and drug dosages
should be made. To the fullest extent of the law, no responsibility is assumed by Elsevier, authors, editors
or contributors for any injury and/or damage to persons or property as a matter of products liability,
negligence or otherwise, or from any use or operation of any methods, products, instructions, or ideas
contained in the material herein.

Previous editions copyrighted 2019, 2016, 2012, 2007, 2003, 1999, 1995, 1991, 1986, 1982, 1975, 1967, 1959, and 1949.

Library of Congress Control Number: 2021947699

Executive Content Strategist: Sonya Seigafuse
Director, Content Development: Laurie Gower
Content Development Specialist: Betsy McCormac
Publishing Services Manager: Julie Eddy
Book Production Specialist: Clay S. Broeker
Design Direction: Brian Salisbury

Printed in India

Last digit is the print number: 9   8   7   6   5   4   3   2   1

PREVIOUS AUTHORS

Vinita Merrill, 1905-1977, Vinita Merrill was born in Oklahoma in 1905 and died in New York City in 1977. Vinita began compilation of *Merrill's* in 1936 while she worked as Technical Director and Chief Technologist in the Department of Radiology and Instructor in the School of Radiography at the New York Hospital. In 1949, while employed as Director of the Educational Department of Picker X-Ray Corporation, she wrote the first edition of the *Atlas of Roentgenographic Positions.* She completed three more editions from 1959 to 1975. Seventy-four years later, Vinita's work lives on in the fifteenth edition of *Merrill's Atlas of Radiographic Positioning & Procedures.*

Philip W. Ballinger, PhD, RT(R), FASRT, FAEIRS, became the author of *Merrill's Atlas* in its fifth edition, which was published in 1982. He served as author through the tenth edition, helping to launch successful careers for thousands of students who have learned radiographic positioning from *Merrill's.* Phil currently serves as Professor Emeritus in Radiologic Sciences and Therapy, Division of the School of Health and Rehabilitation Sciences, at The Ohio State University. In 1995, he retired after a 25-year career as Radiography Program Director and, after ably guiding *Merrill's Atlas* through six editions, he retired as *Merrill's* author. Phil continues to be involved in professional activities such as speaking engagements at state, national, and international meetings.

Eugene D. Frank, MA, RT(R), FASRT, FAEIRS, began working with Phil Ballinger on the eighth edition of *Merrill's Atlas* in 1995. He became the coauthor in its ninth, 50th anniversary edition, published in 1999. He served as lead author for the eleventh and twelfth editions and mentored three coauthors. Gene retired from the Mayo Clinic/Foundation in Rochester, Minnesota, in 2001 after 31 years of employment. He was Associate Professor of Radiology in the College of Medicine and Director of the Radiography Program. He also served as Director of the Radiography Program at Riverland Community College, Austin, Minnesota, for 6 years before fully retiring in 2007. He is a Fellow of the ASRT and AEIRS. In addition to *Merrill's*, he is the coauthor of two radiography textbooks, *Quality Control in Diagnostic Imaging* and *Radiography Essentials for Limited Practice.* He continues to help radiography programs by teaching courses for sabbaticals and helps equip x-ray departments in West Africa with equipment.

Barbara J. Smith, MS, RT(R)(QM), FASRT, FAEIRS, is an instructor in the Radiologic Technology program at Portland Community College, where she has taught for 34 years. The Oregon Society of Radiologic Technologists inducted her as a Life Member in 2003. She presents at state, regional, national, and international meetings, was a trustee with the American Registry of Radiologic Technologists (ARRT), and is involved in professional activities at these levels. Her publication activities include articles, book reviews, and chapter contributions. Currently, she serves as chair of the Oregon Radiation Advisory Committee. As coauthor for four editions, Barb's role with the *Merrill's* team was working with the contributing authors and editing Volume 3.

THE MERRILL'S TEAM

Jeannean Hall Rollins, MRC, BSRT(R) (CV)(M), is an Associate Professor in the Medical Imaging and Radiation Sciences department at Arkansas State University, where she has taught for 30 years. She presents regularly at national meetings. Her publication activities include articles, book reviews, and chapter contributions. The fifteenth edition is Jeannean's first as the lead author and fifth time on the *Merrill's* team. She is also sharing responsibility for revising the workbook with Dr. Tammy Curtis on this edition. Her first contribution to *Merrill's Atlas* was on the tenth edition as coauthor of the trauma radiography chapter. Prior to becoming a coauthor on the textbook, Jeannean was responsible for revising the workbook, *Mosby's Radiography Online,* and the *Evolve Instructor Electronic Resources* that accompany *Merrill's Atlas.*

Bruce W. Long, MS, RT(R)(CV), FASRT, FAEIRS, is Associate Professor Emeritus of the Indiana University Radiologic and Imaging Sciences Programs, where he taught for 35 years. A Life Member of the Indiana Society of Radiologic Technologists, he frequently presented at state and national professional meetings. His publication activities include 28 articles in national professional journals and two books, *Orthopaedic Radiography* and *Radiography Essentials for Limited Practice,* in addition to being coauthor of the *Atlas.* The fifteenth edition is Bruce's fifth on the *Merrill's* team, with two editions as lead author.

Tammy Curtis, PhD, RT(R)(CT)(CHES), is a Professor and Director of the Radiologic Sciences Program at Northwestern State University, where she has taught for 20 years. She presents at the state, regional, and national levels and is involved in professional activities at the state and national levels. Her publication activities include articles, book reviews, and book contributions. Previously, Tammy served on the advisory board and submitted several projects to the *Atlas.* In particular, for the twelfth edition, Tammy submitted an updated photo and biography of the original author, Vinita Merrill, which she discovered after a 3-year search of historical records. The fifteenth edition is Tammy's first as a coauthor of the textbook and third time as part of the *Merrill's* team. In addition, she is sharing the workbook revision responsibilities with Jeannean Rollins for the fifteenth edition. Her previous role on the *Merrill's* team was to update the workbook and work with the coauthors of the textbook to review content for all three volumes.

ADVISORY BOARD

This edition of *Merrill's Atlas* benefits from the expertise of a special advisory board. The following board members have provided professional input and advice and have helped the authors make decisions about *Atlas* content throughout the preparation of the fifteenth edition.

Kellie Cranfill, MSRS, RT(R)(BD)
Program Director of the IU Radiologic & Imaging Sciences Programs
Program Director for the IU Radiography Program
Assistant Professor of Clinical Radiologic & Imaging Sciences
Indiana University Purdue University at Indianapolis (IUPUI)
Indianapolis, IN

Kimberly Cross, MSRS, RT(R)(CT)
Clinical Coordinator and Assistant Program Director
Emory University Medical Imaging Program
Emory Department of Radiology and Imaging Sciences
Atlanta, Georgia

Parsha Y. Hobson, MPA, RT(R)
Professor, Program Director, and Chairperson
Radiography, Public Health, Health Sciences, and Health Information
Passaic County Community College
Paterson, New Jersey

James G. Murrell, EdD, RT(R)(M)(QM) (CT), CRT(R)(F), FAEIRS
Campus Director and Executive Program Director
Gurnick Academy of Medical Arts
Los Angeles, California

Christine Preachuk, RT(R), CAE
Manager
Diagnostic Imaging Program for X-Ray and Mammography
Health Sciences Centre, Shared Health Manitoba
Winnipeg, Canada

Marilyn J. Lewis Thompson, MBA, RT(R) (M)
Clinical Coordinator
Saint Luke's School of Radiologic Technology
Saint Luke's Hospital of Kansas City
Kansas City, Missouri

CHAPTER CONTENT EXPERTS

J. Tyler Carter, MSHS, RT(R)(CT) (ARRT)
Chief Technologist
Piggott Community Hospital
Paragould, Arkansas

Derek Carver, MEd, RT(R)(MR) (ARRT)
Department of Radiology
Boston Children's Hospital
Boston, Massachusetts

Jennifer G. Chiu, EdD, MBA, RT(R) (CT)(ARRT)
Associate Professor and Program
   Director
St. John's University
Queens, New York

Rex T. Christensen, MHA, RT(R)(MR) (CT)(ARRT), CIIP, MRSO
Associate Professor
Radiologic Sciences
Weber State University
Ogden, Utah

Steven G. Hayes Jr., MSRS, RT(R) (ARRT)
Instructor
Radiologic Sciences
Ivy Tech Community College
Indianapolis, Indiana

Garrett Johnson, BSRS RT(R)(ARRT)
Radiologic Technologist
St. Bernard's Medical Center
Jonesboro, Arkansas

Raymond J. Johnson, BS, CNMT
Radiology/Nuclear Medicine
John Peter Smith Health Network
Fort Worth, Texas

Rebecca H. Keith, MS, RT(R)(CT) (ARRT)
Assistant Professor
Radiography/MRI
Tidewater Community College
Virginia Beach, Virginia

Machele D. Michels, RT(R)(T)(CT) (ARRT), CMD
Certified Medical Dosimetrist
Radiation Oncology
Mayo Clinic
Rochester, Minnesota

Zaidalynet Morales, MS, RT(R)(CT) (ARRT)
Associate Professor
St. John's University
Queens, New York

Cheryl Morgan-Duncan, MAS, RT(R)(M)(ARRT)
Assistant Professor and Clinical
   Coordinator
Radiography Program
Passaic County Community College
Staff Mammographer
St. Joseph's University Medical Center
Paterson, New Jersey

Elizabeth Nelson, MSRS, RT(R)(MR) (ARRT), MRSO
Lead MRI Technologist
Highland Clinic, APMC
Shreveport, Louisiana

Susanna L. Ovel, RT, RDMS, RVT
Senior Sonographer and Clinical
   Instructor
Medical Imaging
Sutter Medical Foundation
Sacramento, California

Carolyn Palazzolo, MBA, MS, RT(R) (CT)(QM)(ARRT)
CT Technologist
Rutland Regional Medical Center
Rutland, Vermont

Lynette Petrie, MEd, RT(R)(CV) (ARRT)
Vascular and Interventional Radiologic
   Technologist
Cape Coral, Florida

Bartram J. Pierce, BS, RT(R)(MR) (ARRT), MRSO
Adjunct Professor
Medical Imaging
Portland Community College
Albany, Oregon

Sharon R. Wartenbee, RT(R)(BD) (ARRT), CBDT, FASRT
Senior Bone Densitometry Technologist
Avera Medical Group McGreevy Clinic
Sioux Falls, South Dakota

Haneen Zeidan, MSRS, RT(R)(M) (ARRT)
Mammography Technologist
Christus Health
Shreveport, Louisiana

PREFACE

Welcome to the fifteenth edition of *Merrill's Atlas of Radiographic Positioning & Procedures.* This edition continues the tradition of excellence begun in 1949, when Vinita Merrill wrote the first edition of what has become a classic text. For more than 70 years, *Merrill's Atlas* has provided a strong foundation in anatomy and positioning for thousands of students around the world who have gone on to successful careers as imaging technologists. *Merrill's Atlas* is also a mainstay for everyday reference in imaging departments all over the world. As the coauthors of the fifteenth edition, we are honored to follow in Vinita Merrill's footsteps.

Learning and Perfecting Positioning Skills

Merrill's Atlas has an established tradition of helping students learn and perfect their positioning skills. After covering preliminary steps in radiography, radiation protection, and terminology in the introductory chapters, the first two volumes of the *Atlas* teach anatomy and positioning in separate chapters for each bone group or organ system. The student learns to position the patient properly so that the resulting radiograph provides the information the physician needs to correctly diagnose the patient's problem. The *Atlas* presents this information for commonly requested projections as well as for those less commonly requested, making it the only reference of its kind in the world.

The third volume provides basic information about a variety of special imaging modalities, such as mobile and surgical imaging, pediatrics, geriatrics, computed tomography (CT), vascular radiology, magnetic resonance imaging (MRI), sonography, nuclear medicine technology, bone densitometry, and radiation therapy.

Merrill's Atlas is not only a comprehensive resource to help students learn but also an indispensable reference as they move into the clinical environment and ultimately into practice as imaging professionals.

New to This Edition

Since the first edition of *Merrill's Atlas* in 1949, many changes have occurred. This new edition incorporates many significant changes designed not only to reflect the technologic progress and advancements in the profession but also to meet the needs of today's radiography students. The major changes in this edition are highlighted as follows.

NEW PATIENT PHOTOGRAPHY

All patient positioning photographs have been replaced in Chapter 6. Additional new patient positioning photographs have been strategically added to replace or better illustrate diagrams. The new photographs show positioning detail to a greater extent and in some cases from a more realistic perspective. In addition, the equipment featured in the new photos is modern, thus providing students with a more realistic visual learning tool. The use of electronic central ray angle indicators enables a better understanding of where the central ray should enter the patient and the exact angle when required.

UPDATED GONADAL SHIELDING GUIDELINES

The most significant recent change in our profession has been the American Association of Physicists in Medicine (AAPM) position statement entitled *AAPM Position Statement on the Use of Patient Gonadal and Fetal Shielding.* The author team, along with the help of the Advisory Board, have made every attempt to abide by this position statement while still considering state law that affect the practice of many technologists and students. The "*Shield gonads*" statement has been removed from Chapters 4 and 8 in accordance with the AAPM recommendations. Additionally, Chapter 1 has been revised to explain how to handle questions from patients regarding gonadal shielding.

COLLIMATION AND EXPOSURE FIELD SIZE

Taking into consideration the recent recommendations to discontinue gonadal shielding for some exams, greater emphasis has been placed on collimation size and field light coverage as radiation protection measures. In addition, collimation parameters are increasingly important because many imaging departments use only a single, large image receptor (IR) size. Proper placement of the radiographic marker in the exposure field is described for routine projections.

UPDATES IN THIS EDITION

Color-coded anatomy diagrams have been added to enhance visual learning and better differentiate anatomic details. New charts have been added to Chapter 2 to assist students to master foundational terms more quickly. Essential projections have been revised to match 2022 ARRT Radiography Exam Content Specifications. Best practices that describe specific skills in each discipline were added to all advanced modality chapters, allowing students more insight into the unique environment of each modality. A new section was added to Chapter 21 regarding the O-arm mobile unit. Chapter 22 was expanded to include mobile radiography for neonates in the neonatal intensive care unit (NICU). NICU exam recommendations for performing routine projection and positions are described and supported with new images. In Chapter 24, three-dimensional (3D) advanced visualization was added to include 3D printing for demonstrating sectional anatomy. Chapter 27 has been significantly reorganized to reflect current practice in vascular, cardiac, and interventional radiography.

Learning Aids for the Student

POCKET GUIDE TO RADIOGRAPHY

The new edition of *Merrill's Pocket Guide to Radiography* complements this revision of *Merrill's Atlas.* Instructions for positioning the patient and the body part for all of the essential projections are presented in a complete yet concise manner. The Coyle method for trauma elbow has been added to this edition. Tabs are included to help the user locate the beginning of each section. Space is provided for the user to write in specifics of department techniques.

RADIOGRAPHIC POSITIONING AND PROCEDURES WORKBOOK

The new edition of this workbook features extensive review and self-assessment exercises that supplement the first 25 chapters in *Merrill's Atlas* in one convenient volume. Relevant material was updated to current practice and integrated into appropriate chapters. Terminology remains consistent to match the Content Specifications for the ARRT Radiography Examination, the ASRT Radiography Curriculum, and the evolution of digital imaging. New questions were developed to assess the newly added content in the textbook that reflects current ARRT content specifications. The features of the previous editions, including anatomy labeling exercises, positioning exercises, and self-tests, are still available. This edition features image evaluations to give students additional opportunities to evaluate radiographs for proper positioning and positioning questions to complement the workbook's strong anatomy review. The comprehensive multiple-choice tests at the end of each chapter help students assess their comprehension of the whole chapter. New exercises in this edition focus on improved understanding of essential projections and the need for appropriate collimated field sizes for digital imaging. Additionally, review and assessment exercises have been expanded for the chapters on pediatrics, reproductive system, mobile, surgical, geriatrics, sectional anatomy, vascular, and interventional radiography. Exercises in these chapters help students learn the theory and concepts of these special techniques with greater ease. Answers to the workbook questions are found on the Evolve website.

Teaching Aids for the Instructor

EVOLVE INSTRUCTOR ELECTRONIC RESOURCES

This comprehensive resource provides valuable tools such as lesson plans, PowerPoint slides, and an electronic test bank for teaching an anatomy and positioning class. The test bank includes more than 1500 questions, each coded by category and level of difficulty. Four exams are already compiled in the test bank to be used "as is" at the instructor's discretion. The instructor also has the option of building new tests as often as desired by pulling questions from the ExamView pool or using a combination of questions from the test bank and questions that the instructor adds.

Evolve may be used to publish the class syllabus, outlines, and lecture notes; set up "virtual office hours" and e-mail communication; share important dates and information through the online class calendar; and encourage student participation through chat rooms and discussion boards. Evolve allows instructors to post exams and manage their grade books online. For more information, visit www.evolve.elsevier.com or contact an Elsevier sales representative.

MOSBY'S RADIOGRAPHY ONLINE

Mosby's Radiography Online: Merrill's Atlas of Radiographic Positioning & Procedures is a well-developed online course companion for the textbook and workbook. This online course includes animations with narrated interactive activities and exercises, as well as multiple-choice assessments that can be tailored to meet the learning objectives of your program or course. The addition of this online course to your teaching resources offers greater learning opportunities while accommodating diverse learning styles and circumstances. This unique program promotes problem-based learning with the goal of developing critical thinking skills that will be needed in the clinical setting.

EVOLVE—ONLINE COURSE MANAGEMENT

Evolve is an interactive learning environment designed to work in coordination with *Merrill's Atlas.* Instructors may use Evolve to provide an Internet-based course component that reinforces and expands on the concepts delivered in class.

We hope you will find this edition of *Merrill's Atlas of Radiographic Positioning & Procedures* the best ever. Input from generations of readers has helped to keep the *Atlas* strong through 14 editions, and we welcome your comments and suggestions. We are constantly striving to build on Vinita Merrill's work, and we trust that she would be proud and pleased to know that the work she began 70 years ago is still so appreciated and valued by the imaging sciences community.

Jeannean Hall Rollins
Bruce W. Long
Tammy Curtis

ACKNOWLEDGMENTS

In preparing for the fifteenth edition, our advisory board continually provided professional expertise and aid in the decision-making on the revision of this edition. The advisory board members are listed on p. ix. We are most grateful for their input and contributions to this edition of the *Atlas*.

Contributors

The group of radiography professionals listed here contributed to this edition of the *Atlas* and made many insightful suggestions. We are most appreciative of their willingness to lend their expertise.

The author team extends special recognition to Jennifer G. Chiu, EdD, MBA, RT(R)(CT)(ARRT), Associate Professor and Program Director at St. John's University in Queens, New York; and Zaidalynet Morales, MS, RT(R)(CT)(ARRT), Associate Professor, also at St. John's University. We are honored to have their expertise as reviewers of all three volumes of this edition. Additionally, they have undertaken the responsibility of revising and updating the *Evolve Instructor Electronic Resources* and *Mosby's Radiography Online: Merrill's Atlas of Radiographic Positioning & Procedures* for this fifteenth edition. We are very thankful and extremely blessed to have their expertise and assistance in maintaining the quality standard that defines *Merrill's Atlas*.

A very special "thank you" to Jon Rollins for agreeing to serve as a positioning model and photography reviewer and editor. Attempting to revise a major textbook during a national quarantine caused many delays, barriers, and obstacles. His willingness to pose for countless hours made the new positioning photos in Chapter 6 possible. Without your support, the team's goals for this fifteenth edition would have not been possible.

Our deepest appreciation to our faith, family, and colleagues, whose support and encouragement remain an indispensable part of this work. Finally, to all of our graduates and students, current and future, this edition is dedicated to you, our greatest teachers and inspiration. Thank you!

CONTENTS

11
CRANIUM

R   L

SUMMARY OF PROJECTIONS

PROJECTIONS, POSITIONS, AND METHODS

Page	Essential	Anatomy	Projection	Position	Method
34	⬥	Skull	Lateral	R or L	
38	⬥	Skull	PA		
38	⬥	Skull	PA axial		CALDWELL
42	⬥	Skull	AP		
42	⬥	Skull	AP axial		REVERSE CALDWELL
44	⬥	Skull	AP axial		TOWNE
50		Skull	PA axial		HAAS
52	⬥	Cranial base	Submentovertical (SMV)		SCHÜLLER
59	⬥	Orbit	Lateral	R or L	
60	⬥	Orbits	PA axial		
61	⬥	Orbits	Parietoacanthial		MODIFIED WATERS
62	⬥	Facial bones	Lateral	R or L	
65	⬥	Facial bones	Parietoacanthial		WATERS
67	⬥	Facial bones	Modified parietoacanthial		MODIFIED WATERS
69		Facial bones	Acanthioparietal		REVERSE WATERS
71	⬥	Facial bones	PA axial		CALDWELL
73	⬥	Nasal bones	Lateral	R and L	
75		Zygomatic arches	Submentovertical		
77		Zygomatic arch	Tangential		
79		Zygomatic arches	AP axial		MODIFIED TOWNE
81	⬥	Mandibular rami	PA		
82	⬥	Mandibular rami	PA axial		
83		Mandibular body	PA		
84		Mandibular body	PA axial		
85	⬥	Mandible	Axiolateral, axiolateral oblique		
88	⬥	Mandible	Submentovertical		
89	⬥	TMJs	AP axial		
91	⬥	TMJs	Axiolateral	R and L	
93	⬥	TMJs	Axiolateral oblique	R and L	
95		Mandible	Panoramic		TOMOGRAPHY
98	⬥	Paranasal sinuses	Lateral	R or L upright	
100	⬥	Frontal and anterior ethmoidal sinuses	PA axial	Upright	CALDWELL
102	⬥	Maxillary sinuses	Parietoacanthial	Upright	WATERS
104		Maxillary and sphenoidal sinuses	Parietoacanthial	Upright with open mouth	WATERS
106	⬥	Ethmoidal and sphenoidal sinuses	Submentovertical	Upright	

Icons in the Essential column indicate projections frequently performed in the United States and Canada. Students should be competent in these projections.

AP, Anteroposterior; *L,* left; *LAO,* left anterior oblique; *PA,* posteroanterior; *R,* right; *RAO,* right anterior oblique.

Skull

The *skull* rests on the superior aspect of the vertebral column. It is composed of 22 separate bones divided into two distinct groups: 8 *cranial* bones and 14 *facial* bones. The cranial bones are divided further into the *calvaria* and the *floor* (Box 11.1). The cranial bones form a protective housing for the brain. The facial bones provide structure, shape, and support for the face. They also form a protective housing for the upper ends of the respiratory and digestive tracts and, with several of the cranial bones, form the orbital sockets for protection of the organs of sight. The *hyoid bone* is commonly discussed with this group of bones.

The bones of the skull are identified in Figs. 11.1–11.3. The 22 primary bones of the skull should be located and recognized in the different views before they are studied in greater detail.

BOX 11.1
Skull Bones

Cranial bones (8)		Facial bones (14)	
Calvaria		Nasal (right and left)	2
Frontal	1	Lacrimal (right and left)	2
Occipital	1	Maxillary (right and left)	2
Right parietal	1	Zygomatic (right and left)	2
Left parietal	1	Palatine (right and left)	2
Floor		Inferior nasal conchae (right and left)	2
Ethmoid	1	Vomer	1
Sphenoid	1	Mandible	1
Right temporal	1		
Left temporal	1		

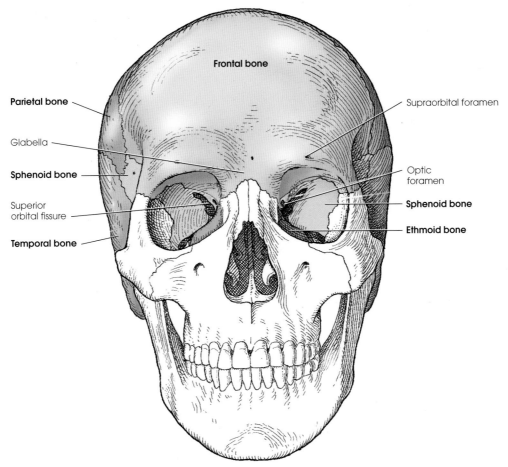

Fig. 11.1 Anterior aspect of cranium.

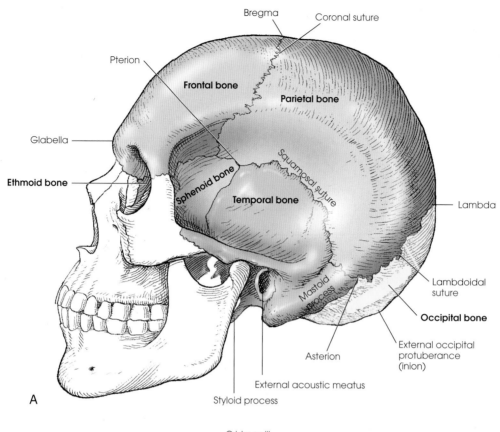

Bregma
Coronal suture
Pterion
Frontal bone
Parietal bone
Glabella
Squamosal suture
Ethmoid bone
Sphenoid bone
Lambda
Temporal bone
Lambdoidal suture
Mastoid process
Occipital bone
External occipital protuberance (inion)
Asterion
External acoustic meatus
Styloid process
A

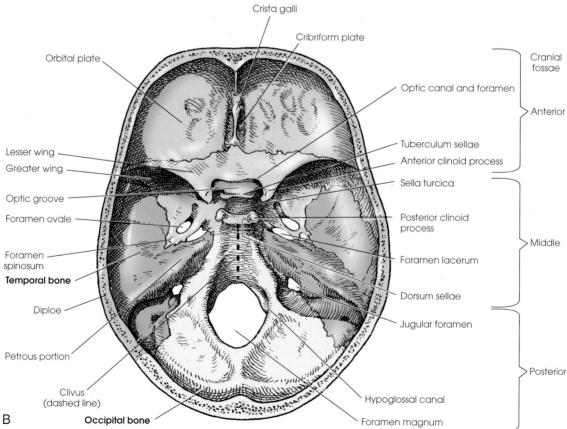

Crista galli
Cribriform plate
Orbital plate
Cranial fossae
Optic canal and foramen
Anterior
Lesser wing
Tuberculum sellae
Greater wing
Anterior clinoid process
Optic groove
Sella turcica
Foramen ovale
Posterior clinoid process
Foramen spinosum
Middle
Temporal bone
Foramen lacerum
Diploe
Dorsum sellae
Jugular foramen
Petrous portion
Clivus (dashed line)
Occipital bone
Hypoglossal canal
Foramen magnum
Posterior
B

Fig. 11.2 (A) Lateral aspect of cranium. (B) Superior aspect of cranial base.

The bones of the cranial vault are composed of two plates of compact tissue separated by an inner layer of spongy tissue called *diploë*. The outer plate, or table, is thicker than the inner table over most of the vault, and the thickness of the layer of spongy tissue varies considerably.

Except for the mandible, the bones of the cranium and face are joined by fibrous joints called *sutures*. The sutures are named *coronal, sagittal, squamosal,* and *lambdoidal* (see Figs. 11.1 and 11.2). The *coronal suture* is found between the frontal and parietal bones. The *sagittal suture* is located on the top of the head between the two parietal bones and just behind the coronal suture line (not visible in Figs. 11.1 and 11.2). The junction of the coronal and sagittal sutures is the *bregma*. Between the temporal bones and the parietal bones are the *squamosal sutures*. Between the occipital bone and the parietal bones is the *lambdoidal suture*. The *lambda* is the junction of the lambdoidal and sagittal sutures. On the lateral aspect of the skull, the junction of the parietal bone, squamosal suture, and greater wing of the sphenoid is the *pterion*, which overlies the middle meningeal artery. At the junction of the occipital bone, parietal bone, and mastoid portion of the temporal bone is the *asterion*.

A

B

Fig. 11.3 (A) Lateral aspect of interior of cranium. (B) Sagittal magnetic resonance imaging of cranium showing contents and position of brain. Note bony protective housing.

5

In a newborn infant, the bones of the cranium are thin and not fully developed. They contain a small amount of calcium, are indistinctly marked, and present six areas of incomplete ossification called *fontanels*, often spelled *fontanelles* (Fig. 11.4). Two of the fontanels are situated in the midsagittal plane (MSP) at the superior and posterior angles of the parietal bones. The *anterior fontanel* is located at the junction of the two parietal bones and the one frontal bone at the bregma. Posteriorly and in MSP is the *posterior fontanel*, located at the point labeled *lambda* in Fig. 11.2. Two fontanels are also on each side at the inferior angles of the parietal bones. Each *sphenoidal fontanel* is found at the site of the pterion; the *mastoid fontanels* are found at the asteria. The posterior and sphenoidal fontanels normally close in the first and third months after birth, and the anterior and mastoid fontanels close during the second year of life.

The cranium develops rapidly in size and density during the first 5 or 6 years, after which a gradual increase occurs until adult size and density are achieved, usually by the age of 12 years. The thickness and degree of mineralization in normal adult crania show comparatively little difference in radiopacity from person to person, and the atrophy of old age is less marked than in other regions of the body.

Internally, the cranial floor is divided into three regions: anterior, middle, and posterior cranial fossae (see Fig. 11.2B). The *anterior cranial fossa* extends from the anterior frontal bone to the lesser wings of the sphenoid. It is associated mainly with the frontal lobes of the cerebrum. The *middle cranial fossa* accommodates the temporal lobes and associated neurovascular structures and extends from the lesser wings of the sphenoid bone to the apices of petrous portions of the temporal bones. The deep depression posterior to the petrous ridges is the *posterior cranial fossa*, which protects the cerebellum, pons, and medulla oblongata (see Fig. 11.3B).

The average or so-called normal cranium is more or less oval in shape, wider in back than in front. The average cranium measures approximately 6 inches (15 cm) at its widest point from side to side, 7 inches (17.8 cm) at its longest point from front to back, and 9 inches (22 cm) at its deepest point from the vertex to the submental region. Crania vary in size and shape, with resultant variation in the position and relationship of internal parts.

Internal deviations from the norm are usually indicated by external deviations and can be estimated with a reasonable degree of accuracy. The length and width of the normally shaped head vary by 1 inch (2.5 cm). Any deviation from this relationship indicates a comparable change in the position and relationship of the internal structures. If the deviation involves more than a 5-degree change, it must be compensated for by a change in part rotation or central ray angulation. This "rule" applies to all images except direct lateral projections. A ½-inch (1.3 cm) change in the 1-inch (2.5-cm) width-to-length measurement indicates an approximately 5-degree change in the direction of the internal parts with reference to MSP.

It is important for the radiographer to understand cranial anatomy from the standpoint of the size, shape, position, and relationship of component parts of the cranium, so that estimations and compensations can be made for deviations from the norm.

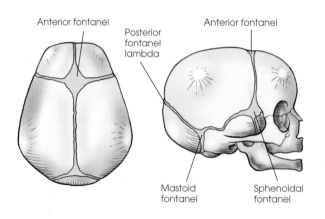

Superior aspect   Lateral aspect

Fig. 11.4 Fontanels of a newborn.

Cranial Bones

FRONTAL BONE

The *frontal bone* has a vertical portion and horizontal portions. The vertical portion, called the *frontal squama*, forms the forehead and the anterior part of the vault. The horizontal portions form the orbital plates (roofs of the orbits), part of the roof of the nasal cavity, and the greater part of the anterior cranial fossa (Figs. 11.5–11.7).

On each side of the MSP of the superior portion of the squama is a rounded elevation called the *frontal eminence*. Below the frontal eminences, just above the *supraorbital margins*, are two arched ridges that correspond in position to the eyebrows. These ridges are called the *superciliary arches*. In the center of the supraorbital margin is an opening for nerves and blood vessels called the *supraorbital foramen*. The smooth elevation between the superciliary arches is termed the *glabella*.

The *frontal sinuses* (Fig. 11.8) are situated between the two tables of the squama on each side of MSP. These irregularly shaped sinuses are separated by a bony wall, which may be incomplete and usually deviates from the midline.

The squama articulates with the parietal bones at the coronal suture, the greater wing of the sphenoid bone at the frontosphenoidal suture, and the nasal bones at the frontonasal suture. The midpoint of the frontonasal suture is termed the *nasion*.

The frontal bone articulates with the right and left parietals, the sphenoid, and the ethmoid bones of the cranium.

The *orbital plates* of the horizontal portion of the frontal bone are separated by a notch called the *ethmoidal notch*. This notch receives the cribriform plate of the ethmoid bone. At the anterior edge of the ethmoidal notch is a small inferior projection of bone, the *nasal spine*, which is the superior-most component of the bony nasal septum. The posterior margins of the orbital plates articulate with the lesser wings of the sphenoid bone.

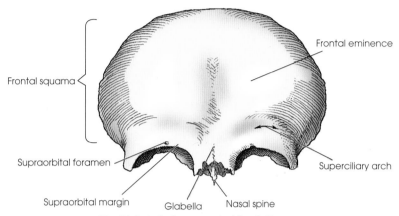

Fig. 11.5 Anterior aspect of frontal bone.

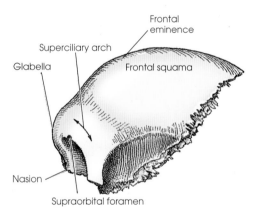

Fig. 11.6 Lateral aspect of frontal bone.

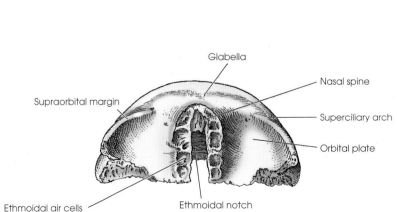

Fig. 11.7 Inferior aspect of frontal bone.

Fig. 11.8 Coronal CT image of frontal sinuses.

(Courtesy Heath Yarbrough, RT(R)(MR)(CT), NEA Baptist Memorial Hospital, Jonesboro, AR.)

ETHMOID BONE

The *ethmoid bone* is a small, cube-shaped bone that consists of a horizontal plate; a vertical plate; and two light, spongy lateral masses called *labyrinths* (Figs. 11.9–11.12). Situated between the orbits, the ethmoid bone forms part of the anterior cranial fossa, the nasal cavity and orbital walls, and the bony nasal septum.

The horizontal portion of the ethmoid bone, called the *cribriform plate*, is received into the ethmoidal notch of the frontal bone. The cribriform plate is perforated by many foramina for the transmission of olfactory nerves. The plate also has a thick, conical process, the *crista galli*, which projects superiorly from its anterior midline and serves as the anterior attachment for the falx cerebri.

The vertical portion of the ethmoid bone is called the *perpendicular plate*. This plate is a thin, flat bone that projects inferiorly from the inferior surface of the cribriform plate and, with the nasal spine, forms the superior portion of the bony septum of the nose.

The *labyrinths* contain the *ethmoidal sinuses*, or air cells. The cells of each side are arbitrarily divided into three groups: the *anterior*, *middle*, and *posterior ethmoidal air cells* (see Fig. 11.12A and B). The walls of the labyrinths form part of the medial walls of the orbits and part of the lateral walls of the nasal cavity. Projecting inferiorly from each medial wall of the labyrinths are two thin, scroll-shaped processes called the *superior* and *middle nasal conchae*.

The ethmoid bone articulates with the frontal and sphenoid bones of the cranium.

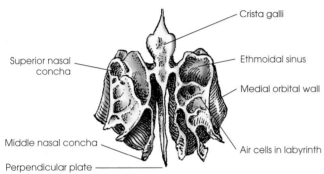
Fig. 11.9 Anterior aspect of ethmoid bone.

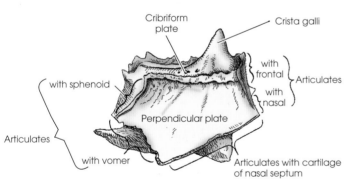
Fig. 11.10 Lateral aspect of ethmoid bone with labyrinth removed.

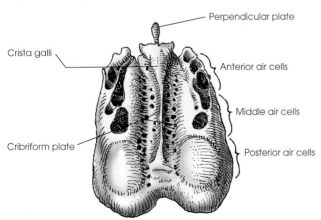
Fig. 11.11 Superior aspect of ethmoid bone.

Fig. 11.12 (A) Coronal CT image of ethmoidal sinuses. (B) Axial CT scan of ethmoidal sinus. *MS,* Maxillary sinuses.

(Courtesy Bryan Harrison, RT(R) (CT), NEA Baptist Memorial Hospital, Jonesboro, AR.)

PARIETAL BONES

The two *parietal bones* are square and have a convex external surface and a concave internal surface (Figs. 11.13 and 11.14). The parietal bones form a large portion of the sides of the cranium. They also form the posterior portion of the cranial roof by their articulation with each other at the sagittal suture in the MSP.

Each parietal bone presents a prominent bulge, called the *parietal eminence*, near the central portion of its external surface.

In radiography, the width of the head should be measured at this point because it is the widest point of the head.

Each parietal bone articulates with the frontal, temporal, occipital, sphenoid, and opposite parietal bones of the cranium.

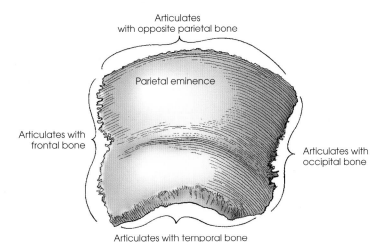

Fig. 11.13 External surface of parietal bone.

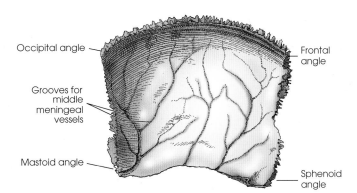

Fig. 11.14 Internal surface of parietal bone.

SPHENOID BONE

The *sphenoid bone* is an irregularly wedge-shaped bone that resembles a bat with its wings extended. It is situated in the base of the cranium anterior to the temporal bones and basilar part of the occipital bone (Figs. 11.15–11.17). The sphenoid bone consists of a body; two lesser wings and two greater wings, which project laterally from the sides of the body; and two pterygoid processes, which project inferiorly from each side of the inferior surface of the body.

The *body* of the sphenoid bone contains the two *sphenoidal sinuses*, which are incompletely separated by a median septum (see Figs. 11.15B and 11.17). The anterior surface of the body forms the posterior bony wall of the nasal cavity. The superior surface presents a deep depression called the *sella turcica* and contains a gland called the *pituitary gland*. The sella turcica lies in the MSP of the cranium at a point ¾ inch (1.9 cm) anterior and ¾ inch (1.9 cm) superior to the level of the *external acoustic meatus* (EAM). The

A

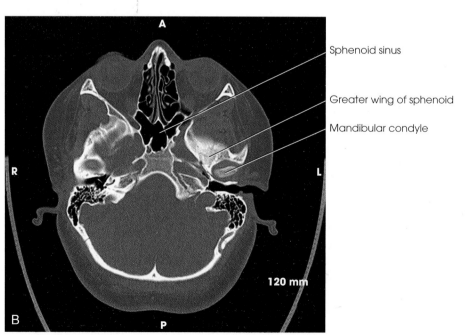

Fig. 11.15 (A) Superior aspect of sphenoid bone. (B) Axial CT scan of sphenoid bone.

(B, Courtesy Bryan Harrison, RT(R)(CT), NEA Baptist Memorial Hospital, Jonesboro, AR.)

sella turcica is bounded anteriorly by the *tuberculum sellae* and posteriorly by the *dorsum sellae*, which bears the *posterior clinoid processes* (see Fig. 11.16B). The slanted area of bone posterior and inferior to the dorsum sellae is continuous with the basilar portion of the occipital bone and is called the *clivus*. The clivus supports the pons. On either side of the sella turcica is a groove, the *carotid sulcus*, in which the internal carotid artery and the cavernous sinus lie.

The *optic groove* extends across the anterior portion of the tuberculum sellae. The groove ends on each side at the *optic canal*. The optic canal is the opening into the apex of the orbit for the transmission of the optic nerve and ophthalmic artery. The actual opening is called the *optic foramen*.

The *lesser wings* are triangular in shape and nearly horizontal in position. They arise, one on each side, from the anterosuperior portion of the body of the sphenoid bone and project laterally, ending in sharp points. The lesser wings form the posteromedial portion of the roofs of the orbits, the posterior portion of the anterior cranial fossa, the upper margin of the *superior orbital fissures,* and the optic canals. The medial ends of their posterior borders form the *anterior clinoid processes*. Each process arises from two roots. The anterior (superior) root is thin and flat, and the posterior (inferior) root, referred to as the *sphenoid strut*, is thick and rounded. The circular opening between the two roots is the *optic canal*.

The *greater wings* arise from the sides of the body of the sphenoid bone and curve laterally, posteriorly, anteriorly, and superiorly. The greater wings form part of the middle cranial fossa, the posterolateral walls of the orbits, the lower margin of the superior orbital sulci, and the greater part of the posterior margin of the inferior orbital sulci. The *foramina rotundum, ovale*, and *spinosum* are paired and are situated in the greater wings. Because these foramina transmit nerves and blood vessels, they are subject to radiologic investigation for the detection of erosive lesions of neurogenic or vascular origin.

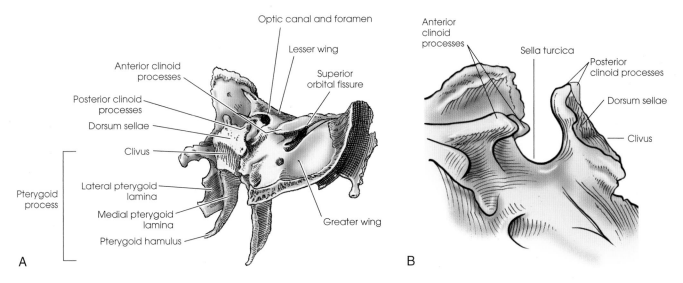

Fig. 11.16 (A) Oblique aspect of upper and lateroposterior aspects of sphenoid bone (right lateral pterygoid lamina removed). (B) Sella turcica of sphenoid bone, lateral view.

Fig. 11.17 Sagittal CT scan of sella turcica and sphenoid sinus.

(Courtesy Natalie Reece, RT(R) (CT)(MR), NEA Baptist Memorial Hospital, Jonesboro, AR.)

The *pterygoid processes* arise from the lateral portions of the inferior surface of the body of the sphenoid bone and the medial portions of the inferior surfaces of the greater wings. These processes project inferiorly and curve laterally. Each pterygoid process consists of two plates of bone, the *medial* and *lateral pterygoid laminae*, which are fused at their supero-anterior parts. The inferior extremity of the medial lamina possesses an elongated, hook-shaped process, the *pterygoid hamulus*, which makes it longer and narrower than the lateral lamina. The pterygoid processes articulate with the palatine bones anteriorly and with the wings of the vomer, where they enter into the formation of the nasal cavity.

The sphenoid bone articulates with each of the other seven bones of the cranium.

OCCIPITAL BONE

The *occipital bone* is situated at the posteroinferior part of the cranium. It forms the posterior half of the base of the cranium and the greater part of the posterior cranial fossa (Figs. 11.18–11.20). The occipital bone has four parts: the *squama*, which is saucer-shaped, being convex externally; *two occipital condyles*, which extend anteriorly, one on each side of the foramen magnum; and the *basilar portion*. The occipital bone also has a large aperture, the *foramen magnum*, through which the inferior portion of the medulla oblongata passes as it exits the cranial cavity and joins the spinal cord.

The *squama* curves posteriorly and superiorly from the foramen magnum and is curved from side to side. It articulates with the parietal bones at the lambdoidal sutures and with the mastoid portions of the temporal bones at the occipitomastoid sutures. On the external surface of the squama, midway between its summit and the foramen magnum, is a prominent process termed the *external occipital protuberance*, or *inion*, which corresponds in position with the *internal occipital protuberance*.

Fig. 11.18 (A) External surface of occipital bone. (B) Coronal CT showing atlantooccipital joint.

(B, Courtesy Siemens Medical Systems, Iselin, NJ.)

The *occipital condyles* project anteriorly, one from each side of the squama, for articulation with the atlas of the cervical spine. Part of each lateral portion curves medially to fuse with the basilar portion and complete the foramen magnum, and part of it projects laterally to form the jugular process. On the inferior surface of the curved parts, extending from the level of the middle of the foramen magnum anteriorly to the level of its anterior margin, reciprocally shaped condyles articulate with superior facets of the atlas. These articulations, known as the *occipitoatlantal joints*, are the only bony articulations between the skull and the neck. The *hypoglossal canals* are found at the anterior ends of the condyles and transmit the hypoglossal nerves. At the posterior end of the condyles are the *condylar canals*, through which the emissary veins pass. The anterior portion of the occipital bone contains a deep notch that forms a part of the *jugular foramen* (see Fig. 11.2B). The jugular foramen is an important large opening in the skull for two reasons: It allows blood to drain from the brain via the internal jugular vein, and it lets three cranial nerves pass through it.

The *basilar portion* of the occipital bone curves anteriorly and superiorly to its junction with the body of the sphenoid. In an adult, the basilar part of the occipital bone fuses with the body of the sphenoid bone, resulting in the formation of a continuous bone. The sloping surface of this junction between the dorsum sellae of the sphenoid bone and the basilar portion of the occipital bone is called the *clivus*.

The occipital bone articulates with the two parietals, the two temporal bones and the sphenoid of the cranium, and the first cervical vertebra.

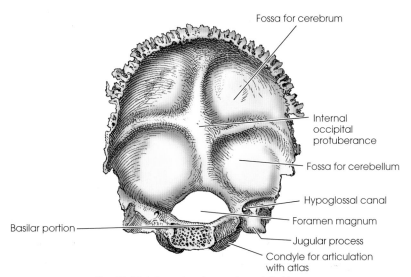

Fig. 11.19 Internal surface of occipital bone.

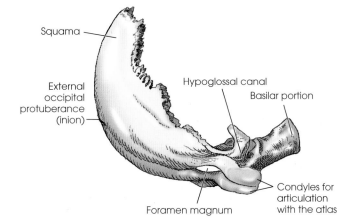

Fig. 11.20 Lateroinferior aspect of occipital bone.

TEMPORAL BONES

The temporal bones are irregular in shape and are situated on each side of the base of the cranium between the greater wings of the sphenoid bone and the occipital bone (Figs. 11.21–11.25). The temporal bones form a large part of the middle fossa of the cranium and a small part of the posterior fossa. Each temporal bone consists of a squamous portion, a tympanic portion, a styloid process, a zygomatic process, and a petromastoid portion (the mastoid and petrous portions) that contains the organs of hearing and balance.

The *squamous portion* is the thin upper portion of the temporal bone. It forms a part of the side wall of the cranium and has a prominent arched process, the *zygomatic process*, which projects anteriorly to articulate with the zygomatic bone of the face and complete the zygomatic arch. On the inferior border of the zygomatic process is a rounded eminence, the *articular tubercle*, which forms the anterior boundary of the *mandibular fossa*. The mandibular fossa receives the condyle of the mandible to form the *temporomandibular joint* (TMJ).

The *tympanic portion* is situated below the squama and in front of the mastoid and petrous portions of the temporal bone. This portion forms the anterior wall, the inferior wall, and part of the posterior walls of the EAM. The EAM is approximately ½ inch (1.3 cm) in length and projects medially, anteriorly, and slightly superiorly.

The *styloid process*, a slender, pointed bone of variable length, projects inferiorly, anteriorly, and slightly medially from the inferior portion of the tympanic part of the temporal bone.

Petromastoid portion

The petrous and mastoid portions together are called the *petromastoid portion*. The mastoid portion, which forms the inferior, posterior part of the temporal bone, is prolonged into the conical *mastoid process* (see Figs. 11.23 and 11.25).

The *mastoid portion* articulates with the parietal bone at its superior border through the parietomastoid suture and with the occipital bone at its posterior border through the occipitomastoid suture, which is contiguous with the lambdoidal suture. The *mastoid process* varies considerably in size, depending on its pneumatization, and is larger in males than in females.

The first of the *mastoid air cells* to develop is situated at the upper anterior part of the process and is termed the *mastoid antrum*. This air cell is quite large and communicates with the tympanic cavity. Shortly before or after birth, smaller air cells begin to develop around the mastoid antrum and continue to increase in number and size until around puberty. The air cells vary considerably in size and number. Occasionally they are absent altogether, in which case the mastoid process is solid bone and is usually small.

The *petrous portion*, often called the *petrous pyramid*, is conical or pyramidal and is the thickest, densest bone in the cranium. This part of the temporal bone contains the organs of hearing and balance. From its base at the squamous and mastoid portions, the petrous portion projects medially and anteriorly between the greater wing of the sphenoid bone and the occipital bone to the body of the sphenoid bone, with which its apex articulates. The internal carotid artery in the *carotid canal* enters the inferior aspect of the petrous portion, passes superior to the cochlea, and then passes medially to exit the *petrous apex*. Near the petrous apex is a ragged foramen called the *foramen lacerum*. The carotid canal opens into this foramen, which contains the internal carotid artery (see Fig. 11.2B). At the center of the posterior aspect of the petrous portion is the *internal acoustic meatus* (IAM), which transmits the vestibulocochlear and facial nerves. The upper border of the petrous portion is commonly referred to as the *petrous ridge*. The top of the ridge lies approximately at the level of an external radiography landmark called the *top of ear attachment* (TEA).

The temporal bone articulates with the parietal, occipital, and sphenoid bones of the cranium.

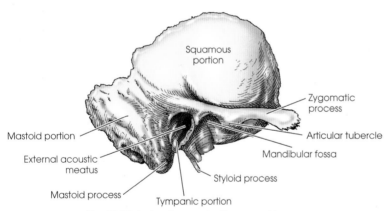

Fig. 11.21 Lateral aspect of temporal bone.

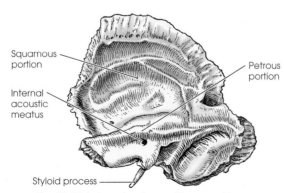

Fig. 11.22 Internal surface of temporal bone.

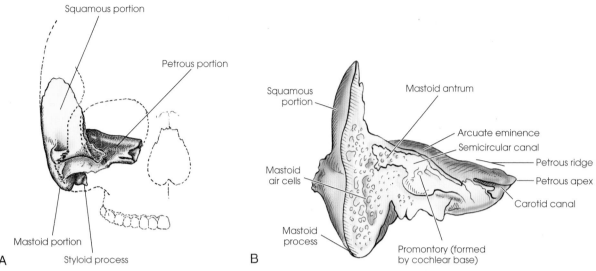

Squamous portion

Petrous portion

Mastoid portion

Styloid process

A

Squamous portion

Mastoid antrum

Arcuate eminence

Semicircular canal

Petrous ridge

Petrous apex

Carotid canal

Mastoid air cells

Mastoid process

Promontory (formed by cochlear base)

B

Fig. 11.23 (A) Anterior aspect of temporal bone in relation to surrounding structures. (B) Coronal section through mastoid and petrous portions of temporal bone.

Mastoid air cells

Auditory ossicles

Cochlea

External auditory meatus

Fig. 11.24 CT scan through temporal bones.

(Courtesy Karl Mockler, RT(R).)

EAM

Mastoid air cells

Petrous portion, temporal bone

Fig. 11.25 Axial CT scan of petrous portion at level of external auditory meatus *(EAM)*.

(Courtesy Kylee Leath, RT(R)(CT), NEA Baptist Memorial Hospital, Jonesboro, AR.)

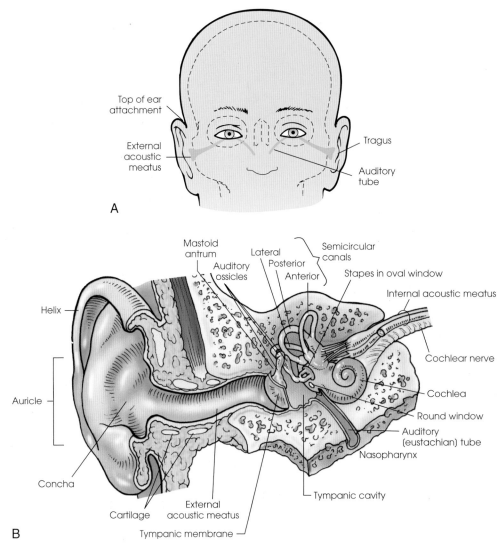

A

B

Fig. 11.26 (A) Frontal view of face showing internal structures of the ear *(shaded area)*. (B) External, middle, and internal ear.

Fig. 11.27 Coronal CT scan through petrous portion of temporal bone showing middle and inner ear.

(Courtesy Karl Mockler, RT(R).)

Fig. 11.28 Coronal CT scan of petromastoid portion of temporal bone showing semicircular canals and mastoid air cells.

(Courtesy Karl Mockler, RT(R).)

Ear

The ear is the organ of hearing and balance (Fig. 11.26). The essential parts of the ear are housed in the petrous portion of the temporal bone. The organs of hearing and equilibrium consist of three main divisions: external ear, middle ear, and internal ear.

EXTERNAL EAR

The *external ear* consists of two parts: (1) the *auricle*, the oval-shaped, fibrocartilaginous, sound-collecting organ situated on the side of the head, and (2) the *EAM*, a sound-conducting canal. The superior attachment of the auricle is the TEA. The TEA is a reference point for positioning the lateral cervical spine. The auricle has a deep central depression, the *concha*, the lower part of which leads into the EAM. At its anterior margin, the auricle has a prominent cartilaginous lip, the *tragus*, which projects posteriorly over the entrance of the meatus. The outer rim of the ear is the *helix*. The EAM is about 1 inch (2.5 cm) long. The outer third of the canal wall is cartilaginous, and the inner two-thirds is osseous. From the meatal orifice, the canal forms a slight curve as it passes medially and anteriorly in line with the axis of the IAM. The EAM ends at the tympanic membrane of the middle ear.

MIDDLE EAR

The *middle ear* is situated between the external ear and the internal ear. The middle ear proper consists of (1) the *tympanic membrane* (or eardrum); (2) an irregularly shaped, air-containing compartment called the *tympanic cavity*; and (3) three small bones called the *auditory ossicles* (see Figs. 11.25 and 11.26). The middle ear communicates with the mastoid antrum and auditory eustachian tube.

The *tympanic membrane* is a thin, concavoconvex, membranous disk with an elliptic shape. The disk, the convex surface of which is directed medially, is situated obliquely over the medial end of the EAM and serves as a partition between the external ear and the middle ear. The function of the tympanic membrane is the transmission of sound vibrations.

The *tympanic cavity* is a narrow, irregularly shaped chamber that lies just posterior and medial to the mandibular fossa. The cavity is separated from the external ear by the tympanic membrane and from the internal ear by the bony labyrinth. The tympanic cavity communicates with the nasopharynx through the *auditory (eustachian) tube*, a passage by which air pressure in the middle ear is equalized with the pressure in the outside air passages. The auditory tube is about 1½ inches (3 cm) long. From its entrance into the tympanic cavity, the auditory tube passes medially and inferiorly to its orifice on the lateral wall of the nasopharynx.

The mastoid antrum is the large air cavity situated in the temporal bone above the mastoid air cells and immediately behind the posterior wall of the middle ear.

The *auditory ossicles,* named for their shape, are the *malleus* (hammer), *incus* (anvil), and *stapes* (stirrup). These three delicate bones are articulated to permit vibratory motion. They bridge the middle ear cavity for the transmission of sound vibrations from the tympanic membrane to the internal ear. The handle of the malleus (the outermost ossicle) is attached to the tympanic membrane, and its head articulates with the incus (the central ossicle). The head of the stapes (the innermost ossicle) articulates with the incus, and its base is fitted into the oval window of the inner ear.

INTERNAL EAR

The *internal ear* contains the essential sensory apparatus of hearing and equilibrium, and lies on the densest portion of the petrous portion immediately below the arcuate eminence. Composed of an irregularly shaped bony chamber called the *bony labyrinth*, the internal ear is housed within the bony chamber and is an intercommunicating system of ducts and sacs known as the *membranous labyrinth*. The bony labyrinth consists of three distinctly shaped parts: (1) a spiral-coiled, tubular part called the *cochlea*, which communicates with the middle ear through the membranous covering of the *round window* (Fig. 11.27); (2) a small, ovoid central compartment behind the cochlea, known as the *vestibule*, which communicates with the middle ear via the *oval window*; and (3) three unequally sized *semicircular canals* that form right angles to one another and are called, according to their positions, the *anterior, posterior,* and *lateral semicircular canals* (Fig. 11.28). From its cranial orifice, the IAM passes inferiorly and laterally for a distance of about ½ inch (1.3 cm). Through this canal, the cochlear and vestibular nerves pass from their fibers in the respective parts of the membranous labyrinth to the brain. The cochlea is used for hearing, and the vestibule and semicircular canals are involved with equilibrium.

Facial Bones

NASAL BONES

The two small, thin *nasal bones* vary in size and shape in different individuals (Figs. 11.29 and 11.30). They form the superior bony wall (called the *bridge* of the nose) of the nasal cavity. The nasal bones articulate in the MSP, where at their posterosuperior surface they also articulate with the perpendicular plate of the ethmoid bone. They articulate with the frontal bone above and with the maxillae at the sides.

LACRIMAL BONES

The two *lacrimal bones*, which are the smallest bones in the skull, are very thin and are situated at the anterior part of the medial wall of the orbits between the labyrinth of the ethmoid bone and the maxilla (see Figs. 11.29 and 11.30). Together with the maxillae, the lacrimal bones form the lacrimal fossae, which accommodate the lacrimal sacs. Each lacrimal bone contains a *lacrimal foramen* through which a tear duct passes. Each lacrimal bone articulates with the frontal and ethmoid cranial bones, and the maxilla and inferior nasal concha facial bones. The lacrimal bones can be seen on PA and lateral projections of the skull.

MAXILLARY BONES

The two *maxillary bones* are the largest of the immovable bones of the face (see Figs. 11.29 and 11.30). Each articulates with all other facial bones except the mandible. Each also articulates with the frontal and ethmoid bones of the cranium. The maxillary bones form part of the lateral walls and most of the floor of the nasal cavity, part of the floor of the orbital cavities, and three-fourths of the roof of the mouth. Their zygomatic processes articulate with the zygomatic bones and assist in the formation of the prominence of the cheeks. The body of each maxilla contains a large, pyramidal cavity called the *maxillary sinus*, which empties into the nasal cavity. An *infraorbital foramen* is located under each orbit and serves as a passage through which the infraorbital nerve and artery reach the nose.

At their inferior borders, the maxillae possess a thick, spongy ridge called the *alveolar process*, which supports the roots of the teeth. In the anterior MSP at their junction with each other, the maxillary bones form a pointed, forward-projecting process called the *anterior nasal spine*. The midpoint of this prominence is called the *acanthion*.

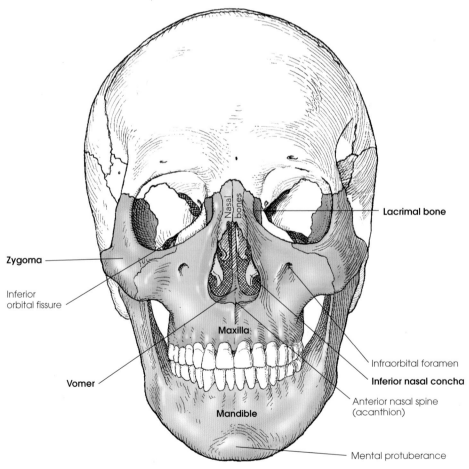

Fig. 11.29 Anterior aspect of skull showing facial bones.

ZYGOMATIC BONES

The zygomatic bones form the prominence of the cheeks and a part of the side wall and floor of the orbital cavities (see Figs. 11.29 and 11.30). A posteriorly extending *temporal process* unites with the zygomatic process of the temporal bone to form the *zygomatic arch*. The zygomatic bones articulate with the frontal bone superiorly, with the zygomatic process of the temporal bone at the side, with the maxilla anteriorly, and with the sphenoid bone posteriorly.

PALATINE BONES

The two palatine bones are L-shaped bones composed of *vertical* and *horizontal plates*. The horizontal plates articulate with the maxillae to complete the posterior fourth of the bony palate, or roof of the mouth (see Fig. 11.3). The vertical portions of the palatine bones extend upward between the maxillae and the pterygoid processes of the sphenoid bone in the posterior nasal cavity. The superior tips of the vertical portions of the palatine bones assist in forming the posteromedial bony orbit.

INFERIOR NASAL CONCHAE

The inferior nasal conchae extend diagonally and inferiorly from the lateral walls of the nasal cavity at approximately its lower third (see Fig. 11.29). They are long, narrow, and extremely thin; they curl laterally, which gives them a scroll-like appearance.

The upper two nasal conchae are processes of the ethmoid bone. The three nasal conchae project into and divide the lateral portion of the respective sides of the nasal cavity into superior, middle, and inferior meatus. They are covered with a mucous membrane to warm, moisten, and cleanse inhaled air.

VOMER

The *vomer* is a thin plate of bone situated in the MSP of the floor of the nasal cavity, where it forms the inferior part of the *nasal septum* (see Fig. 11.29). The anterior border of the vomer slants superiorly and posteriorly from the anterior nasal spine to the body of the sphenoid bone, with which its superior border articulates. The superior part of its anterior border articulates with the perpendicular plate of the ethmoid bone; its posterior border is free.

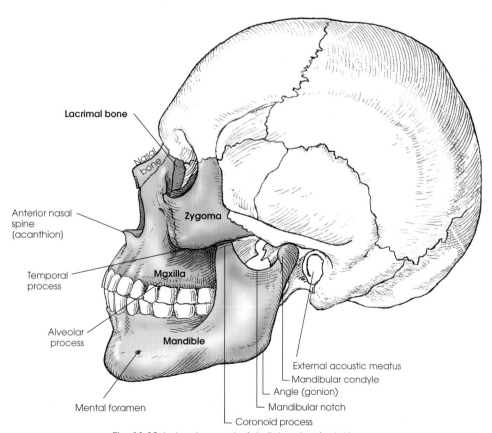

Fig. 11.30 Lateral aspect of skull showing facial bones.

MANDIBLE

The *mandible*, the largest and densest bone of the face, consists of a curved horizontal portion, called the *body*, and two vertical portions, called the *rami*, which unite with the body at the *angle* of the mandible, or *gonion* (Fig. 11.31). At birth, the mandible consists of bilateral pieces held together by a fibrous symphysis that ossifies during the first year of life. At the site of ossification is a slight ridge that ends below in a triangular prominence, the *mental protuberance*. The *symphysis* is the most anterior and central part of the mandible. This is where the left and right halves of the mandible have fused.

The superior border of the body of the mandible consists of spongy bone, called the *alveolar portion*, which supports the roots of the teeth. Below the second premolar tooth, approximately halfway between the superior and inferior borders of the bone, is a small opening on each side for the transmission of nerves and blood vessels. These two openings are called the *mental foramina*.

The rami project superiorly at an obtuse angle to the body of the mandible, and their broad surface forms an angle of approximately 110 to 120 degrees. Each ramus presents two processes at its upper extremity—one coronoid and one condylar—which are separated by a concave area called the *mandibular notch*. The anterior process, the *coronoid process*, is thin, tapered, and projects to a higher level than the posterior process. The *condylar process* consists of a constricted area, the *neck*, above which is a broad, thick, almost transversely placed *condyle* that articulates with the mandibular fossa of the temporal bone (Fig. 11.32). This articulation, the TMJ, slants posteriorly approximately 15 degrees and inferiorly and medially approximately 15 degrees. Radiographic projections, produced from the opposite side, must reverse these directions. In other words, the central ray angulation must be superior and anterior to coincide with the long axis of the joint. The TMJ is situated immediately in front of the EAM.

A

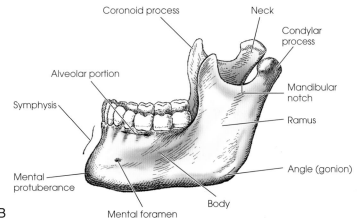

B

Fig. 11.31 (A) Anterior aspect of mandible. (B) Lateral aspect of mandible.

Fig. 11.32 CT scan of mandibular condyle situated in mandibular fossa. (A) Coronal. (B) Sagittal.

(Courtesy Karl Mockler, RT(R).)

HYOID BONE

The *hyoid bone* is a small, U-shaped structure situated at the base of the tongue, where it is held in position in part by the stylohyoid ligaments extending from the styloid processes of the temporal bones (Fig. 11.33). Although the hyoid bone is an accessory bone of the axial skeleton, it is described in this chapter because of its connection with the temporal bones. The hyoid is the only bone in the body that does not articulate with any other bone.

The hyoid bone is divided into a *body*, two *greater cornua*, and two *lesser cornua*. The bone serves as an attachment for certain muscles of the larynx and tongue and is easily palpated just above the larynx.

ORBITS

Each orbit is composed of *seven* different bones (Fig. 11.34). Three of these are cranial bones: *frontal*, *sphenoid*, and *ethmoid*. The other four bones are the facial bones: *maxilla*, *zygoma*, *lacrimal*, and *palatine*. The circumference of the orbit, or outer rim area, is composed of three of the seven bones—frontal, zygoma, and maxilla. The remaining four bones compose most of the posterior aspect of the orbit.

Articulations of the Skull

The sutures of the skull are connected by toothlike projections of bone interlocked with a thin layer of fibrous tissue. These articulations allow no movement and are classified as *fibrous* joints of the *suture* type. The articulations of the facial bones, including the joints between the roots of the teeth and the jawbones, are *fibrous gomphoses*. The exception is the point at which the rounded condyle of the mandible articulates with the mandibular fossa of the temporal bone to form the TMJ. The TMJ articulation is a *synovial* joint of the *hinge* and *gliding* type. The atlantooccipital joint is a *synovial ellipsoidal* joint that joins the base of the skull (occipital bone) with the atlas of the cervical spine. The seven joints of the skull are summarized in Table 11.1.

TABLE 11.1
Joints of the Skull

Joint	Structural Classification		Movement
	Tissue	Type	
Coronal suture	Fibrous	Suture	Immovable
Sagittal suture	Fibrous	Suture	Immovable
Lambdoidal suture	Fibrous	Suture	Immovable
Squamosal suture	Fibrous	Suture	Immovable
Temporomandibular	Synovial	Hinge and gliding	Freely movable
Alveolar sockets	Fibrous	Gomphosis	Immovable
Atlantooccipital	Synovial	Ellipsoidal	Freely movable

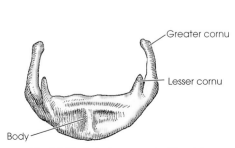
Fig. 11.33 Anterior aspect of hyoid.

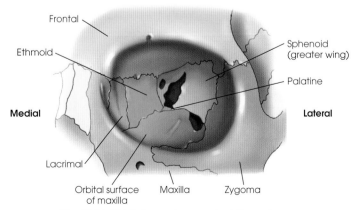
Fig. 11.34 Orbit. Seven bones of orbit are shown.

Sinuses

The air-containing cavities situated in the frontal, ethmoidal, and sphenoidal bones of the cranium and the maxillary bones of the face are called the *paranasal sinuses* because of their formation from the nasal mucosa and their continued communication with the nasal fossae (Fig. 11.35). Although the functions of the sinuses are not agreed on by all anatomists, these cavities are believed to do the following:

- Serve as a resonating chamber for the voice
- Decrease the weight of the skull by containing air
- Help warm and moisten inhaled air
- Act as shock absorbers in trauma (as airbags do in automobiles)
- Possibly control the immune system

The sinuses begin to develop early in fetal life, at first appearing as small sacculations of the mucosa of the nasal meatus and recesses. As the pouches, or sacs, grow, they gradually invade the respective bones to form the air sinuses and cells. The maxillary sinuses are usually sufficiently well developed and aerated at birth, to be shown radiographically. The other groups of sinuses develop more slowly; by age 6 or 7 years, the frontal and sphenoidal sinuses are distinguishable from the ethmoidal air cells. The paranasal sinuses are not completely developed until the age of 17 or 18 years. When fully developed, each of the sinuses communicates with the others and with the nasal cavity.

An understanding of the actual size, shape, and position of the sinuses within the skull is made possible by studying the sinuses on computed tomography (CT) head images (Fig. 11.36).

MAXILLARY SINUSES

The largest sinuses, the maxillary sinuses, are paired and are located in the body of each maxilla (see Figs. 11.35 and 11.36). Although the maxillary sinuses appear rectangular in the lateral image, they are approximately pyramidal in shape and have only three walls. The apices are directed inferiorly and laterally. The two maxillary sinuses vary considerably in size and shape but are usually symmetric. In adults, each maxillary sinus is approximately 1½ inches (3.5 cm) high and 1 to 1⅓ inches (2.5 to 3.3 cm) wide. The sinus is often divided into subcompartments by partial septa, and occasionally it is divided into two sinuses by a complete septum. The sinus floor presents several elevations that correspond to the roots of the subjacent teeth. The maxillary sinuses communicate with the middle nasal meatus at the superior aspect of the sinus.

Fig. 11.35 (A) Anterior aspect of paranasal sinuses, showing lateral relationship to each other and to surrounding parts. (B) Schematic drawing of paranasal sinuses, showing AP relationship to each other and surrounding parts.

FRONTAL SINUSES

The frontal sinuses, the second largest sinuses, are paired and are normally located between the tables of the vertical plate of the frontal bone (see Figs. 11.35 and 11.36). The frontal sinuses vary greatly in size and form. Occasionally they are absent. One or both may be approximately ¾ to 1 inch (2 to 2.5 cm) in the vertical or lateral dimension. The sinuses often extend beyond the frontal region of the bone, most frequently into the orbital plates. The *intersinus septum* is usually deviated from the midline; for this reason, the frontal sinuses are rarely symmetric. Multiple septa are sometimes present. Similar to maxillary sinuses, the frontal sinuses drain into the middle nasal meatus.

ETHMOIDAL SINUSES

The two ethmoidal sinuses are located within the lateral masses of the labyrinths of the ethmoid bone. They are composed of a varying number of air cells that are divided into three main groups: anterior, middle, and posterior (see Figs. 11.35 and 11.36). The anterior and middle ethmoidal cells range in number from two to eight, and each group opens into the middle nasal meatus. The posterior cells range in number from two to six or more and drain into the superior nasal meatus.

SPHENOIDAL SINUSES

The sphenoidal sinuses are normally paired and occupy the body of the sphenoid bone (see Figs. 11.35 and 11.36). Anatomists state that often only one sphenoidal sinus is present; however, more than two sphenoidal sinuses are never present. The sphenoidal sinuses vary considerably in size and shape and are usually asymmetric. They lie immediately below the sella turcica and extend between the dorsum sellae and the posterior ethmoidal air cells. The sphenoidal sinuses open into the sphenoethmoidal recess of the nasal cavity.

Text continued on p. 29

Fig. 11.36 (A) Coronal CT image of frontal sinuses (FS). (B) Coronal CT image of ethmoidal and maxillary sinuses *(MS)*. (C) Axial CT image of MS. (D) Axial CT image of ethmoidal and sphenoid sinuses *(SS)*. (E) Sagittal CT image of SS.

(Courtesy NEA Baptist Memorial Hospital, Jonesboro, AR.)

SUMMARY OF ANATOMY

Skull
Cranial bones (8)
Facial bones (14)

Cranial bones
Calvaria
  Frontal
  Right parietal
  Left parietal
  Occipital
Floor
  Right temporal
  Left temporal
  Sphenoid
  Ethmoid
Diploë

Sutures
Coronal suture
Sagittal suture
Squamosal sutures
Lambdoidal suture
Bregma
Lambda
Pterion
Asterion

Fontanels
Anterior fontanel
Posterior fontanel
Sphenoidal fontanels (2)
Mastoid fontanels (2)

Fossae
Anterior cranial fossa
Middle cranial fossa
Posterior cranial fossa

Frontal bone
Frontal squama
Frontal eminence
Supraorbital margins
Superciliary arches
Supraorbital foramen
Glabella
Frontal sinuses
Nasion
Orbital plates
Ethmoidal notch
Nasal spine

Ethmoid bone
Cribriform plate
Crista galli
Perpendicular plate
Labyrinths
Anterior air cells
Middle air cells
Posterior air cells
Ethmoidal sinuses
Superior nasal conchae
Middle nasal conchae

Parietal bones (R & L)
Parietal eminence

Sphenoid bone
Body
  Sphenoidal sinuses
  Sella turcica
    Tuberculum sellae
    Dorsum sellae
    Posterior clinoid
      processes
  Clivus
Carotid sulcus
Optic groove
  Optic canals
  Optic foramen
Lesser wings
  Superior orbital fissures
  Anterior clinoid
    processes
  Sphenoid strut
Greater wings
  Foramen rotundum
  Foramen ovale
  Foramen spinosum
  Pterygoid processes
    Medial pterygoid
      lamina
    Lateral pterygoid
      lamina
    Pterygoid hamulus

Occipital bone
Foramen magnum
Squama
  External occipital protuberance
    (inion)
  Internal occipital protuberance
  Occipital condyles
  Hypoglossal canals
  Condylar canals
  Jugular foramen
  Basilar portion

Temporal bones (R & L)
Squamous portions
  Zygomatic process
  Articular tubercle
  Mandibular fossa
Tympanic portions
  External acoustic meatus
    (EAM)
  Styloid process
Petromastoid portions
  Mastoid portions
    Mastoid process
    Mastoid antrum
    Mastoid air cells
  Petrous portions (petrous
    pyramids)
    Carotid canals
    Petrous apex
    Foramen lacerum
    Internal acoustic meatus
      (IAM)
    Petrous ridge
    Top of ear attachment
      (TEA)

Ear
External ear
  Auricle
    Concha
    Tragus
    Helix
  EAM
Middle ear
  Tympanic membrane
  Tympanic cavity
  Auditory (eustachian)
    tube
Auditory ossicles
  Malleus
  Incus
  Stapes
Internal ear
  Arcuate eminence
  Bony labyrinth
    Cochlea
    Round window
    Vestibule
    Oval window
    Semicircular canals
    Anterior
    Posterior
    Lateral
  Membranous labyrinth

Facial bones (14)
Nasal (R & L)
Lacrimal (R & L)
Maxillary (R & L)
Zygomatic (R & L)
Palatine (R & L)
Inferior nasal conchae
  (R & L)
Vomer (1)
Mandible (1)
Hyoid bone
Diploë

Lacrimal bones (R & L)
Lacrimal foramen

Maxillary bones (R & L)
Maxillary sinuses
Infraorbital foramen
Alveolar process
Anterior nasal spine
Acanthion

Zygomatic bones (R & L)
Temporal process
Zygomatic arch

Palatine bones (R & L)
Vertical plates
Horizontal plates

**Inferior nasal conchae
(R & L)**
Vomer (1)
Nasal septum

Mandible (1)
Body
  Alveolar portion
  Mental foramina
Angle (gonion)
Rami
  Coronoid process
  Condylar process
    Condyle
    Neck
    Temporomandibular
    joint (TMJ)
  Mandibular notch
Mental protuberance
  (mentum)
Symphysis

Hyoid bone
Body
Greater cornua
Lesser cornua

Paranasal sinuses
Maxillary sinuses
Frontal sinuses
  Intersinus septum
Ethmoidal sinuses
  Anterior ethmoidal cells
  Middle ethmoidal cells
  Posterior ethmoidal
    cells
Sphenoidal sinuses

Articulations
Coronal suture
Sagittal suture
Lambdoidal sutures
Squamosal sutures
Temporomandibular (TMJ)
Alveolar sockets
Atlantooccipital

Morphology
Mesocephalic
Brachycephalic
Dolichocephalic

Orbit
Base
Apex
Optic foramen
Superior orbital fissures
Inferior orbital fissures

Eye
Eyeball
Conjunctiva
Sclera
Cornea
Retina
  Rods
  Cones

SUMMARY OF PATHOLOGY

Condition	Definition
Fracture	Disruption in continuity of bone
Basal	Fracture located at the base of the skull
Blowout	Fracture of the floor of the orbit
Contrecoup	Fracture to one side of a structure caused by trauma to the other side
Depressed	Fracture causing a portion of the skull to be pushed into the cranial cavity
Le Fort	Bilateral horizontal fractures of the maxillae
Linear	Irregular or jagged fracture of the skull
Tripod	Fracture of the zygomatic arch and orbital floor or rim and dislocation of the frontozygomatic suture
Mastoiditis	Inflammation of the mastoid antrum and air cells
Metastasis	Transfer of cancerous lesion from one area to another
Osteomyelitis	Inflammation of bone due to a pyogenic infection
Osteopetrosis	Increased density of atypically soft bone
Osteoporosis	Loss of bone density
Paget disease	Thick, soft bone marked by bowing and fractures
Polyp	Growth or mass protruding from a mucous membrane
Sinusitis	Inflammation of one or more of the paranasal sinuses
TMJ syndrome	Dysfunction of temporomandibular joint (TMJ)
Tumor	New tissue growth where cell proliferation is uncontrolled
Acoustic neuroma	Benign tumor arising from Schwann cells of eighth cranial nerve (also termed "schwannoma")
Multiple myeloma	Malignant neoplasm of plasma cells involving the bone marrow and causing destruction of the bone
Osteoma	Tumor composed of bony tissue
Pituitary adenoma	Tumor arising from the pituitary gland, usually in the anterior lobe

Eponymous (named) pathologies are listed in nonpossessive form to conform to the *AMA manual of style: a guide for authors and editors.* 10th ed. Oxford: Oxford University Press; 2009.

SAMPLE EXPOSURE TECHNIQUE CHART ESSENTIAL PROJECTIONS

These techniques were accurate for the equipment used to produce each exposure. However, use caution when applying them in your department because "there is considerable variability in image receptor response owing to varying scatter sensitivity, the use of grids with different grid ratios, collimation, beam filtration, the choice of kilovoltage, source-to-image distance, and image receptor size."[a]

CRANIUM

Part	cm	kVp[b]	SID[c]	Collimation	CR[d] mAs	CR[d] Dose (mGy)[f]	DR[e] mAs	DR[e] Dose (mGy)[f]
Skull								
Lateral[g]	15	85	40"	11" × 9" (28 × 23 cm)	6.3[h]	0.794	3.2[h]	0.399
PA[g]	20	85	40"	8" × 10" (20 × 25 cm)	12.5[h]	1.781	6.3[h]	0.891
PA axial (Caldwell)[g]	20	85	40"	8" × 11" (20 × 28 cm)	14[h]	2.008	7.1[h]	1.014
AP[g]	20	85	40"	8" × 10" (20 × 25 cm)	12[h]	1.781	6.3[h]	0.893
AP axial[g]	20	85	40"	8" × 11" (20 × 28 cm)	14[h]	2.005	7.1[h]	1.014
AP axial (Towne)[g]	22	85	40"	8.5" × 12" (21.3 × 30 cm)	20[i]	3.030	10[i,j]	1.507
PA axial (Haas)[g]	21	85	40"	8.5" × 12" (21.3 × 30 cm)	20[i]	2.950	10[i]	1.467
Cranial base								
SMV[g]	23	85	40"	8" × 11" (20 × 28 cm)	28[i]	4.330	14[i]	2.169
Facial bones								
Lateral[g]	15	80	40"	7" × 7" (18 × 18 cm)	6.3[h]	0.701	3.2[h]	0.354
Parietoacanthial (Waters)[g]	24	85	40"	7.5" × 8" (18.8 × 20 cm)	16[h]	2.470	8[h]	1.231
Acanthioparietal (reverse Waters)[g]	24	85	40"	7.5" × 8" (18.8 × 20 cm)	16[h]	2.470	8[h]	1.231
PA axial (Caldwell)[g]	20	85	40"	7.5" × 8" (18.8 × 20 cm)	14[h]	1.958	7.1[h]	0.988
Nasal bones								
Lateral[j]	6	70	40"	3" × 5" (8 × 13 cm)	5.0[h]	0.282	2.5[h]	1.408
Zygomatic arches								
SMV[g]	23	80	40"	8" × 5" (20 × 13 cm)	16[i]	2.094	8[i]	1.041
Tangential[g]	20	80	40"	3" × 5" (8 × 13 cm)	14[i]	1.294	7.1[i]	0.653
AP axial[g]	17	80	40"	8.5" × 7" (21.3 × 18 cm)	20[i]	2.270	6.3[i]	1.126
Mandibular rami								
PA[g]	17	80	40"	8" × 5" (20 × 13 cm)	12.5[h]	1.367	6.3[h]	0.686
PA axial[g]	17	80	40"	8" × 5" (20 ×13 cm)	14[h]	1.532	7[h]	0.773
Mandible								
Axiolateral oblique[g]	13	80	40"	8" × 6" (20 × 15 cm)	12.5[h]	1.266	6.3[h]	0.635

SAMPLE EXPOSURE TECHNIQUE CHART ESSENTIAL PROJECTIONS—cont'd

CRANIUM

Part	cm	kVp[b]	SID[c]	Collimation	CR[d] mAs	CR[d] Dose (mGy)[f]	DR[e] mAs	DR[e] Dose (mGy)[f]
TMJ								
AP axial[g]	21	80	40″	8.5″ × 7″ (21.3 × 18 cm)	20[h]	2.480	10[h]	1.233
Axiolateral oblique[g]	15	80	40″	4″ × 4″ (10 × 10 cm)	16[i]	1.501	8[i]	0.748
Paranasal sinuses								
Lateral[g]	15	85	40″	6″ × 6″ (15 × 15 cm)	6.3[h]	0.721	3.2[h]	0.363
Frontal and anterior ethmoidal sinuses								
PA axial (Caldwell)[g]	20	85	40″	6″ × 6″ (15 × 15 cm)	14[h]	1.807	7.1[h]	0.912
Maxillary sinuses								
Parietoacanthial (Waters)[g]	24	85	40″	6″ × 6″ (15 × 15 cm)	16[h]	2.280	8[h]	1.133
Maxillary and sphenoidal sinuses								
Parietoacanthial (open-mouth Waters)[g]	24	85	40″	6″ × 6.5″ (15 × 16.3 cm)	14[h]	2.003	7.1[h]	1.011
Ethmoidal and sphenoidal sinuses								
SMV[g]	23	85	40″	6.5″ × 6.5″ (16.3 × 16.3 cm)	28[i]	3.900	14[i]	1.948

This chart was created in collaboration with Dennis Bowman, AS, RT(R), Clinical Instructor, Community Hospital of the Monterey Peninsula, Monterey, CA. http://digitalradiographysolutions.com/.

[a]ACR-AAPM-SIMM Practice Parameter for Digital Radiography, revised 2017.
[b]kVp values are for a high-frequency generator.
[c]40 inches minimum; 44 to 48 inches recommended to improve spatial resolution (mAs increase needed, but no increase in patient dose will result).
[d]AGFA CR MD 4.0 General IP, CR 75.0 reader, 400 speed class, with 6:1 (178LPI) grid when needed.
[e]GE Definium 8000, with 13:1 grid when needed.
[f]All doses are skin entrance for an average adult (160- to 200-pound male, 150- to 190-pound female) at part thickness indicated.
[g]Bucky/Grid.
[h]Small focal spot.
[i]Large focal spot.
[j]Nongrid.

ABBREVIATIONS USED IN CHAPTER 11	
AML	Acanthiomeatal line
EAM	External acoustic meatus
GML	Glabellomeatal line
IAM	Internal acoustic meatus
IOML	Infraorbitomeatal line
IPL	Interpupillary line
MML	Mentomeatal line
OID	Object-to-IR distance
OML	Orbitomeatal line
TEA	Top of ear attachment
TMJ	Temporomandibular joint

See Addendum B for a summary of all abbreviations used in Volume 2.

Skull Topography

The basic localization points and planes of the skull (all of which can be seen or palpated) used in radiographic positioning are illustrated in Figs. 11.37 and 11.38.

Accurate positioning of the skull requires a full understanding of these landmarks, *which should be studied thoroughly before positioning of the skull is learned.* The planes, points, lines, and abbreviations most frequently used in skull positioning are as follows:

- Midsagittal plane (MSP)
- Interpupillary line (IPL)
- Acanthion
- Outer canthus
- Infraorbital margin
- EAM
- Orbitomeatal line (OML)
- Infraorbitomeatal line (IOML)
- Acanthiomeatal line (AML)
- Mentomeatal line (MML)

In an adult, an average 7-degree angle difference exists between the OML and the IOML, and an average 8-degree angle difference exists between the OML and the glabellomeatal line. The degree difference between the cranial positioning lines must be recognized. Often the relationship of the patient, image receptor (IR), and central ray is the same, but the angle that is described may vary depending on the cranial line of reference.

Fig. 11.37 Anterior landmarks.

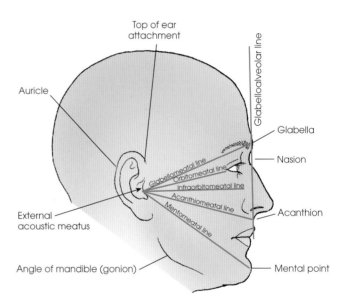

Fig. 11.38 Lateral landmarks.

Skull Morphology

All radiographic images of the skull are based on the normal size and shape of the cranium. Rules have been established for centering and adjustment of localization points and planes and for the exact degree of central ray angulation for each projection. Although the heads of many patients fall within the limits of normality and can be radiographed satisfactorily using established positions, numerous skulls vary enough in shape that the standard procedure must be adjusted to obtain an undistorted image.

In the typically shaped head (Fig. 11.39), the petrous pyramids project anteriorly and medially at an angle of 47 degrees from the MSP of the skull. The superior borders of these structures are situated in the base of the cranium.

Depending on its shape, the atypical cranium requires more or less rotation of the head or an increase or decrease in angulation of the central ray compared with the typical, or *mesocephalic*, skull (see Fig. 11.39). In the *brachycephalic* skull (Fig. 11.40), which is short from front to back, broad from side to side, and shallow from vertex to base, the internal structures are higher with reference to the IOML, and their long axes are more frontal in position (i.e., the petrous pyramids form a wider angle with the MSP). The petrous pyramids lie at an average angle of 54 degrees. In the *dolichocephalic* skull (Fig. 11.41), which is long from front to back, narrow from side to side, and deep from vertex to base, the internal structures are lower with reference to the IOML, and their long axes are less frontal in position (i.e., the petrous pyramids form a narrower angle with the MSP). The petrous pyramids form an average angle of 40 degrees in the dolichocephalic skull.

Asymmetry must also be considered. The orbits are not always symmetric in size and shape, the lower jaw is often asymmetric, and the nasal bones and cartilage are frequently deviated from the MSP. Many deviations are not as obvious as these, but if the radiographer adheres to the fundamental rules of positioning, relatively little difficulty is encountered. Varying the position of the part or the degree of central ray angulation to compensate for structural variations becomes a simple procedure if care and precision are used initially.

The radiographic positions depicted in this chapter show the patient seated at the vertical grid device or lying on a radiographic table. Whether the radiographer elects to perform the examination with the patient in the recumbent or upright position depends on four variables: (1) the equipment available, (2) the age and condition of the patient, (3) the preference of the radiographer and/or radiologist, and (4) whether upright images would increase diagnostic value, such as showing air-fluid levels in paranasal sinuses.

Comparable images of the skull and facial bones can usually be obtained with the patient either upright or recumbent, as long as the patient/part positioning and central ray are correctly aligned with the IR. For radiography of the paranasal sinuses, *the upright position is essential* for demonstration of air/fluid levels. Therefore, unless specifically noted in the text, the photographic illustration does *not* constitute a recommendation for performing the examination with the patient in the upright or recumbent position. Line drawings illustrating both table and upright radiography are included for most radiographic positions in this chapter.

Fig. 11.39 Mesocephalic skull.

Fig. 11.40 Brachycephalic skull.

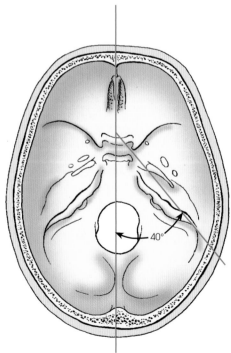

Fig. 11.41 Dolichocephalic skull.

Technical Considerations

GENERAL BODY POSITION

The position of the body is important in radiography of the cranium to obtain quality images (Fig. 11.42). If the body is not correctly adjusted, great strain is placed on the muscles, making it difficult for the patient to maintain the correct head position. This is especially true when recumbent positions are used for skull radiography. An uncomfortable body position can contribute to positioning errors during skull, facial bone, and sinus radiography, such as rotation and tilt. Rotation results from lateral misplacement of MSP. Tilt results from longitudinal angulation of MSP of the head in relation to MSP of the entire body (Fig. 11.43). Some guidelines to alleviate strain and facilitate accurate positioning are as follows:

- To prevent rotation of the head, place the patient's body so that its long axis, depending on the image, either coincides with or is parallel to the midline of the radiographic table.
- To prevent tilt (superior or inferior pull on the head), align the long axis of the cervical vertebrae with the level of the midpoint of the foramen magnum.
- Support any elevated part, such as the patient's shoulder or hip, on a pillow or sandbags to relieve strain.
- For recumbent examinations of hyposthenic or asthenic patients, elevate the patient's chest on a small pillow to raise the cervical vertebrae to the correct level for the lateral, PA, and oblique projections (Figs. 11.44 and 11.45).
- For recumbent examination of obese or hypersthenic patients, elevate the patient's head on a radiolucent pad to obtain the correct part-IR relationship (Figs. 11.46 and 11.47).
- While adjusting the body, stand in a position that facilitates estimation of the approximate part position. For example, stand so that the longitudinal axis of the radiographic table is visible as the MSP of the body is being centered. This allows the anterior surface of the forehead to be viewed while the degree of body rotation for a lateral projection of the skull is adjusted. As a result, the body can be adjusted in such a way that it does not interfere with the final adjustment of the head, and the final position is comfortable for the patient.
- When the body is correctly placed and adjusted so that the long axis of the cervical vertebrae is supported at the level of the foramen magnum, the final position of the head requires only minor adjustments. The average patient can maintain this relatively comfortable position without the aid of elaborate immobilization devices, although the following techniques may be helpful:
  - If necessary, apply a head clamp with equal pressure on the two sides of the head.

Fig. 11.42 Correct parietoacanthial (Waters) without rotation or tilt.

Fig. 11.43 Incorrect parietoacanthial (Waters) with rotation and tilt. *Red lines* show rotation, evidenced by the unequal distances from the lateral orbital margins to lateral skull borders. Tilt is shown by the *yellow line*, demonstrating MSP of the head is not aligned with long axis of collimated field.

- If such a clamp is not available, use a strip of adhesive tape where it will not be projected onto the image. The portion of the tape touching the hair should have the adhesive side covered with a second piece of tape so that the hairs are not pulled out when the tape is removed. Do *not* place adhesive tape directly on the patient's skin.

- When the area to be exposed is small, immobilize the head with sandbags placed against the sides or vertex.
- Correct basic body positions and compensatory adjustments for recumbent radiography are illustrated in Figs. 11.44–11.51.

CLEANLINESS

The hair and face are naturally oily and leave a residue, even with the most hygienic patients. If the patient is sick, the residue is worse. During positioning of the skull, the patient's hair, mouth, nose, and eyes come in direct contact with the vertical grid device, tabletop, or IR. For medical asepsis, a paper towel or a cloth sheet may be placed between the imaging surface and the patient. As part of standard procedure, the contacted area should be cleaned with a disinfectant before and after positioning.

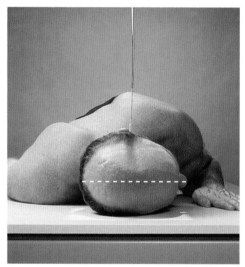

Fig. 11.44 Horizontal sagittal plane *(dashed lines)*.

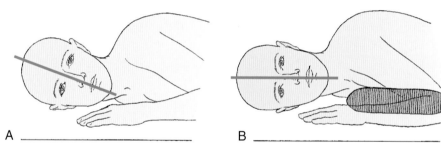

Fig. 11.45 Adjusting sagittal planes to horizontal position. (A) Asthenic or hyposthenic patient. (B) Angulation corrected.

Fig. 11.46 Horizontal sagittal plane.

Fig. 11.47 Adjusting sagittal plane to horizontal position. (A) Hypersthenic patient. (B) Angulation corrected.

Radiation Protection

Protection of the patient from unnecessary radiation is a professional responsibility of the radiographer (see Chapter 1 for specific guidelines). In this chapter, radiation shielding of the patient is not specified or illustrated. The federal government has reported that placing a lead shield over a patient's pelvis does not significantly reduce gonadal exposure during imaging of the skull, facial bones, or sinuses.[1] However, lead shields may be used to reassure the patient, if requested, and shielding the abdomen of a pregnant woman is recommended by the authors of this atlas.

Infants and children may receive radiation shielding of the thyroid and thymus glands and the gonads, if the procedure is not compromised. The protective lead shielding used to cover the thyroid and thymus glands may assist in immobilizing pediatric patients.

The most effective way to protect the patient from unnecessary radiation is to restrict the radiation beam by using *proper collimation*. Taking care to ensure that the patient is properly instructed and immobilized also reduces the likelihood of having to repeat the procedure, further limiting the radiation exposure received by the patient.

Fig. 11.48 Perpendicular sagittal plane *(dashed lines)*.

Fig. 11.49 Adjusting orbitomeatal line to vertical position. (A) Hypersthenic or round-shouldered patient. (B) Angulation corrected.

Fig. 11.50 Perpendicular sagittal plane *(dashed lines)*.

Fig. 11.51 Adjusting orbitomeatal line to vertical position. (A) Correction for hyposthenic patient. (B) Correction for hypersthenic patient.

Cranium

▲ LATERAL PROJECTION
Right or left position

Image receptor + grid: Positioned by manufacturer or department protocol for proper anatomy display orientation; CR plate: 10 × 12 inches (24 × 30 cm) crosswise.

Position of patient
- Place the patient in the anterior oblique position, seated upright or recumbent.
- If recumbent anterior oblique position is used, have the patient rest on the forearm and flex the knee of the elevated side.

Position of part
- Adjust the patient's head so that the MSP is parallel to the plane of the IR. If necessary, place a support under the side of the mandible to prevent it from sagging.

- Adjust the flexion of the patient's neck so that the IOML is perpendicular to the front edge of the IR. The IOML should also be parallel to the long axis of the IR.
- Position the head to place the IPL perpendicular to the IR (Figs. 11.52 and 11.53). Patient's head usually rests on the auricle of the ear.
- Immobilize the head.
- *Respiration:* Suspend.

Central ray
- Perpendicular, entering 2 inches (5 cm) superior to the EAM.
- Center the IR to the central ray.

Collimation
Adjust radiation field to extend 1 inch (2.5 cm) beyond the skin line of the skull. Check for light at vertex, anterior, posterior, and base of the skull borders. Place the side marker in the collimated exposure field.

Structures shown
Superimposed halves of the cranium with the details of the side adjacent to the IR. The sella turcica, anterior clinoid processes, dorsum sellae, and posterior clinoid processes are well shown in the lateral projection (Figs. 11.54 and 11.55).

EVALUATION CRITERIA
The following should be clearly seen:
- Evidence of proper collimation and presence of the side marker placed clear of anatomy of interest
- Entire cranium without rotation or tilt, demonstrated by:
  - Superimposed orbital roofs and greater wings of sphenoid
  - Superimposed mastoid regions and EAM
  - Superimposed TMJs
  - Sella turcica in profile
- No overlap of cervical spine by mandible
- Bony detail of cranium and surrounding soft tissues

Fig. 11.52 (A) Lateral skull, recumbent position. (B) Table radiography diagram: lateral skull.

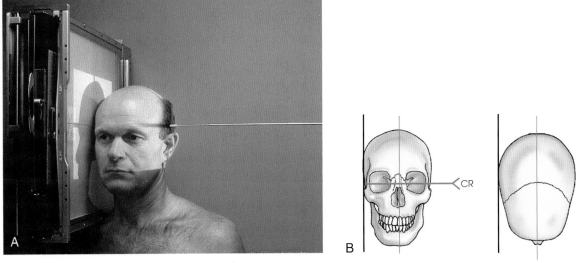

Fig. 11.53 (A) Lateral skull, upright position. (B) Upright radiography diagram: lateral skull.

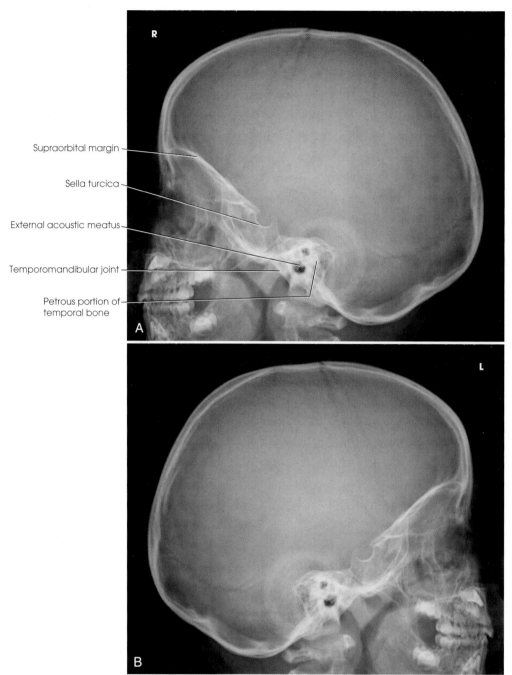

Supraorbital margin

Sella turcica

External acoustic meatus

Temporomandibular joint

Petrous portion of
temporal bone

Fig. 11.54 Skull images on pediatric patient. (A) Right lateral. (B) Left lateral.

(Courtesy St. Bernard's Medical Center, Jonesboro, AR.)

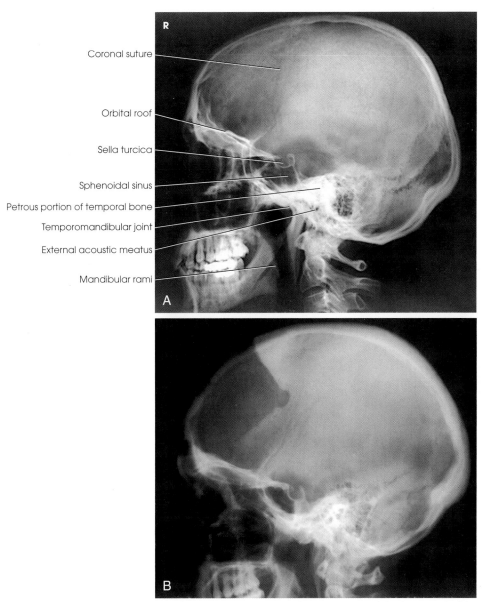

Coronal suture

Orbital roof

Sella turcica

Sphenoidal sinus

Petrous portion of temporal bone

Temporomandibular joint

External acoustic meatus

Mandibular rami

Fig. 11.55 Skull images on adult patients. (A) Right lateral. (B) Right lateral showing surgical removal of frontal bone.

♠ PA PROJECTION AND PA AXIAL PROJECTION
CALDWELL METHOD

Image receptor + grid: Positioned by manufacturer or department protocol for proper anatomy display orientation; CR plate: 10 × 12 inches (24 × 30 cm) lengthwise.

Position of patient
- Place the patient in a prone or seated position.
- Center MSP of the patient's body to the midline of the grid.
- Rest the patient's forehead and nose on the table or against the upright bucky.
- Flex the patient's elbows, and place the arms in a comfortable position.

Position of part
- Adjust the flexion of the patient's neck so that the OML is perpendicular to the plane of the IR.
- If the patient is recumbent, support the chin on a radiolucent sponge if needed.
- If the patient is obese or hypersthenic, a small radiolucent sponge may need to be placed under (or in front of) the forehead.
- Align MSP perpendicular to the IR. This is accomplished by adjusting the lateral margins of the orbits or the EAM equidistant from the tabletop.
- Immobilize the patient's head, and center the IR to the nasion.
- *Respiration:* Suspend.

Central ray
- For the PA projection, when the frontal bone is of primary interest, direct the central ray perpendicular to exit the nasion (Fig. 11.56).
- For the PA axial projection, Caldwell method, direct the central ray to exit the nasion at an angle of 15 degrees caudad (Figs. 11.57–11.59).
- Center the IR to the central ray.
- To show the superior orbital fissures, direct the central ray through the mid-orbits at an angle of 20 to 25 degrees caudad.
- To show the rotundum foramina, direct the central ray to the nasion at an angle of 25 to 30 degrees caudad. (The Waters method, presented in the Sinus Radiography section, is also used to show the rotundum foramina.)

Collimation
- Adjust radiation field to extend 1 inch (2.5 cm) beyond the skin line of the skull. Check for light at vertex and on both sides. Place the side marker in the collimated exposure field.

Fig. 11.56 PA skull: central ray angulation of 0 degree for frontal bone.

Fig. 11.57 PA axial skull: Caldwell method with central ray angulation of 15 degrees.

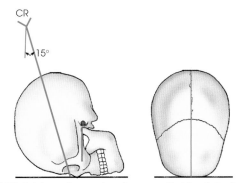

Fig. 11.58 Table radiography diagram: Caldwell method.

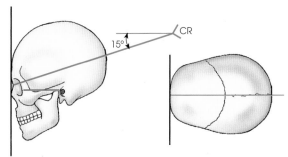

Fig. 11.59 Upright radiography diagram: Caldwell method.

(R) Parietal bone

Frontal bone

Dorsum sella

Supraorbital margin

Petrous ridge

Crista galli

Ethmoidal sinus

Fig. 11.60 PA skull with perpendicular central ray.

(Courtesy St. Bernard's Medical Center, Jonesboro, AR.)

Frontal sinus

Crista galli

Superior orbital margin

Superior orbital fissure

Ethmoidal sinus

Petrous ridge

Inferior orbital margin

Fig. 11.61 PA axial skull: Caldwell method with 15-degree caudal central ray angulation.

Structures shown

For the PA projection with a perpendicular central ray (Fig. 11.60), the orbits are filled by the margins of the petrous pyramids. Other structures shown include the posterior ethmoidal air cells, crista galli, frontal bone, and frontal sinuses. The dorsum sellae is seen as a curved line extending between the orbits, just above the ethmoidal air cells.

When the central ray is angled 15 degrees caudad to the nasion for the PA axial projection, Caldwell method, many of the same structures that appear in the PA projection are seen (Fig. 11.61); however, the petrous ridges are projected into the lower third of the orbits. The Caldwell method also shows the anterior ethmoidal air cells. Schüller,[2] who first described this positioning for the skull, recommended a caudal angle of 25 degrees.

Stretcher and bedside examinations
Lateral decubitus position

- When the patient cannot be turned to the prone position for the PA or PA axial Caldwell projection, and cervical spinal injury has been ruled out, elevate one side enough to place the patient's head in a true lateral position, and support the shoulder and hip on pillows or sandbags if needed.
- Elevate the patient's head on a suitable support, and adjust its height to center MSP of the head to a vertically positioned grid.
- Adjust the patient's head so that the OML is perpendicular to the plane of the IR (Fig. 11.62).
- Direct the *horizontal* central ray perpendicular, or 15 degrees caudad, to exit the nasion.

The following should be clearly seen:
- Evidence of proper collimation and presence of the side marker placed clear of anatomy of interest
- Entire cranium without rotation or tilt, demonstrated by:
  - Equal distances from lateral borders of skull to lateral borders of orbits on both sides
  - Symmetric petrous ridges
  - MSP of cranium aligned with long axis of collimated field
- PA axial (Caldwell) demonstrates petrous pyramids lying in lower third of orbit
- PA projection shows orbits filled by petrous ridges
- Entire cranial perimeter showing three distinct tables of squamous bone
- Bony detail of frontal bone and surrounding soft tissues

Fig. 11.62 PA skull with patient semisupine.

AP PROJECTION AND AP AXIAL PROJECTION
REVERSE CALDWELL METHOD

Image receptor + grid: Positioned by manufacturer or department protocol for proper anatomy display orientation; CR plate: 10 × 12 inches (24 × 30 cm) lengthwise.

When the patient cannot be positioned for a PA or PA axial projection, a similar but magnified image can be obtained with an AP projection. The AP axial is often referred to as a *reverse Caldwell.*

Position of patient and part
- Position the patient supine with the MSP of the body centered to the grid.
- Ensure that MSP and OML are perpendicular to the IR.

Central ray
- Perpendicular (Fig. 11.63) or directed to the nasion at an angle 15 degrees cephalad (Fig. 11.64).
- Center IR to the central ray.

Collimation
- Adjust radiation field to extend 1 inch (2.5 cm) beyond the skin line of the skull. Check for light above the vertex and on both sides of the face. Place the side marker in the collimated exposure field.

Structures shown
The structures shown on the AP projection are the same as the structures shown on the PA projection. On the AP projection (Fig. 11.65), the orbits are considerably magnified because of the increased object–to–image receptor distance (OID). Similarly, because of the magnification, the distance from the lateral margin of the orbit to the lateral margin of the temporal bone measures less on the AP projection than on the PA projection.

The following should be clearly seen:
- Evidence of proper collimation and presence of the side marker placed clear of anatomy of interest
- Entire cranium without rotation or tilt, demonstrated by:
  - □ Equal distances from lateral borders of skull to lateral borders of orbits on both sides
  - □ Symmetric petrous ridges
  - □ MSP of cranium aligned with long axis of collimated field
- Petrous pyramids lying in lower third of orbit with a cephalad central ray angulation of 15 degrees and filling orbits with a 0-degree central ray angulation
- Entire cranial perimeter showing three distinct areas of squamous bone
- Bony detail of frontal bone and surrounding soft tissues

Fig. 11.63 AP skull.

Fig. 11.64 AP axial, reverse Caldwell, skull with 15-degree cephalad central ray.

Fig. 11.65 AP skull with perpendicular central ray.

Cranium

 AP AXIAL PROJECTION

TOWNE METHOD

Image receptor + grid: Positioned by manufacturer or department protocol for proper anatomy display orientation; CR plate: 10 × 12 inches (24 × 30 cm) lengthwise.

NOTE: Although this technique is most commonly referred to as the Towne method,[3] numerous authors have described slightly different variations. In 1912 Grashey[4] published the first description of the AP axial projection of the cranium. In 1926 Altschul[5] and Towne[3] described the position. Altschul recommended strong depression of the chin and direction of the central ray through the foramen magnum at a caudal angle of 40 degrees. Towne (citing Chamberlain) recommended that with the patient's chin depressed, the central ray should be directed through the MSP from a point about 3 inches (7.6 cm) above the eyebrows to the foramen magnum. Towne gave no specific central ray angulation, but the angulation would depend on the flexion of the neck.

Position of patient

- With the patient supine or seated upright, center MSP of the patient's body to the midline of the grid.
- Place the patient's arms in a comfortable position, and adjust the shoulders to lie in the same horizontal plane.
- To ensure the patient's comfort without increasing the IR distance, examine the hypersthenic or obese patient in the seated-upright position, if possible.
- The skull can be brought closer to the IR by having the patient lean back lordotically and rest the shoulders against the vertical grid device. When this is impossible, the desired projection of the occipitobasal region may be obtained by using the PA axial projection described by Haas (pp. 50-51). The Haas method is the reverse of the AP axial projection and produces a comparable result.

Position of part

- Adjust the patient's head so that MSP is perpendicular to the midline of the IR.
- Flex the patient's neck enough to place the OML perpendicular to the plane of the IR.
- When the patient cannot flex the neck to this extent, adjust the neck so that the IOML is perpendicular and then increase the central ray angulation by 7 degrees (Figs. 11.66–11.69).
- Position the IR center at or near the level of the foramen magnum.
- For a localized image of the dorsum sellae and petrous pyramids, adjust the IR so that its midpoint coincides with the central ray. The IR is centered at or slightly below the level of the occlusal plane.
- Recheck the position and immobilize the head.
- *Respiration:* Suspend.

Fig. 11.66 AP axial skull: Towne method, upright position.

Fig. 11.67 AP axial skull: Towne method, supine position.

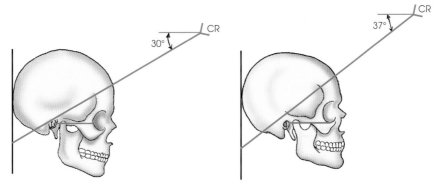

Fig. 11.68 Upright radiography diagram: AP axial skull: Towne method. Same radiographic result with central ray directed 30 degrees to OML or 37 degrees to IOML.

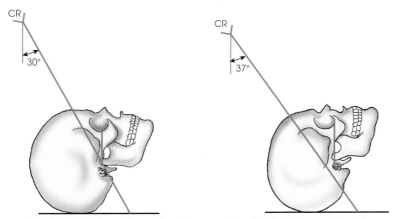

Fig. 11.69 Table radiography diagram: AP axial skull: Towne method.

Central ray

- Directed through the foramen magnum at a caudal angle of 30 degrees to the OML or 37 degrees to the IOML. The central ray enters approximately 2½ inches (6.3 cm) above the glabella and passes through the level of the EAM.

Collimation

- Adjust the radiation field to extend 1 inch (2.5 cm) beyond the skin line of the skull. Check for light at the vertex and on both sides. Place the side marker in the collimated exposure field.

Structures shown

A symmetric image of the petrous pyramids, the posterior portion of the foramen magnum, the dorsum sellae, and the posterior clinoid processes projected within the foramen magnum, the occipital bone, and the posterior portion of the parietal bones (Fig. 11.70).

EVALUATION CRITERIA

The following should be clearly seen:

- Evidence of proper collimation and presence of the side marker placed clear of anatomy of interest
- Entire cranium, without rotation or tilt, demonstrated by:
  - Equal distances from lateral borders of skull to lateral margins of foramen magnum on both sides
  - Symmetric petrous pyramids
  - MSP of cranium aligned with long axis of collimated field
- Dorsum sellae and posterior clinoid processes visible within foramen magnum
- Bony detail of occipital bone and surrounding soft tissues

Parietal bone

Occipital bone

Foramen magnum

Petrous ridge

Posterior clinoid process

Dorsum sellae

Fig. 11.70 AP axial skull: Towne method with 30-degree central ray angulation to OML.

Pathologic condition or trauma

To show the entire foramen magnum, the caudal angulation of the central ray is increased from 40 to 60 degrees to the OML (Figs. 11.71–11.75).

Lateral decubitus position

For pathologic conditions, trauma, or a deformity such as a strongly accentuated dorsal kyphosis when the patient cannot be examined in a direct supine or prone position, the following steps should be taken:

- Adjust and support the body in a semi-recumbent position; this allows the head to be placed in a true lateral position.

- Immobilize the IR and grid in a vertical position behind the patient's occiput.
- Direct the *horizontal* central ray 30 degrees caudally to the OML (Fig. 11.76).

Fig. 11.71 AP axial skull, Towne method, on a trauma patient. OML and IOML lines are not perpendicular, which would require CR angulation greater than 37 degrees.

Fig. 11.72 AP axial skull: central ray angulation of 40 to 45 degrees.

Occipital bone

Foramen magnum

Petrous ridge

Posterior arch of C1

Mandibular condyle

Fig. 11.73 AP axial skull: central ray angulation of 45 degrees.

Fig. 11.74 AP axial foramen magnum, supine position.

Fig. 11.75 AP axial foramen magnum: 55-degree caudal central ray.

Posterior arch of C1

Dens

Fig. 11.76 AP axial skull, with the patient's head in lateral decubitus position and with IR and grid vertical.

Fig. 11.77 PA axial skull: Haas method.

PA AXIAL PROJECTION

HAAS METHOD

Haas[6] devised this projection for obtaining an image of the sellar structures projected within the foramen magnum on hypersthenic, obese, or other patients who cannot be adjusted correctly for the AP axial (Towne) projection.

> **Image receptor + grid:** Positioned by manufacturer or department protocol for proper anatomy display orientation; CR plate: 10 × 12 inches (24 × 30 cm) lengthwise.

Position of patient

- Adjust the patient in the prone or seated-upright position, and center MSP of the body to the midline of the grid.
- Flex the patient's elbows, place the arms in a comfortable position, and adjust the shoulders to lie in the same horizontal plane.

Position of part

- Rest the patient's forehead and nose on the table, with MSP perpendicular to the midline of the grid.
- Adjust the flexion of the neck so that the OML is perpendicular to the IR (Figs. 11.77–11.79).
- Immobilize the head.
- For a localized image of the sellar region or the petrous pyramids, or both, adjust the position of the IR so that the midpoint coincides with the central ray; shift the IR cephalad approximately 3 inches (7.6 cm) to include the vertex of the skull.
- *Respiration:* Suspend.

Central ray

- Directed at a cephalad angle of 25 degrees to the OML to enter a point 1½ inches (3.8 cm) below the external occipital protuberance (inion) and to exit approximately 1½ inches (3.8 cm) superior to the nasion. The central ray can be varied to show other cranial anatomy.

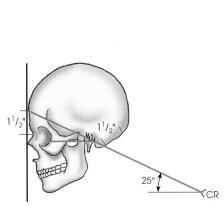

Fig. 11.78 Upright radiography diagram: PA axial skull: Haas method diagram.

Fig. 11.79 Table radiography diagram: PA axial skull: Haas method diagram.

Collimation

- Adjust the radiation field to extend 1 inch (2.5 cm) beyond the skin line of the skull. Check for light above the vertex and on both sides. Place the side marker in the collimated exposure field.

Structures shown

The occipital region of the cranium, a symmetric image of the petrous pyramids, and the dorsum sellae and posterior clinoid processes within the foramen magnum (Figs. 11.80 and 11.81).

EVALUATION CRITERIA

The following should be clearly seen:

- Evidence of proper collimation and presence of the side marker placed clear of anatomy of interest
- Entire cranium, without rotation or tilt, demonstrated by:
  - □ Equal distances from lateral borders of skull to lateral margins of foramen magnum on both sides
  - □ Symmetric petrous pyramids
  - □ MSP of cranium aligned with long axis of collimated field
- Dorsum sellae and posterior clinoid processes within the foramen magnum
- Bony detail of occipital bone and surrounding soft tissues

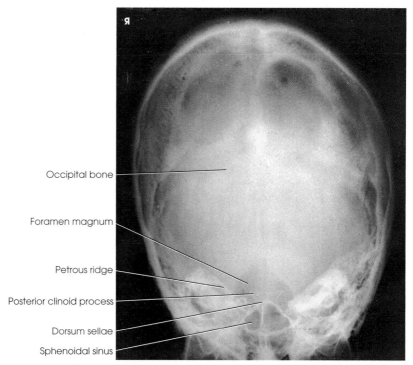

Occipital bone

Foramen magnum

Petrous ridge

Posterior clinoid process

Dorsum sellae

Sphenoidal sinus

Fig. 11.80 PA axial skull: Haas method, with 25-degree cephalad CR.

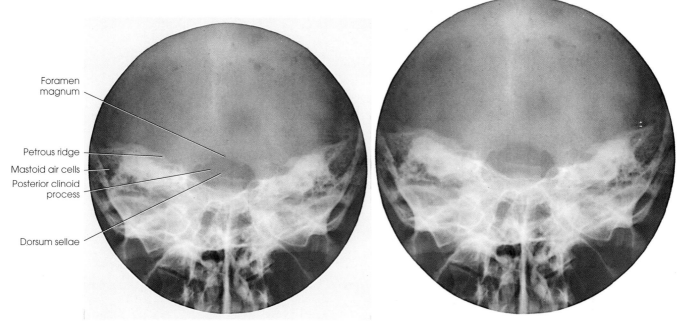

Foramen magnum

Petrous ridge

Mastoid air cells

Posterior clinoid process

Dorsum sellae

Fig. 11.81 PA axial sella turcica: Haas method, using cylindric extension cone that restricts the exposure field to small area. Beam restriction decreases scatter radiation and increases visibility of detail of sellar structures.

⚑ SUBMENTOVERTICAL PROJECTION
SCHÜLLER METHOD

Image receptor + grid: Positioned by manufacturer or department protocol for proper anatomy display orientation; CR plate: 10 × 12 inches (24 × 30 cm) lengthwise.

Position of patient

The success of the submentovertical (SMV) projection of the cranial base depends on placing the IOML as nearly parallel with the plane of the IR as possible and directing the central ray perpendicular to the IOML. The following steps are taken:

- Place the patient in the supine or the seated-upright position; the latter is more comfortable. If a chair that supports the back is used, the upright position allows greater freedom in positioning the patient's body to place the IOML parallel with the IR. If the patient is seated far enough away from the vertical grid device, the head can usually be adjusted without placing great pressure on the neck.
- When the patient is placed in the supine position, elevate the torso on firm pillows or a suitable pad to allow the head to rest on the vertex with the neck in hyperextension.
- Flex the patient's knees to relax the abdominal muscles.
- Place the patient's arms in a comfortable position, and adjust the shoulders to lie in the same horizontal plane.

- Do not keep the patient in the final adjustment longer than is absolutely necessary, because the supine position places considerable strain on the neck.

Position of part

- With MSP of the patient's body centered to the midline of the grid, extend the patient's neck to the greatest extent as can be achieved, placing the IOML as parallel as possible to the IR.
- Adjust the patient's head so that MSP is perpendicular to the IR (Figs. 11.82–11.85).

NOTE: Patients placed in the supine position for the cranial base may have increased intracranial pressure. As a result, they may be dizzy or unstable for a few minutes after having been in this position. Use of the upright position may alleviate some of this pressure.

Fig. 11.82 SMV cranial base, patient upright.

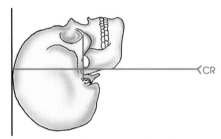

Fig. 11.83 Upright radiography diagram: SMV skull.

Fig. 11.84 SMV cranial base, patient supine.

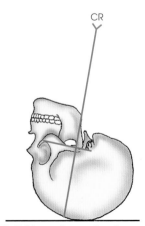

Fig. 11.85 Table radiography diagram: SMV skull.

- Immobilize the patient's head. In the absence of a head clamp, place a suitably backed strip of adhesive tape across the tip of the chin and anchor it to the sides of the radiographic unit if needed. (The part of the tape touching the skin should be covered.)
- *Respiration:* Suspend.

Central ray

- Directed through the sella turcica perpendicular to the IOML. The central ray enters MSP of the throat between the angles of the mandible and passes through a point ¾ inch (1.9 cm) anterior to the level of the EAM.
- Center the IR to the central ray. The IR should be parallel to the IOML.

Collimation

- Adjust the radiation field to extend 1 inch (2.5 cm) beyond the shadow of the tip of the nose and 1 inch (2.5 cm) beyond the lateral borders. Place the side marker in the collimated exposure field.

Structures shown

Symmetric images of the petrosae, the mastoid processes, the foramina ovale and spinosum (which are best shown in this projection), the carotid canals, the sphenoidal and ethmoidal sinuses, the mandible, the bony nasal septum, the dens of the axis, and the occipital bone. The maxillary sinuses are superimposed over the mandible (Fig. 11.86).

SMV projection is also used to demonstrate the zygomatic arches, mandible, ethmoidal, and sphenoidal sinuses with an adjustment in exposure factors (see sections on Facial Bone Radiography and Sinus Radiography later in this chapter).

The following should be clearly seen:

- Evidence of proper collimation and presence of the side marker placed clear of anatomy of interest
- Entire cranium, without tilt or rotation, demonstrated by:
  - Equal distances from the lateral borders of the skull to the mandibular condyles on both sides
  - Symmetric petrosae
- IOML is parallel to IR (full neck extension), demonstrated by:
  - Mental protuberance superimposed over anterior frontal bone
  - Mandibular condyles anterior to petrosae
- Bony details of the cranial base and surrounding soft tissues.

NOTE: Schüller[7] described and illustrated the basal projections—SMV and verticosubmental (VSM)—but Pfeiffer[8] gave specific directions for the central ray angulation.

Maxillary sinus
Ethmoidal air cells
Mandible
Sphenoidal sinus
Foramen spinosum
Mandibular condyle
Dens (odontoid process)
Petrosa
Mastoid process
Occipital bone

Fig. 11.86 SMV cranial base.

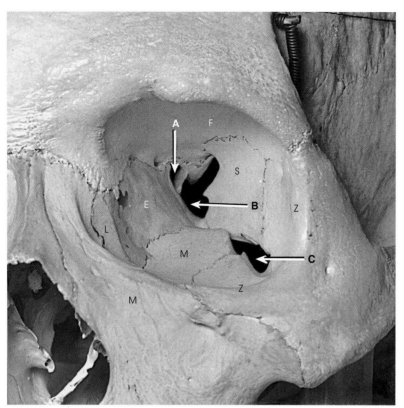

Fig. 11.87 Bones of left orbit of dry specimen. *A,* Optic canal and foramen. *B,* Superior orbital fissure. *C,* Inferior orbital fissure. *E,* Ethmoid; *F,* frontal; *L,* lacrimal; *M,* maxilla; *S,* sphenoid; *Z,* zygomatic (palatine not shown).

The orbits are cone-shaped, bony-walled cavities situated on each side of the MSP of the head (Fig. 11.87). They are formed by the seven previously described and illustrated bones of the cranium (frontal, ethmoid, and sphenoid) and the face (lacrimal, palatine, maxillary, and zygomatic). Each orbit has a roof, a medial wall, a lateral wall, and a floor. The easily palpable, quadrilateral-shaped anterior circumference of the orbit is called its *base.* The *apex* of the orbit corresponds to the *optic foramen.* The long axis of each orbit is directed obliquely, posteriorly, and medially at an average angle of 37 degrees to the MSP of the head and superiorly at an angle of about 30 degrees from the OML (Fig. 11.88).

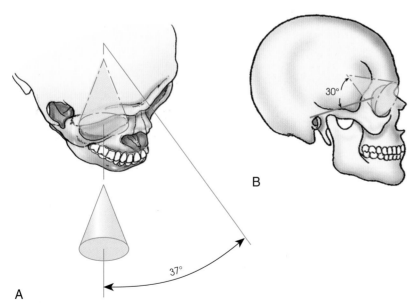

Fig. 11.88 Cone-shaped orbit. (A) Average angle of 37 degrees from midsagittal plane. (B) Average angle of 30 degrees superior to OML.

The orbits serve primarily as bony sockets for the eyeballs and the structures associated with them, but they also contain blood vessels and nerves that pass through openings in their walls to other regions. The major and frequently radiographed openings are the previously described optic foramina and the superior and inferior orbital sulci.

The *superior orbital fissure* is the cleft between the greater and lesser wings of the sphenoid bone. From the body of the sphenoid at a point near the orbital apex, this sulcus extends superiorly and laterally between the roof and the lateral wall of the orbit. The *inferior orbital fissure* is the narrow cleft extending from the lower anterolateral aspect of the sphenoid body anteriorly and laterally between the floor and lateral wall of the orbit. The anterior margin of the cleft is formed by the orbital plate of the maxilla, and its posterior margin is formed by the greater wing of the sphenoid bone and the zygomatic bone.

Because the walls of the orbits are thin, they are subject to fracture. When a person is forcibly struck squarely on the eyeball (e.g., by a fist, by a piece of sporting equipment), the resulting pressure directed to the eyeball forces the eyeball into the cone-shaped orbit and "blows out" the thin, delicate bony floor of the orbit (Figs. 11.89 and 11.90). The injury must be diagnosed and treated accurately so that the person's vision is not jeopardized. Blowout fractures may be shown radiographically using the parietoacanthial projection (Waters method) or CT.

Fig. 11.89 Parietoacanthial orbits using Waters method and showing blowout fracture of right orbit *(arrows)*.

Fig. 11.90 Coronal CT of complex blowout fracture, zygoma fracture *(red circle)*, and additional maxilla fracture *(arrowhead)*. Associated blood/soft tissue in maxillary sinus *(*)*.

(Courtesy Priscilla Rounds, RT(R), NEA Baptist Memorial Hospital, Jonesboro, AR.)

The organ of vision, or eye (Latin, *oculus*; Greek, *ophthalmos*), consists of the following: eyeball; optic nerve, which connects the eyeball to the brain; blood vessels; and accessory organs such as extrinsic muscles, lacrimal apparatus, and eyelids (Figs. 11.91 and 11.92).

The *eyeball* is situated in the anterior part of the orbital cavity. Its posterior segment (about two thirds of the bulb) is adjacent to the soft parts that occupy the remainder of the orbital cavity (chiefly muscles, fat, and connective tissue). The anterior portion of the eyeball is exposed and projects beyond the base of the orbit. Bone-free radiographic images of the anterior segment of the eye can be obtained. The exposed part of the eyeball is covered by a thin mucous membrane known as the *conjunctiva*, portions of which line the eyelids. The conjunctival membrane is kept moist by tear secretions from the lacrimal gland. These secretions prevent drying and friction irritation during movements of the eyeball and eyelids.

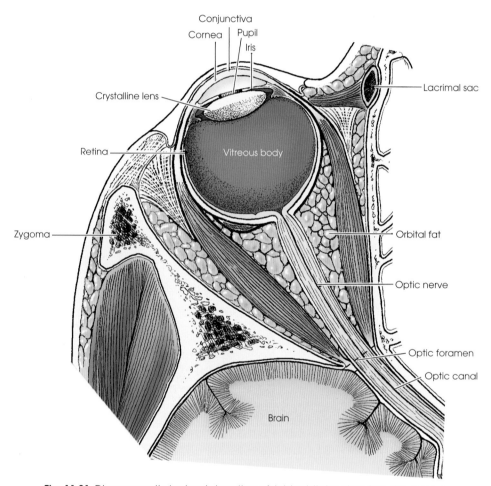

Fig. 11.91 Diagrammatic horizontal section of right orbital region: top-down view.

The outer, supporting coat of the eyeball is a firm, fibrous membrane consisting of a posterior segment called the *sclera* and an anterior segment called the *cornea*. The opaque, white sclera is commonly referred to as the "white of the eye." The cornea is situated in front of the *iris*, with its center point corresponding to the pupil. The corneal part of the membrane is transparent, allowing the passage of light into the eyeball, and it serves as one of the four refractive media of the eye.

The inner coat of the eyeball is called the *retina*. This delicate membrane is contiguous with the optic nerve. The retina is composed chiefly of nervous tissue and several million minute receptor organs, called *rods* and *cones*, which transmit light impulses to the brain. The rods and cones are important radiographically because they play a role in the ability of the radiologist or radiographer to see the fluoroscopic image. Their function is described in discussions of fluoroscopy in radiography physics and imaging textbooks.

Fig. 11.92 Diagrammatic sagittal section of right orbital region.

LOCALIZATION OF FOREIGN BODIES WITHIN ORBIT OR EYE

Ultrasonography and CT (Fig. 11.93) have been increasingly used to locate foreign bodies in the eye. (Magnetic resonance imaging [MRI] is not used for foreign body localization because movement of a metallic foreign object by the magnetic field could lead to hemorrhage or other serious complications.) Whether an ultrasound or a radiographic approach is used, accurate localization of foreign particles lodged within the orbit or eye requires the use of a precision localization technique.

Image Quality

The highest possible spatial resolution is essential for detecting and localizing minute foreign particles within the orbit or eyeball. Optimal image quality requires the following:

1. Reduce geometric unsharpness as much as possible by using minimal OID and a small focal spot at a SID that is as long as is consistent with the exposure factors required.
2. Minimize secondary radiation by close collimation.
3. Eliminate motion by firmly immobilizing the patient's head and by having the patient gaze steadily at a fixed object, immobilizing the eyeballs.

4. Minimize possibility of artifacts by thoroughly cleaning IRs just prior to imaging. An artifact can cast an image that simulates the appearance of a foreign body located within the orbit or eye.

PRELIMINARY EXAMINATION

Lateral projections, PA projections, and bone-free studies are performed to determine whether a radiographically demonstrable foreign body is present. For these images, the patient may be placed in the recumbent position or may be seated upright before a vertical grid device. These projections may be used for metallic foreign body screening before MRI procedures are performed or to evaluate trauma to the bony orbits.

Fig. 11.93 (A) Lateral localizer CT image showing multiple buckshot in the face. (B) Axial CT image of same patient, showing shotgun pellets within the eye *(arrows)*.

⚜ LATERAL PROJECTION
Right or left position

A nongrid technique is recommended to reduce magnification and eliminate possible artifacts in or on the radiographic table and grid. The following steps are taken:

- Position patient in an upright or recumbent anterior oblique position and place the outer canthus of the affected eye adjacent to and centered over the midpoint of the IR.
- Adjust the patient's head to place the MSP parallel with the plane of the IR and the IPL perpendicular to the IR plane. Adjust neck flexion to place IOML perpendicular to the front IR edge.
- *Respiration* Suspend.

Central ray

- Perpendicular through the outer canthus.
- Instruct the patient to look straight ahead for the exposure (Figs. 11.94 and 11.95).

EVALUATION CRITERIA

The following should be clearly shown:
- Entire orbit(s)
- No rotation, demonstrated by:
  - □ Superimposed orbital roofs
- Close beam restriction centered to orbital region
- Bony orbit and soft tissues of the eye for localization of foreign bodies

Fig. 11.94 Lateral projection for orbital foreign body localization.

Superior orbital margin

Nasal bone

Fig. 11.95 Lateral projection showing foreign body *(white speck)*.

Fig. 11.96 PA axial projection for orbital foreign body localization.

★ PA AXIAL PROJECTION

A nongrid (very high resolution) technique is recommended to reduce magnification and eliminate possible artifacts in or on the radiographic table and grid. The following steps are taken:

- Rest the patient's forehead and nose on the IR and center the IR ¾ inch (1.9 cm) distal to the nasion.
- Adjust the patient's head so that the MSP and OML are perpendicular to the plane of the IR.
- *Respiration:* Suspend.

Central ray

- Directed through the center of the orbits at a caudal angulation of 30 degrees. This angulation is used to project the petrous portions of the temporal bones below the inferior margin of the orbits (Figs. 11.96 and 11.97).
- Instruct the patient to close the eyes and to concentrate on holding them still for the exposure.

EVALUATION CRITERIA

The following should be clearly shown:
- Entire orbit(s)
- Petrous pyramids lying below orbital shadows
- No rotation of cranium, demonstrated by:
  □ Symmetric visualization of the orbits
- Close beam restriction centered to orbital region
- Bony details of orbit and soft tissues of the eye for localization of foreign bodies

Fig. 11.97 PA axial projection showing foreign body *(arrow)* in the right eye.

▲ PARIETOACANTHIAL PROJECTION

MODIFIED WATERS METHOD

Some physicians prefer to have the PA projection performed with the patient's head adjusted in a modified Waters position so that the petrous margins are displaced by part adjustment rather than by central ray angulation. The following steps are taken:

- With the IR centered at the level of the center of the orbits, rest the patient's chin on the IR holder.
- Adjust the patient's head so that the MSP is perpendicular to the plane of the IR.
- Adjust the flexion of the patient's neck so that the OML forms an angle of 50 degrees with the plane of the IR.
- *Respiration:* Suspend.

Central ray

- Perpendicular through the mid-orbits (Figs. 11.98 and 11.99).
- Instruct the patient to close the eyes and to concentrate on holding them still for the exposure.

EVALUATION CRITERIA

The following should be clearly shown:

■ Entire orbit(s)
■ Petrous pyramids lying well below orbital shadows
■ No rotation, demonstrated by:
   ☐ Symmetric visualization of orbits
■ Close beam restriction centered to the orbital region
■ Bony orbit and soft tissues of the eye for localization of foreign bodies

Fig. 11.98 Parietoacanthial projection, modified Waters method, for orbital foreign body localization.

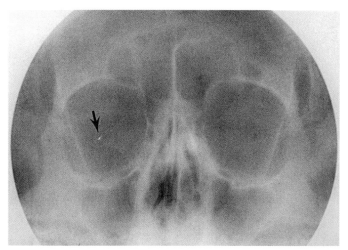

Fig. 11.99 Parietoacanthial projection, modified Waters method, showing foreign body (*arrow*).

⚕ LATERAL PROJECTION
Right or left position

Image receptor + grid: Positioned by manufacturer or department protocol for proper anatomy display orientation; CR plate: 10 × 12 inches (24 × 30 cm) lengthwise.

Position of patient
- Place the patient in a recumbent anterior oblique or seated anterior oblique position before a vertical grid device. This is the same basic position that is used for the lateral skull position.

Position of part
- Adjust the patient's head so that MSP is parallel with the IR and the IPL is perpendicular to the IR.
- Adjust the flexion of the patient's neck so that the IOML is perpendicular to the front edge of the IR (Figs. 11.100–11.102).
- Immobilize the head.
- *Respiration:* Suspend.

Fig. 11.100 Lateral facial bones.

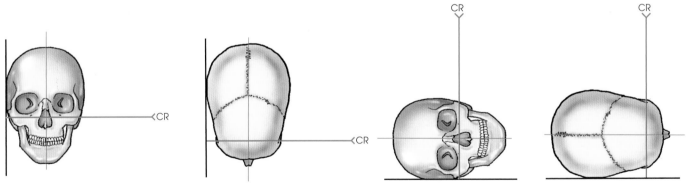

Fig. 11.101 Upright radiography diagram: lateral facial bones.

Fig. 11.102 Table radiography diagram: lateral facial bones.

Facial Bones

Central ray
- Perpendicular and entering the lateral surface of the zygomatic bone halfway between the outer canthus and the EAM.
- Center IR to the central ray.

Collimation
- Adjust radiation field to extend 1 inch (2.5 cm) beyond the shadow of the tip of the nose, superiorly to 1 inch (2.5 cm) above the supraorbital margins, inferiorly to the gonion, and posteriorly to the EAM. The exposure field should be set no larger than 6 × 10 inches (15 × 24 cm). Place the side marker in the collimated exposure field.

Structures shown
A lateral image of the bones of the face, with the right and left sides superimposed (Fig. 11.103).

EVALUATION CRITERIA
The following should be clearly seen:
- Evidence of proper collimation and presence of the side marker placed clear of anatomy of interest
- All facial bones in their entirety, with the zygomatic bone in the center
- No rotation or tilt of the facial bones, demonstrated by:
  - ☐ Almost perfectly superimposed mandibular rami
  - ☐ Superimposed orbital roofs
  - ☐ Sella turcica in profile
- Soft tissue and bony trabecular detail

Fig. 11.103 Lateral facial bones.

Frontal sinus

Nasal bone
Sella turcica

Maxillary sinus

External acoustic meatus
Maxilla

Mandible

♠ PARIETOACANTHIAL PROJECTION
WATERS METHOD[9]

Image receptor + grid: Positioned by manufacturer or department protocol for proper anatomy display orientation; CR plate: 10 × 12 inches (24 × 30 cm) lengthwise.

Position of patient
- Place the patient in the prone or seated-upright position.
- Center MSP of the patient's body to the midline of the grid device.

Position of part
- Rest the patient's head on the tip of the extended chin. Hyperextend the neck so that the OML forms a 37-degree angle with the plane of the IR.
- The MML is approximately perpendicular to the plane of the IR; the average patient's nose is about ¾ inch (1.9 cm) away from the grid device.
- Adjust the head so that MSP is perpendicular to the plane of the IR (Figs. 11.104–11.106).
- Center the IR at the level of the acanthion.
- Immobilize the head.
- *Respiration:* Suspend.

Central ray
- Perpendicular to exit the acanthion

Collimation
- Adjust the radiation field to 1 inch (2.5 cm) beyond the shadows of the lateral sides of the face, superiorly to include the supraorbital margins and inferiorly to the level of the chin. The exposure field should be no larger than 8 × 10 inches (18 × 24 cm). Place the side marker in the collimated exposure field.

Structures shown
The orbits, maxillae, and zygomatic arches (Fig. 11.107).

EVALUATION CRITERIA
The following should be clearly seen:
- Evidence of proper collimation and presence of the side marker placed clear of anatomy of interest
- Entire orbits and facial bones
- No rotation or tilt, demonstrated by:
  □ Distances between the lateral borders of the skull and the orbits equal on each side
  □ MSP of head aligned with long axis of collimated field
- Petrous ridges projected immediately below maxillary sinuses
- Soft tissue and bony trabecular detail

Fig. 11.104 Parietoacanthial facial bones: Waters method.

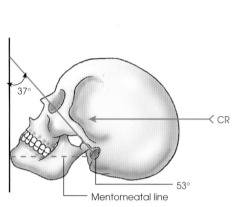

Fig. 11.105 Upright radiography diagram: parietoacanthial facial bones: Waters method.

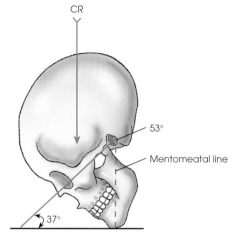

Fig. 11.106 Table radiography diagram: parietoacanthial facial bones: Waters method.

Orbit

Zygomatic arch

Maxillary sinus

Maxilla

Petrous ridge

Mandibular angle

Fig. 11.107 Parietoacanthial facial bones: Waters method.

(Courtesy St. Bernard's Medical Center, Jonesboro, AR.)

Fig. 11.108 Modified parietoacanthial facial bones: modified Waters method.

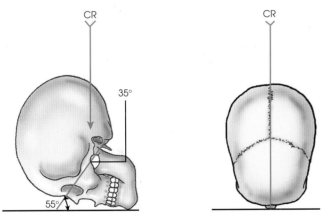

Fig. 11.109 Table radiography diagram, modified parietoacanthial facial bones: modified Waters method with OML adjusted to 55 degrees.

MODIFIED PARIETOACANTHIAL PROJECTION
MODIFIED WATERS METHOD

Although the parietoacanthial projection (Waters method) is widely used, many institutions modify the projection by radiographing the patient using less extension of the patient's neck. This modification, although sometimes called a "shallow" Waters, actually increases the angulation of the OML by placing it more perpendicular to the plane of the IR. The patient's head is positioned as described using the Waters method, but the neck is extended to a lesser degree. In the modification, the OML is adjusted to form an approximately 55-degree angle with the plane of the IR (Figs. 11.108–11.110). The resulting radiographic image shows the facial bones with less axial angulation than with the Waters method (see Fig. 11.107). With the modified Waters method, the petrous ridges are projected immediately below the inferior border of the orbits at a level midway through the maxillary sinuses (Fig. 11.111).

The modified Waters method is a good projection to show blowout fractures. This method places the orbital floor perpendicular to the IR and parallel to the central ray, showing inferior displacement of the orbital floor and the commonly associated opacified maxillary sinus.

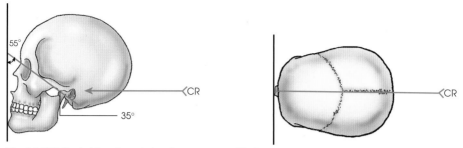

Fig. 11.110 Upright radiography diagram, modified parietoacanthial facial bones: modified Waters method with OML adjusted to 55 degrees.

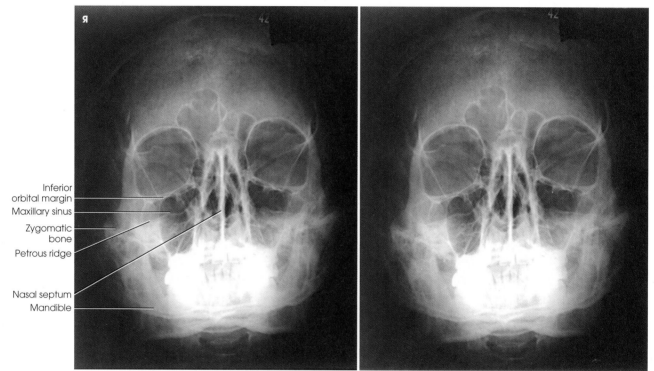

Inferior orbital margin
Maxillary sinus
Zygomatic bone
Petrous ridge

Nasal septum
Mandible

Fig. 11.111 Modified parietoacanthial facial bones: modified Waters method.

ACANTHIOPARIETAL PROJECTION
REVERSE WATERS METHOD

Image receptor + grid: Positioned by manufacturer or department protocol for proper anatomy display orientation; CR plate: 10 × 12 inches (24 × 30 cm) lengthwise.

The *reverse* Waters method is used to show the facial bones when the patient cannot be placed in the prone position. (See the sections on the trauma method in Chapter 12, p. 142.)

Position of patient
- With the patient in the supine position, center MSP of the body to the midline of the grid.

Position of part
- Bringing the patient's chin up, adjust the extension of the neck so that the OML forms a 37-degree angle with the plane of the IR (Fig. 11.112). If necessary, place a support under the patient's shoulders to help extend the neck.

- The MML is approximately perpendicular to the plane of the IR.
- Adjust the head so that MSP is perpendicular to the plane of the IR.
- Immobilize the head.
- *Respiration:* Suspend.

Central ray
- Perpendicular to enter the acanthion and centered to the IR

Collimation
- Adjust the radiation field to extend about 1 inch (2.5 cm) beyond the lateral sides of the face, superiorly just to the skin shadow, and inferiorly to the chin. The exposure field should be no larger than 8 × 10 inches (18 × 24 cm). Place the side marker in the collimated exposure field.

Structures shown
The *reverse* Waters method shows the superior facial bones. The image is similar to that obtained with the Waters method, but the facial structures are considerably magnified (Fig. 11.113).

The following should be clearly seen:
- Evidence of proper collimation and presence of the side marker placed clear of anatomy of interest
- Entire orbits and facial bones
- No rotation or tilt, demonstrated by:
  - Distances between lateral borders of the skull and orbits equal on each side
  - MSP of head aligned with long axis of collimated field
- Petrous ridges projected below maxillary sinuses
- Soft tissue and bony trabecular detail

Fig. 11.112 Table radiography. Acanthioparietal facial bones: reverse Waters method with neck extended. MML is perpendicular to IR.

Facial Bones

Cranium

ALTERNATIVE ACANTHIOPARIETAL PROJECTION

Many patients, including those being evaluated for acute injury, are often unable to hyperextend the neck far enough to place the OML 37 degrees to the IR and the MML perpendicular to the plane of the IR. In these patients, the acanthioparietal projection, or the reverse Waters projection, can be achieved by adjusting the central ray so that it enters the acanthion while remaining parallel with the MML (Fig. 11.114).

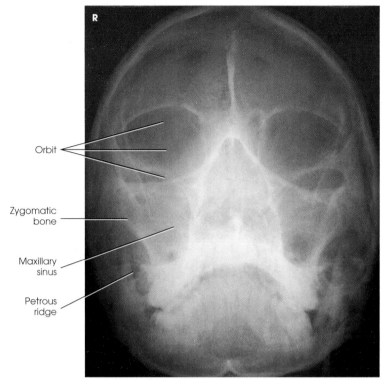

Orbit

Zygomatic bone

Maxillary sinus

Petrous ridge

Fig. 11.113 Acanthioparietal facial bones: reverse Waters method.

CR

30°

Mentomeatal line

Fig. 11.114 Table radiography. Acanthioparietal facial bones: reverse Waters method with the CR parallel to MML.

70

☀ PA AXIAL PROJECTION
CALDWELL METHOD

Image receptor + grid: Positioned by manufacturer or department protocol for proper anatomy display orientation; CR plate: 10 × 12 inches (24 × 30 cm) lengthwise.

Position of patient
- Place the patient in a prone or a seated position.
- Center MSP of the patient's body to the midline of the grid.
- Rest the patient's forehead and nose on the table or against the upright bucky.
- Flex the patient's elbows, and place the arms in a comfortable position.

Position of part
- Adjust the flexion of the patient's neck so that the OML is perpendicular to the plane of the IR.
- If the patient is obese or hypersthenic, a small radiolucent sponge may need to be placed in front of the forehead.
- Align MSP of the head perpendicular to the IR by adjusting the lateral margins of the orbits or the EAM equidistant from the tabletop.
- Immobilize the head, and center the IR to the nasion (Fig. 11.115).
- *Respiration:* Suspend.

Central ray
- Direct the central ray to exit the nasion at an angle of 15 degrees caudad.
- To show the orbital rims, in particular, the orbital floors, use a 30-degree caudal angle (sometimes referred to as the *exaggerated Caldwell*).
- Center the IR to the central ray.

Collimation
- Adjust the radiation field to extend about 1 inch (2.5 cm) beyond the lateral sides of the face, superiorly to include the supraorbital margins, and inferiorly to the chin. The exposure field should be no larger than 8 × 10 inches (18 × 24 cm). Place the side marker in the collimated exposure field.

Structures shown
The orbital rims, maxillae, nasal septum, zygomatic bones, and anterior nasal spine. When the central ray is angled 15 degrees caudad to the nasion, the petrous ridges are projected into the lower third of the orbits (Fig. 11.116). When the central ray is angled 30 degrees caudad, the petrous ridges are projected below the inferior margins of the orbits.

Fig. 11.115 Upright radiography, PA axial facial bones: Caldwell method.

Facial Bones

EVALUATION CRITERIA

The following should be clearly seen:
- Evidence of proper collimation and presence of the side marker placed clear of anatomy of interest
- Entire orbits and facial bones
- No rotation or tilt, demonstrated by:
  - Equal distances from lateral borders of skull to lateral borders of orbits on both sides
  - MSP of head aligned with long axis of collimated field
- Symmetric petrous ridges lying in lower third of orbit
- Bony detail and surrounding soft tissues

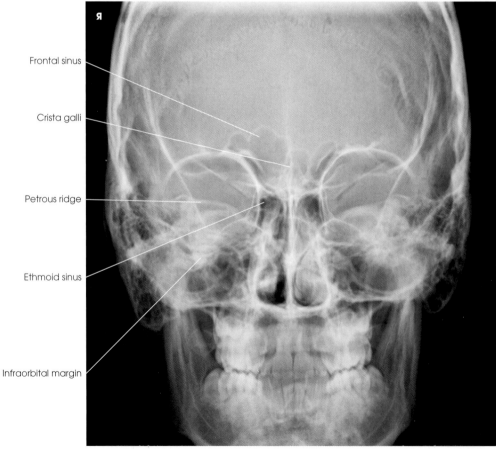

Frontal sinus

Crista galli

Petrous ridge

Ethmoid sinus

Infraorbital margin

Fig. 11.116 PA axial facial bones: Caldwell method.

(Courtesy St. Bernard's Medical Center, Jonesboro, AR.)

⚕ LATERAL PROJECTION
Right and left positions

Image receptor: Positioned by manufacturer or department protocol for proper anatomy display orientation; CR plate: 10 × 12 inches (24 × 30 cm), crosswise for two exposures on one IR.

Position of patient

- With the patient in a recumbent or upright anterior oblique position, adjust the rotation of the body so that MSP of the head can be placed horizontally.

Position of part

- Adjust the head so that MSP is parallel with the tabletop and the IPL is perpendicular to the tabletop.
- Adjust the flexion of the patient's neck so that the IOML is parallel with the transverse axis of the IR (Figs. 11.117 and 11.118).
- Support the mandible to prevent rotation.
- *Respiration:* Suspend.

Placement of image receptor

- When using a crosswise IR, slide the unmasked half of the IR under the frontonasal region and center it to the nasion (see Fig. 11.117). This centering allows space for the identification marker to be projected across the upper part of the IR. Tape the side marker (R or L) in position.

Fig. 11.117 Lateral nasal bones.

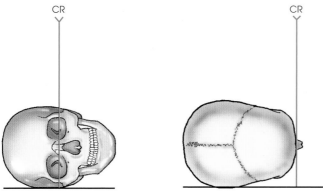

Fig. 11.118 Table radiography diagram: lateral nasal bones.

Nasal Bones

Central ray

- Perpendicular to the bridge of the nose at a point 1 inch (2.5 cm) distal to the nasion (see Fig. 11.118).

Collimation

- Adjust the radiation field to extend from the glabella to 1 inch (2.5 cm) inferior to the acanthion and 1 inch (2.5 cm) beyond the tip of the nose. The exposure field should be no larger than 3 × 3 inches (8 × 8 cm). Place the side marker in the collimated exposure field.

Structures shown

Nasal bone and soft tissues of the nose closer to the IR (Fig. 11.119). Both sides are examined for comparison.

EVALUATION CRITERIA

The following should be clearly seen:

- Evidence of proper collimation and presence of the side marker placed clear of anatomy of interest
- Nasal bones, anterior nasal spine, and frontonasal suture
- No rotation of nasal bones and soft tissue
- Soft tissue and bony trabecular detail

Frontonasal suture

Nasal bone

Anterior nasal spine of maxilla

Fig. 11.119 Nasal bones. (A) Right lateral. (B) Left lateral.

(Courtesy St. Bernard's Medical Center, Jonesboro, AR.)

Fig. 11.120 SMV zygomatic arches, patient upright.

Fig. 11.121 Upright radiography diagram: SMV zygomatic arches.

Fig. 11.122 Table radiography diagram: SMV zygomatic arches.

SUBMENTOVERTICAL PROJECTION

This projection is similar to the SMV projection described in the Skull Radiography section.

> **Image receptor + grid:** Positioned by manufacturer or department protocol for proper anatomy display orientation; CR plate: 10 × 12 inches (24 × 30 cm) crosswise.

Position of patient

- Place the patient in a seated upright or supine position.
- When the supine position is used, elevate the patient's trunk on several firm pillows or a suitable pad to allow complete extension of the neck. Flex the patient's knees to relax the abdominal muscles.
- Center MSP of the patient's body to the midline of the grid device.

Position of part

- Hyperextend the patient's neck completely so that the IOML is as parallel with the plane of the IR as possible.
- Rest the patient's head on its vertex, and adjust the head so that MSP is perpendicular to the plane of the IR (Figs. 11.120–11.122).
- *Respiration:* Suspend.

Zygomatic Arches

Central ray

- Perpendicular to the IOML and entering MSP of the throat at a level approximately 1 inch (2.5 cm) posterior to the outer canthi.
- Center the IR to the central ray.

Collimation

- Adjust radiation field to extend 1 inch (2.5 cm) beyond the lateral sides of the face, superiorly to the chin, and inferiorly to the gonions. The exposure field should be no larger than 10 inches (24 cm) wide and 8 inches (18 cm) long. Place the side marker in the collimated exposure field.

Structures shown

Bilateral symmetric SMV images of the zygomatic arches are shown, projected free of superimposed structures (Fig. 11.123). Unless very flat or traumatically depressed, the arches, being farther from the IR, are projected beyond the prominent parietal eminences by the divergent x-ray beam.

EVALUATION CRITERIA

The following should be clearly seen:

- Evidence of proper collimation and presence of the side marker placed clear of anatomy of interest
- Zygomatic arches free from overlying structures
- No rotation or tilt of head, demonstrated by:
  - □ Zygomatic arches symmetric and without foreshortening
- Soft tissue and bony trabecular detail

Fig. 11.123 (A) SMV projection showing normal zygomatic arch *(right)* and fracture *(arrow)* of left zygomatic arch. (B) SMV zygomatic arches.

(Courtesy St. Bernard's Medical Center, Jonesboro, AR.)

Fig. 11.124 Tangential zygomatic arch, patient upright.

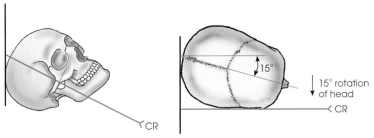

Fig. 11.125 Upright radiography diagram: tangential zygomatic arch.

Fig. 11.126 Table radiography diagram: tangential zygomatic arch.

TANGENTIAL PROJECTION

Image receptor + grid: Positioned by manufacturer or department protocol for proper anatomy display orientation; CR plate: 10 × 12 inches (24 × 30 cm) lengthwise.

Position of patient

• Seat the patient with the back against a vertical grid device, or place the patient in the supine position with the trunk elevated on several firm pillows and the knees flexed to permit complete extension of the neck.

Position of part
Seated position

• Hyperextend the patient's neck, and rest the head on its vertex.
• Adjust the position of the patient's head so that the IOML is as parallel as possible with the plane of the IR.
• Rotate MSP of the head approximately 15 degrees toward the side being examined.
• Tilt the top of the head approximately 15 degrees away from the side being examined. This rotation and tilt ensure that the central ray is tangent to the lateral surface of the skull. The central ray skims across the lateral portion of the mandibular angle and the parietal bone to project the zygomatic arch onto the IR.
• Center the zygomatic arch to the IR (Figs. 11.124–11.126).

Supine position

- Rest the patient's head on its vertex.
- Elevate the upper end of the IR on sandbags, or place it on an angled sponge of suitable size.
- Adjust the elevation of the IR and the extension of the patient's neck so that the IOML is placed as nearly parallel with the plane of the IR as possible.
- Rotate and tilt MSP of the head approximately 15 degrees toward the side being examined (similar to the upright position).
- If the IOML is parallel with the plane of the IR, center the IR to the zygomatic arch; if not, displace the IR so that the midpoint of the IR coincides with the central ray (see Fig. 11.126).
- Attach a strip of adhesive tape to the inferior surface of the chin; draw the tape upward, and anchor it to the edge of the table or IR stand. This usually affords sufficient support. Do not put the adhesive surface directly on the patient's skin.
- *Respiration:* Suspend.

Central ray

- Perpendicular to the IOML and centered to the zygomatic arch at a point approximately 1 inch (2.5 cm) posterior to the outer canthus.
- Centered to the IR.

Collimation

- Adjust the radiation field to 1 inch (2.5 cm) beyond the skin shadow of the affected cheek, superiorly to the tip of the nose, and inferiorly to the gonion. The exposure field should be no larger than 6 × 10 inches (18 × 24 cm). Place the side marker in the collimated exposure field.

Structures shown

A tangential image of one zygomatic arch is seen free of superimposition (Fig. 11.127). This projection is particularly useful in patients with depressed fractures or flat cheekbones.

Temporal process of zygomatic bone

Zygomatic arch

Temporal bone

Fig. 11.127 Tangential zygomatic arch.

(Courtesy St. Bernard's Medical Center, Jonesboro, AR.)

AP AXIAL PROJECTION
MODIFIED TOWNE METHOD

Image receptor + grid: Positioned by manufacturer or department protocol for proper anatomy display orientation; CR plate: 10 × 12 inches (24 × 30 cm) crosswise.

Position of patient
- Place the patient in the seated-upright or supine position.
- Center MSP of the body to the midline of the grid.

Position of part
- Adjust the patient's head so that MSP is perpendicular to the midline of the grid.
- Adjust the flexion of the neck so that the OML is perpendicular to the plane of the IR (Figs. 11.128–11.130).
- *Respiration:* Suspend.

Central ray
- Directed to enter the glabella approximately 1 inch (2.5 cm) above the nasion at an angle of 30 degrees caudad.
- If the patient is unable to flex the neck sufficiently, adjust the IOML perpendicular with the IR and direct the central ray 37 degrees caudad.
- Center the IR to the central ray.

Collimation
- Adjust the radiation field to 1 inch (2.5 cm) beyond the skin shadow of the affected cheek, superiorly to the tip of the nose, and inferiorly to the gonion. The exposure field should be no larger than 6 × 10 inches (18 × 24 cm). Place the side marker in the collimated exposure field.

Structures shown
A symmetric AP axial projection of both zygomatic arches is shown. The arches should be projected free of superimposition (Fig. 11.131).

EVALUATION CRITERIA
The following should be clearly seen:
- Evidence of proper collimation and presence of the side marker placed clear of anatomy of interest
- No overlap of zygomatic arches by mandible
- No rotation or tilt, demonstrated by:
  - ☐ Symmetric arches
  - ☐ Zygomatic arches projected lateral to mandibular rami
  - ☐ MSP of head aligned with long axis of collimated field
- Soft tissue and bony trabecular detail

Fig. 11.128 AP axial zygomatic arches: modified Towne method.

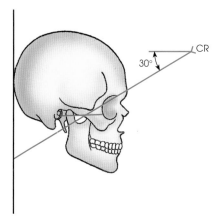

Fig. 11.129 Upright radiography diagram: modified Towne method.

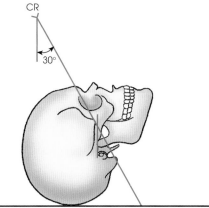

Fig. 11.130 Table radiography diagram: modified Towne method.

Zygomatic Arches

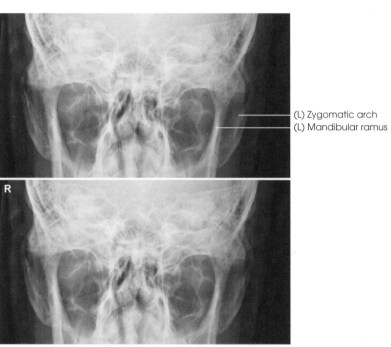

(L) Zygomatic arch
(L) Mandibular ramus

Fig. 11.131 AP axial zygomatic arches: modified Towne method.

✤ PA PROJECTION

Image receptor + grid: Positioned by manufacturer or department protocol for proper anatomy display orientation; CR plate: 10 × 12 inches (24 × 30 cm) lengthwise.

Position of patient

- Place the patient in the prone position, or seat the patient before a vertical grid device.

Position of part

- Rest the patient's forehead and nose on the IR. Adjust the OML to be perpendicular to the plane of the IR.
- Adjust the head so that its MSP is perpendicular to the plane of the IR (Fig. 11.132).
- Immobilize the head.
- *Respiration:* Suspend.

Central ray

- Perpendicular to exit the acanthion.
- Center the IR to the central ray.

Collimation

- Adjust the radiation field to extend 1 inch (2.5 cm) beyond the lateral sides, above the TMJs and below the chin. The exposure field should be no larger than 8 × 10 inches (18 × 24 cm). Place the side marker in the collimated exposure field.

Structures shown

The mandibular body and rami (Fig. 11.133). The central part of the body is not well shown because of the superimposed spine. This radiographic approach is usually employed to show medial or lateral displacement of fragments in fractures of the rami.

EVALUATION CRITERIA

The following should be clearly seen:

- Evidence of proper collimation and presence of the side marker placed clear of anatomy of interest
- Entire mandible
- No rotation or tilt, demonstrated by:
    - ☐ Mandibular body and rami symmetric on each side
    - ☐ MSP of head aligned with long axis of collimated field
- Soft tissue and bony trabecular detail

Fig. 11.132 PA mandibular rami.

Mastoid air cells

Condyle

Ramus

Body

Fig. 11.133 PA mandibular rami.

(Courtesy St. Bernard's Medical Center, Jonesboro, AR.)

⚹ PA AXIAL PROJECTION

Image receptor + grid: Positioned by manufacturer or department protocol for proper anatomy display orientation; CR plate: 10 × 12 inches (24 × 30 cm) lengthwise.

Position of patient
- Place the patient in the prone position, or seat the patient before a vertical grid device.

Position of part
- Rest the patient's forehead and nose on the IR holder.
- Adjust the OML to be perpendicular to the plane of the IR.
- Adjust the patient's head so that MSP is perpendicular to the plane of the IR (Fig. 11.134).
- Immobilize the patient's head.
- *Respiration:* Suspend.

Central ray
- Directed 20 or 25 degrees cephalad to exit at the acanthion.
- Center the IR to the central ray.

Collimation
- Adjust the radiation field to extend 1 inch (2.5 cm) beyond the lateral sides, above the TMJs and below the chin. The exposure field should be no larger than 8 × 10 inches (18 × 24 cm). Place the side marker in the collimated exposure field.

Structures shown
The mandibular body and rami (Fig. 11.135). The central part of the body is not well shown because of the superimposed spine. This radiographic approach is usually employed to show medial or lateral displacement of fragments in fractures of the rami.

EVALUATION CRITERIA
The following should be clearly seen:
- Evidence of proper collimation and presence of the side marker placed clear of anatomy of interest
- Entire mandible
- No rotation or tilt, demonstrated by:
  - □ Mandibular body and rami symmetric on each side
  - □ MSP of head aligned with long axis of collimated field
- Condylar processes
- Soft tissue and bony trabecular detail

Fig. 11.134 PA axial mandibular rami.

Fig. 11.135 PA axial mandibular body and rami.

PA PROJECTION

Image receptor + grid: Positioned by manufacturer or department protocol for proper anatomy display orientation; CR plate: 10 × 12 inches (24 × 30 cm) lengthwise.

Position of patient

- Place the patient in the prone position, or seat the patient before a vertical grid device.

Position of part

- With MSP of the patient's head centered to the midline of the IR, rest the head on the nose and chin so that the anterior surface of the mandibular symphysis is parallel with the plane of the IR. This position places the AML nearly perpendicular to the IR plane.
- Adjust the patient's head so that MSP is perpendicular to the plane of the IR (Fig. 11.136).
- *Respiration:* Suspend.

Central ray

- Perpendicular to the level of the lips.
- Center the IR to the central ray.

Collimation

- Adjust the radiation field to extend 1 inch (2.5 cm) beyond the lateral sides, above the TMJs and below the chin. The exposure field should be no larger than 8 × 10 inches (18 × 24 cm). Place the side marker in the collimated exposure field.

Structures shown

The mandibular body (Fig. 11.137).

The following should be clearly seen:

- Evidence of proper collimation and presence of the side marker placed clear of anatomy of interest
- Entire mandible
- No rotation or tilt, demonstrated by:
  - ☐ Mandibular body symmetric on each side
  - ☐ MSP of head aligned with long axis of collimated field
- Soft tissue and bony trabecular detail

Fig. 11.136 PA mandibular body.

Ramus

Symphysis

Body

Angle

Fig. 11.137 PA mandibular body.

Mandibular Body

PA AXIAL PROJECTION

Image receptor + grid: Positioned by manufacturer or department protocol for proper anatomy display orientation; CR plate: 10 × 12 inches (24 × 30 cm) lengthwise.

Position of patient

• Place the patient in the prone position, or seat the patient before a vertical grid device.

Position of part

• With MSP of the patient's head centered to the midline of the IR, rest the head on the nose and chin so that the anterior surface of the mandibular symphysis is parallel with the plane of the IR. This position places the AML nearly perpendicular to the plane of the IR.
• Adjust the patient's head so that MSP is perpendicular to the plane of the IR (Fig. 11.138).
• *Respiration:* Suspend.

Central ray

• Directed midway between the TMJs at an angle of 30 degrees cephalad. Zanelli[10] recommended that better contrast around the TMJs could be obtained if the patient was instructed to fill the mouth with air for this projection.
• Center the IR to the central ray.

Collimation

• Adjust the radiation field to extend 1 inch (2.5 cm) beyond the lateral sides, above the TMJs and below the chin. The exposure field should be no larger than 8 × 10 inches (18 × 24 cm). Place the side marker in the collimated exposure field.

Structures shown

The mandibular body and TMJs (Fig. 11.139).

The following should be clearly seen:
■ Evidence of proper collimation and presence of the side marker placed clear of anatomy of interest
■ Entire mandible
■ TMJs just inferior to the mastoid process
■ No rotation or tilt, demonstrated by:
  □ Symmetric rami
  □ MSP of head aligned with long axis of collimated field
■ Soft tissue and bony trabecular detail

Fig. 11.138 PA axial mandibular body.

Mastoid process
Condyle
Coronoid process
Ramus
Body
Symphysis

Fig. 11.139 PA axial mandibular body.

✿ AXIOLATERAL AND AXIOLATERAL OBLIQUE PROJECTIONS

The goal of these projections is to place the desired portion of the mandible parallel with the IR.

> **Image receptor + grid:** Positioned by manufacturer or department protocol for proper anatomy display orientation; CR plate: 10 × 12 inches (24 × 30 cm) lengthwise.

Position of patient

- Place the patient in the seated, semi-prone, or semisupine position.

Position of part

- Place the patient's head in a lateral position with the IPL perpendicular to the IR. The mouth should be closed with the teeth together.
- Extend the patient's neck enough that the long axis of the mandibular body is parallel with the transverse axis of the IR to prevent superimposition of the cervical spine.
- If the projection is to be performed on the tabletop, position the IR so that the complete body of the mandible is on the IR.
- Adjust the rotation of the patient's head to place the area of interest parallel to the IR, as follows.

  Ramus
- Keep the patient's head in a true lateral position (Fig. 11.140).

  Body
- Rotate the patient's head 30 degrees toward the IR (Fig. 11.141).

  Symphysis
- Rotate the patient's head 45 degrees toward the IR (Fig. 11.142).
- *Respiration:* Suspend.

NOTE: When the patient is in the semisupine position, place the IR on a wedge device or wedge sponge (Fig. 11.143). Ensure that combined CR angle and midsagittal plane tilt equals 25 degrees.

Central ray

- Directed 25 degrees cephalad to pass directly through the mandibular region of interest (see the note on p. 87).
- Center the IR to the central ray for projections done on upright grid units.

Collimation

- Adjust the radiation field to extend 1 inch (2.5 cm) beyond the anterior and inferior skin shadows and above the TMJ. The exposure field should be no larger than 8 × 10 inches (18 × 24 cm). Place the side marker in the collimated exposure field.

Structures shown

Each projection shows the region of the mandible that was parallel with the IR (Figs. 11.144–11.146).

Fig. 11.140 Axiolateral mandibular ramus.

Fig. 11.141 Axiolateral oblique mandibular body.

Fig. 11.142 Axiolateral oblique mandibular symphysis.

Fig. 11.143 Semisupine axiolateral oblique mandibular body and symphysis.

Coronoid process
Ramus
Body
Hyoid bone
Angle

Fig. 11.144 Axiolateral oblique mandibular body.

EVALUATION CRITERIA

The following should be clearly seen:
- Evidence of proper collimation and presence of the side marker placed clear of anatomy of interest
- Soft tissue and bony trabecular detail

Ramus and body
- No overlap of the ramus by the opposite side of the mandible
- No elongation or foreshortening of ramus or body

- No superimposition of the ramus by the cervical spine

Symphysis
- No overlap of the mentum region by the opposite side of the mandible
- No foreshortening of the mentum region

NOTE: To reduce the possibility of projecting the shoulder over the mandible when radiographing muscular or hypersthenic patients, adjust MSP of the patient's skull with an approximately 15-degree angle, open inferiorly. The cephalad angulation of 10 degrees of the central ray maintains the optimal 25-degree central ray/part angle relationship.

Temporomandibular joint
Condyle
Coronoid process
Ramus
Body
Angle

Fig. 11.145 Axiolateral mandibular ramus.

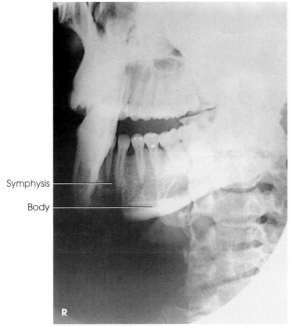

Symphysis
Body

Fig. 11.146 Axiolateral oblique mandibular symphysis.

⚜ SUBMENTOVERTICAL PROJECTION

Image receptor + grid: Positioned by manufacturer or department protocol for proper anatomy display orientation; CR plate: 10 × 12 inches (24 × 30 cm) lengthwise.

Position of patient

- Place the patient upright in front of a vertical grid device or in the supine position. When the patient is supine, elevate the shoulders on firm pillows to permit complete extension of the neck.
- Flex the patient's knees to relax the abdominal muscles and relieve strain on the neck muscles.
- Center MSP of the body to the midline of the grid device.

Position of part

- With the neck fully extended, rest the head on its vertex and adjust the head so that MSP is vertical.
- Adjust the IOML as parallel as possible with the plane of the IR (Fig. 11.147).
- When the neck cannot be extended enough that the IOML is parallel with the IR plane, angle the *grid device* and place it parallel to the IOML.
- Immobilize the head.
- *Respiration:* Suspend.

Central ray

- Perpendicular to the IOML and centered midway between the angles of the mandible.

Collimation

- Adjust the radiation field to extend 1 inch (2.5 cm) beyond the lateral sides and above the tip of the nose. The exposure field should be no larger than 8 × 10 inches (18 × 24 cm). Place the side marker in the collimated exposure field.

Structures shown

SMV projection of the mandibular body shows the coronoid and condyloid processes of the rami (Fig. 11.148).

EVALUATION CRITERIA

The following should be clearly seen:

- Evidence of proper collimation and presence of the side marker placed clear of anatomy of interest
- No rotation or tilt, demonstrated by:
  - □ Distance between the lateral border of the skull and the mandible equal on both sides
  - □ MSP of head aligned to long axis of collimated field
- Condyles of the mandible anterior to the pars petrosal
- Symphysis extending almost to the anterior border of the face so that the mandible is not foreshortened
- Soft tissue and bony trabecular detail

Fig. 11.147 SMV mandible.

Symphysis
Body
Coronoid process
Ramus
Condyle
Petrous ridge

Fig. 11.148 SMV mandible.

Fig. 11.149 AP axial TMJs.

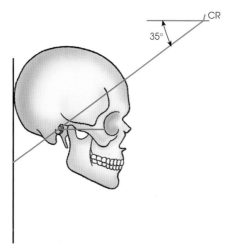

Fig. 11.150 Upright radiography diagram: AP axial TMJs.

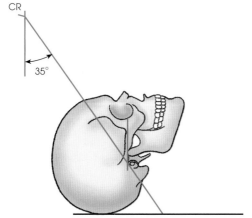

Fig. 11.151 Table radiography diagram: AP axial TMJs.

⚜ AP AXIAL PROJECTION

For radiography of the TMJs in the closed-mouth position, the *posterior teeth*, rather than the incisors, must be in contact. Occlusion of the incisors places the mandible in a position of protrusion, and the condyles are carried out of the mandibular fossae. In the open-mouth position, the mouth should be opened as wide as possible but not with the mandible protruded (jutted forward).

Because of the danger of fragment displacement, the open-mouth position should not be attempted in patients with recent injury. Trauma patients are examined without any stress movement of the mandible.

> **Image receptor + grid:** Positioned by manufacturer or department protocol for proper anatomy display orientation; CR plate: 10 × 12 inch (24 × 30 cm) lengthwise.

Position of patient
- Place the patient in a supine or seated-upright position with the posterior skull in contact with the upright bucky.

Position of part
- Adjust the patient's head so that MSP is perpendicular to the plane of the IR.
- Flex the patient's neck so that the OML is perpendicular to the plane of the IR (Figs. 11.149–11.151).
- *Respiration:* Suspend.

Temporomandibular Articulations

Central ray
- Directed 35 degrees caudad, centered midway between the TMJs, and entering at a point approximately 3 inches (7.6 cm) above the nasion.
- Expose one image with the mouth closed; when not contraindicated, expose one image with the mouth open.
- Center the IR to the central ray.

Collimation
- Adjust the radiation field to extend 1 inch (2.5 cm) beyond the lateral sides, superiorly to the glabella, and inferiorly to the lips. The exposure field should be no larger than 8 × 10 inches (18 × 24 cm). Place the side marker in the collimated exposure field.

Structures shown
The condyles of the mandible and the mandibular fossae of the temporal bones (Figs. 11.152 and 11.153).

EVALUATION CRITERIA
The following should be clearly seen:
- Evidence of proper collimation and presence of the side marker placed clear of anatomy of interest
- No rotation of head
- Minimal superimposition of petrosa on the condyle in the closed-mouth examination
- Condyle and temporomandibular articulation below pars petrosa in the open-mouth position
- Soft tissue and bony trabecular detail

Fig. 11.152 AP axial TMJs: mouth closed.

Fig. 11.153 AP axial TMJs: mouth open.

Fig. 11.154 Axiolateral TMJ: mouth closed.

Fig. 11.155 Upright radiography diagram: axiolateral TMJ.

Fig. 11.156 Table radiography diagram: axiolateral TMJ.

� AXIOLATERAL PROJECTION
Right and left positions

This projection is sometimes called the *modified Schüller method* because it consists of approximately the same positioning details and CR orientation as the Schüller method for the petromastoid portion of the temporal bone, seen in the 10th edition of *Merrill's Atlas.*

Image receptor + grid: Positioned by manufacturer or department protocol for proper anatomy display orientation; CR plate: 10 × 12 inches (24 × 30 cm) crosswise.

Position of patient
- Put a mark on each cheek at a point ½ inch (1.3 cm) anterior to the EAM and 1 inch (2.5 cm) inferior to the EAM to localize the TMJ if needed.
- Place the patient in a semiprone position, or seat the patient before a vertical grid device.

Position of part
- Center a point ½ inch (1.3 cm) anterior to the EAM to the IR, and place the patient's head in the lateral position with the affected side closest to the IR.
- Adjust the patient's head so that MSP is parallel with the plane of the IR and the IPL is perpendicular to the IR plane (Figs. 11.154–11.156).
- Immobilize the head.
- *Respiration:* Suspend.
- After making the exposure with the patient's mouth closed, change the IR; then, unless contraindicated, have the patient open the mouth widely (Fig. 11.157).
- Recheck the patient's position, and make the second exposure.

Central ray

- Directed to the midpoint of the IR at an angle of 25 or 30 degrees caudad. The central ray enters about ½ inch (1.3 cm) anterior and 2 inches (5 cm) superior to the upside EAM.

Collimation

- Adjust the radiation field to extend 1 inch (2.5 cm) beyond the anterior skin line, posterior and inferior to the TMJs. The exposure field should be no larger than 8 × 10 inches (18 × 24 cm). Place the side marker in the collimated exposure field.

Structures shown

The TMJ when the mouth is open and closed (Figs. 11.158 and 11.159). Examine both sides for comparison.

Fig. 11.157 Axiolateral TMJ with mouth open.

EVALUATION CRITERIA

The following should be clearly seen:

- Evidence of proper collimation and presence of the side marker placed clear of anatomy of interest
- TMJ anterior to the EAM
- Condyle in mandibular fossa in the closed-mouth examination
- Condyle inferior to the articular tubercle in the open-mouth examination if the patient is normal and able to open the mouth widely
- Soft tissue and bony trabecular detail

Fig. 11.158 Axiolateral TMJ, mouth closed. Mandibular condyle *(small dots)* and mandibular fossa *(large dots)* are shown. Mandibular condyle of side away from the IR is also seen *(arrow)*.

External acoustic meatus

Fig. 11.159 Axiolateral TMJ, mouth open. Mandibular fossa *(arrow)* and mandibular condyle *(arrowheads)* are shown.

Fig. 11.160 Axiolateral oblique TMJ.

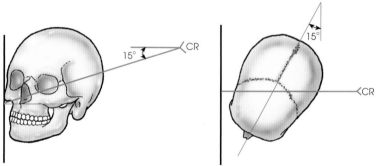

Fig. 11.161 Upright radiography diagram: axiolateral oblique TMJ.

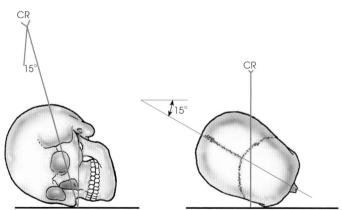

Fig. 11.162 Table radiography diagram: axiolateral oblique TMJ.

▲ AXIOLATERAL OBLIQUE PROJECTION
Right and left positions

This projection is sometimes called the *modified Law method* because it consists of approximately the same positioning details and CR orientation as the modified Law method for the petromastoid portion of the temporal bone, seen in the 10th edition of *Merrill's Atlas*.

> **Image receptor + grid:** Positioned by manufacturer or department protocol for proper anatomy display orientation; CR plate: 10 × 12 inches (24 × 30 cm) crosswise.

Position of patient

- Place the patient in a semiprone position, or seat the patient before a vertical grid device.
- In TMJ examinations, make one exposure with the mouth closed, and when not contraindicated, make one exposure with the mouth open.
- Examine both sides for comparison.

Position of part

- Center a point ½ inch (1.3 cm) anterior to the EAM to the IR, and rest the patient's cheek on the grid device.
- Rotate MSP of the head approximately 15 degrees toward the IR.
- Adjust the IPL perpendicular to the plane of the IR.
- Adjust the flexion of the patient's neck so that the AML is parallel with the transverse axis of the IR (Figs. 11.160–11.162).
- Immobilize the head.
- *Respiration:* Suspend.
- After making the exposure with the mouth closed, change the IR and instruct the patient to open the mouth widely.
- Recheck the position of the AML, and make the second exposure.

Central ray

- Directed 15 degrees caudad and exiting through the TMJ closest to the IR. The central ray enters about 1½ inches (3.8 cm) superior to the upside EAM.

Collimation

- Adjust the radiation field to extend from the outer canthus to the posterior edge of the auricle and from the mid-parietal region to the inferior edge of the auricle. The exposure field should be no larger than 5 × 5 inches (12.5 × 12.5 cm). Place the side marker in the collimated exposure field.

Structures shown

Open-mouth and closed-mouth positions show the condyles and necks of the mandible. The images also show the relationship between the mandibular fossa and the condyle. The open-mouth position shows the mandibular fossa and the inferior and anterior excursion of the condyle. Both sides are examined for comparison (Fig. 11.163). The closed-mouth position shows fractures of the neck and condyle of the ramus.

EVALUATION CRITERIA

The following should be clearly seen:

- Evidence of proper collimation and presence of the side marker placed clear of anatomy of interest
- Temporomandibular articulation
- Condyle lying in the mandibular fossa in the closed-mouth examination
- Condyle lying inferior to the articular tubercle in the open-mouth projection if the patient is normal and is able to open the mouth widely
- Soft tissue and bony trabecular detail

Mandibular fossa

Articular tubercle

External acoustic meatus

Condyle

Fig. 11.163 Axiolateral oblique TMJ. (A) Mouth open, right side. (B) Mouth open, left side (same patient), showing more movement on left side.

Panoramic Tomography of the Mandible

Panoramic tomography, *pantomography*, and *rotational tomography* are terms used to designate the technique employed to produce tomograms of curved surfaces. This technique of body-section radiography provides a panoramic image of the entire mandible, including the TMJ, and of both dental arches on one long, narrow image. Digital panorex units are capable of providing several images necessary for orthodontic and dental treatments, including three-dimensional images, cephalometric analysis, and surgical implant treatment planning.

Two types of equipment are available for pantomography. In the first type, the patient and the IR are rotated before a stationary x-ray tube. This type of machine consists of (1) a specially designed chair mounted on a turntable and (2) a second turntable to support a 4 × 10 inches (10 × 24 cm) IR. The seated and immobilized patient and the IR are electronically rotated in opposite directions at coordinated speeds. The x-ray tube remains stationary. In one machine, the exposure is interrupted in the midline.

In the second type of unit, the x-ray tube and the IR rotate in the same direction around the seated and immobilized patient (Fig. 11.164). The x-ray tube and IR drum are attached to an overhead carriage that is supported by the vertical stand assembly. The chair of this unit is fixed to the base but can be removed to accommodate patients in wheelchairs. The attached head holder and radiolucent bite device center and immobilize the patient's head. A scale on the head holder indicates the jaw size. The latest digital technology offers 33 panoramic options.

In both types of equipment, the beam of radiation is sharply collimated at the tube aperture by a lead diaphragm with a narrow vertical slit. A corresponding slit diaphragm is fixed between the patient and the IR so that the patient and the IR (or the tube and the IR) rotate. Each narrow area of the part is recorded on the IR without overlap and without fogging from scattered and secondary radiation.

The scan (exposure) time varies from 10 to 20 seconds in different makes of equipment. Because of the slit diaphragm, however, radiation exposure to the patient at each fraction of a second is restricted to the skin surface that is passing before the narrow vertical slit aperture.

Panoramic tomography provides a distortion-free lateral image of the entire mandible (Fig. 11.165). It also affords the most comfortable way to position patients who have sustained severe mandibular or TMJ trauma, before and after splint wiring of the teeth. It must be supplemented with an AP, PA, or VSM projection to establish fragment position.

This tomographic technique is useful for general survey studies of various dental and facial bone abnormalities. It is also used to supplement rather than replace conventional periapical images, although digital units are capable of providing standard bitewing images as well as lateral TMJ images.

Fig. 11.164 Digital panograph unit.

(Courtesy Gendex.)

Fig. 11.165 Panoramic digital tomogram.

(Courtesy Gendex.)

Technical Considerations

The most important technical consideration for demonstration of potential pathology of the paranasal sinuses is to image the patient in the *upright* position whenever possible. The upright position is best for demonstration of air-fluid levels and to differentiate fluid from other pathologic conditions, as shown by the research by Cross[11] and Flecker.[12] Appropriate exposure factors are also necessary so that air, fluid, soft tissue, and bony tissues are all well visualized. An appropriate kVp and mAs combination and a well-collimated radiation field will ensure optimum digital image quality at the lowest possible patient dose.

The paranasal sinuses vary not only in size and form but also in position. The cells of one group frequently encroach on and resemble those of another group.

This characteristic of the sinuses, together with their proximity to the vital intracranial organs, makes accurate radiographic demonstration of their anatomic structure of prime importance. The patient's head must be carefully placed in a sufficient number of positions so that the projections of each group of cavities are as free of superimposed bony structures as possible. The images must be of such quality that it is possible to distinguish the cells of several groups of sinuses and their relationship to surrounding structures.

Unless sinus images are almost perfect technically, they are of little diagnostic value. For this reason, a precise technical procedure is necessary in radiography of the paranasal sinuses. The first requirements are a small focal spot and IRs that are free of artifacts. As mentioned previously, the image contrast must markedly distinguish the sinuses from surrounding structures. The head must be carefully positioned and rigidly immobilized, and respiration must be suspended for the exposures.

The effect of body position and central ray angulation is shown in radiographs of a coconut held in position by head clamps. Fig. 11.166 shows a sharply defined air-fluid level. This coconut was placed in the vertical position, and the central ray was directed horizontally. Fig. 11.167 was also taken with the coconut in the vertical position, but the central ray was directed upward at an angle of 45 degrees to show gradual fading of the fluid line when the central ray is *not* horizontal. This effect is much more pronounced in actual practice because of structural irregularities. Fig. 11.168 was made with the coconut in the horizontal position and the central ray directed vertically. The resultant radiograph shows a homogeneous density throughout the cavity of the coconut, with no evidence of an air-fluid level.

Fig. 11.166 Coconut, vertical position: horizontal central ray. Air-fluid level is shown *(arrow)*.

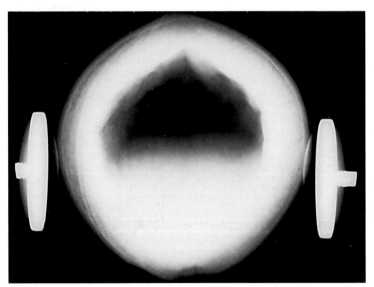

Fig. 11.167 Coconut, vertical position: central ray angled 45 degrees upward. Air-fluid level is not as sharp.

Exudate contained in the sinuses is not fluid in the usual sense of the word but is commonly a heavy, semigelatinous material. The exudate, rather than flowing freely, clings to the walls of the cavity and takes several minutes, depending on its viscosity, to shift position. For this reason, when the position of a patient is changed or the patient's neck is flexed or extended to position the head for special projections, *several minutes* should be allowed for the exudate to gravitate to the desired location before the exposure is made.

Although numerous sinus projections are possible, with each serving a special purpose, many are used only when required to show a specific lesion. The consensus is that five standard projections adequately show all of the paranasal sinuses in most patients. The following steps are observed in preparing for these projections:

- Use a suitable protractor to check and adjust the position of the patient's head to ensure accurate positioning.
- Have the patient remove all potential artifacts, such as dentures, hairpins, earrings and other facial piercings, and necklaces before proceeding with the examination.
- Because the patient's face is in contact with the IR holder or the IR itself for many of the images, these items should be cleaned before the patient is positioned.

Even with the most hygienic patients, the hair and face are naturally oily and leave a residue. If a patient is sick, the residue is worse. During positioning of the patient's head, the hair, mouth, nose, and eyes come in direct contact with the vertical grid device, tabletop, or IR. Medical asepsis can be promoted by placing a paper towel or sheet between the imaging surface and the patient. As standard procedure, the contacted area should be cleaned with a disinfectant before and after positioning.

Fig. 11.168 Coconut, horizontal position: vertical central ray. No evidence of air-fluid level is seen.

🕊 LATERAL PROJECTION
Right or left position

Image receptor + grid: Positioned by manufacturer or department protocol for proper anatomy display orientation; CR plate: 10 × 12 inches (24 × 30 cm) lengthwise.

Position of patient

- Seat the patient before a vertical grid device with the body placed in the RAO or LAO position so that the head can be adjusted in a true lateral position. This is the same basic position that is used for the lateral skull and facial bone positions.

Position of part

- Rest the side of the patient's head on the vertical grid device, and adjust the head in a true lateral position. MSP of the head is parallel with the plane of the IR, and the IPL is perpendicular to the plane of the IR.
- The IOML is positioned horizontally to ensure proper extension of the head. This position places the IOML perpendicular to the front edge of the vertical grid device (Fig. 11.169).
- *Respiration:* Suspend.

Central ray

- Directed *horizontal,* enter the patient's head ½ to 1 inch (1.3 to 2.5 cm) posterior to the outer canthus.
- Center the IR to the central ray.
- Immobilize the head.

Collimation

- Adjust the radiation field to extend 1 inch (2.5 cm) beyond the tip of the nose, superiorly to 3 inches (7.6 cm) above the nasion, inferiorly to the occlusal plane, and posteriorly to the auricle. The exposure field should be no larger than 8 × 10 inches (18 × 24 cm). Place the side marker in the collimated exposure field.

Structures shown

The AP and superoinferior dimensions of the paranasal sinuses, their relationship to surrounding structures, and the thickness of the outer table of the frontal bone (Fig. 11.170).

When the lateral projection is to be used for preoperative measurements, it should be made at a 72-inch (183-cm) SID to minimize magnification and distortion.

The following should be clearly seen:
- Evidence of proper collimation and presence of the side marker placed clear of anatomy of interest
- All four sinus groups, but the sphenoidal sinus is best demonstrated
- No rotation or tilt of sinus anatomy, as demonstrated by:
  - ☐ Sella turcica in profile
  - ☐ Superimposed orbital roofs
  - ☐ Superimposed mandibular rami
- Soft tissue, bony trabecular detail, and air-fluid levels, if present

NOTE: If the patient is unable to assume the upright body position, a lateral projection can be obtained using the dorsal decubitus position. The horizontal beam enables fluid levels to be seen. Positioning of the part is the same except for the IOML, which is vertical rather than horizontal.

Fig. 11.169 Lateral sinuses.

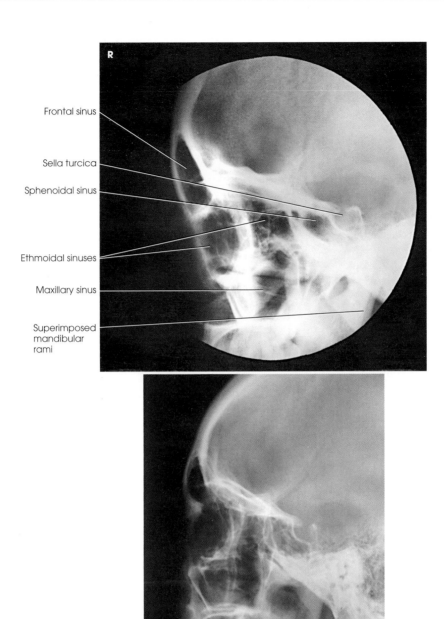

Frontal sinus

Sella turcica

Sphenoidal sinus

Ethmoidal sinuses

Maxillary sinus

Superimposed
mandibular
rami

Fig. 11.170 Lateral sinuses.

⚜ PA AXIAL PROJECTION
CALDWELL METHOD

Because sinus images should always be obtained with the patient in the upright body position and with a *horizontal* direction of the central ray, the Caldwell method is easily modified when a vertical grid device capable of angular adjustment is used. For the modification, all anatomic landmarks and localization planes remain unchanged.

Image receptor + grid: Positioned by manufacturer or department protocol for proper anatomy display orientation; CR plate: 10 × 12 inches (24 × 30 cm) lengthwise.

Position of patient

- Seat the patient facing a vertical grid device.
- Center MSP of the patient's body to the midline of the grid.

Position of part
Angled grid technique

- Before positioning the patient, tilt the vertical grid device down so that an angle of 15 degrees is obtained (Fig. 11.171A).
- Rest the patient's nose and forehead on the vertical grid device, and center the nasion to the IR.
- Adjust the MSP and OML of the patient's head perpendicular to the plane of the IR.
- This positioning places the OML perpendicular to the angled IR and 15 degrees from the horizontal central ray.
- Immobilize the head.
- *Respiration:* Suspend.

Vertical grid technique

- When the vertical grid device cannot be angled, extend the patient's neck slightly, rest the tip of the nose on the grid device, and center the nasion to the IR.
- Position the patient's head so that the OML forms an angle of 15 degrees with the horizontal central ray. For support, place a radiolucent sponge between the forehead and the grid device (see Figs. 11.171B and 11.172).
- Adjust the MSP of the patient's head perpendicular to the plane of the IR.
- Immobilize the head.
- *Respiration:* Suspend.

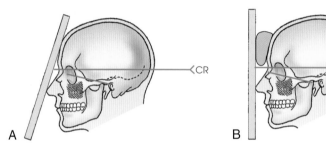

Fig. 11.171 Diagram of PA axial sinuses: Caldwell method. (A) IR tilted 15 degrees. (B) Same projection with vertical IR.

Fig. 11.172 PA axial sinuses: Caldwell method.

Central ray

- Directed *horizontal* to exit the nasion. The 15-degree relationship between the central ray and the OML remains the same for both techniques.
- Center the IR to the central ray.

NOTE: The *angled grid technique* is preferred because it brings the IR closer to the sinuses, increasing resolution. Angulation of the grid device provides a natural position for placement of the patient's nose and forehead.

Collimation

- Adjust the radiation field to extend 1 inch (2.5 cm) beyond the lateral skin shadows, superiorly to include just the shadow of the top of the head, and inferiorly to the occlusal plane. The exposure field should be no larger than 8 × 10 inches (18 × 24 cm). Place the side marker in the collimated exposure field.

Structures shown

The frontal sinuses lying superior to the frontonasal suture, the anterior ethmoidal air cells lying on each side of the nasal fossae and immediately inferior to the frontal sinuses, and the sphenoidal sinuses projected through the nasal fossae just inferior to or between the ethmoidal air cells (Fig. 11.173). The dense petrous pyramids extend from the inferior third of the orbit inferiorly to obscure the superior third of the maxillary sinus. This projection is used primarily to show the frontal sinuses and anterior ethmoidal air cells.

The following should be clearly seen:
- Evidence of proper collimation and presence of the side marker placed clear of anatomy of interest
- Frontal sinuses lying above the frontonasal suture and the anterior ethmoidal air cells lying above the petrous ridges
- No rotation or tilt, demonstrated by:
  - □ Equal distance between the lateral border of the skull and the lateral border of the orbits
  - □ Petrous ridge symmetric on both sides
  - □ MSP of head aligned with long axis of collimated field
- Petrous ridge lying in the lower third of the orbit
- Soft tissue, bony trabecular detail, and air-fluid levels, if present

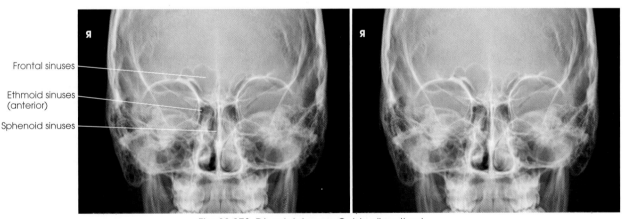

Frontal sinuses
Ethmoid sinuses (anterior)
Sphenoid sinuses

Fig. 11.173 PA axial sinuses: Caldwell method.

PARIETOACANTHIAL PROJECTION
WATERS METHOD

Image receptor + grid: Positioned by manufacturer or department protocol for proper anatomy display orientation; CR plate: 10 × 12 inches (24 × 30 cm) lengthwise.

For the Waters method,[13,14] the goal is to hyperextend the patient's neck just enough to place the dense petrosae immediately below the maxillary sinus floors (Fig. 11.174). When the neck is extended too little, the petrosae are projected over the inferior portions of the maxillary sinuses and obscure underlying pathologic conditions (Fig. 11.175). When the neck is extended too much, the maxillary sinuses are foreshortened, and the antral floors are not shown.

Position of patient
- Place the patient seated in an upright position, facing the vertical grid device.
- Center the MSP plane of the patient's head to the midline of the grid device.

Position of part
- Because this position is uncomfortable for the patient to hold, have the IR and equipment in position so that the examination can be performed quickly.
- Hyperextend the patient's neck to approximately the correct position, and then center the IR to the acanthion.

- Rest the patient's chin on the vertical grid device and adjust it so that the MSP is perpendicular to the plane of the IR.
- Using a protractor as a guide, adjust the head so that the OML forms an angle of 37 degrees from the plane of the IR (see Figs. 11.174 and 11.176). As a positioning check for the average-shaped skull, the MML line should be approximately perpendicular to the IR plane.
- Immobilize the head.
- *Respiration:* Suspend.

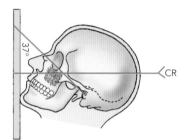

Fig. 11.174 Proper positioning diagram. Petrous ridges are projected below maxillary sinuses.

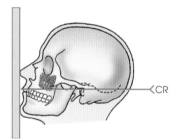

Fig. 11.175 Improper positioning diagram. Petrous ridges are superimposed on maxillary sinuses.

Fig. 11.176 Parietoacanthial sinuses: Waters method.

Central ray
• *Horizontal* to the IR and exiting the acanthion

Collimation
• Adjust the radiation field to extend 1 inch (2.5 cm) beyond the lateral skin shadows, superiorly to include just the shadow of the top of the head, and inferiorly to the occlusal plane. The exposure field should be no larger than 8 × 10 inches (18 × 24 cm). Place the side marker in the collimated exposure field.

Structures shown
The maxillary sinuses, with the petrous ridges lying inferior to the floor of the sinuses (Fig. 11.177). The frontal and ethmoidal air cells are distorted.

The Waters method is also used to show the foramen rotundum. The images of these structures are seen, one on each side, just inferior to the medial aspect of the orbital floor and superior to the roof of the maxillary sinuses.

The following should be clearly seen:
■ Evidence of proper collimation and presence of the side marker placed clear of anatomy of interest
■ Maxillary sinuses
■ OML in proper position (sufficient neck extension), as demonstrated by:
  □ Petrous pyramids lying immediately *inferior* to the floor of the maxillary sinuses
■ No rotation or tilt, demonstrated by:
  □ Equal distance between the lateral border of the skull and the lateral border of the orbit on both sides
  □ Orbits and maxillary sinuses symmetric on each side
  □ MSP of head aligned with long axis of collimated field
■ Soft tissue, bony trabecular detail, and air-fluid levels, if present

Frontal sinuses
Ethmoid sinuses
(R) Maxillary sinus
Petrous ridge
Mastoid air cells

Fig. 11.177 (A) Parietoacanthial sinuses: Waters method. (B) Same projection.

Maxillary and Sphenoidal Sinuses

PARIETOACANTHIAL PROJECTION
OPEN-MOUTH WATERS METHOD

Image receptor + grid: Positioned by manufacturer or department protocol for proper anatomy display orientation; CR plate: 10 × 12 inches (24 × 30 cm) lengthwise.

This method provides an excellent demonstration of the sphenoidal sinuses projected through the open mouth. For patients who cannot be placed in position for the SMV projection, the *open-mouth Waters method* and lateral projections may be the only techniques to show the sphenoidal sinuses. Because the open-mouth position is uncomfortable for the patient to hold, the radiographer must have the IR and equipment in position to perform the examination quickly.

Position of part
- Hyperextend the patient's neck to approximately the correct position, and then position the IR to the acanthion.
- Rest the patient's chin on the vertical grid device, and adjust it so that MSP is perpendicular to the plane of the IR.
- Using a protractor as a guide, adjust the patient's head so that the OML forms an angle of 37 degrees from the plane of the IR. The MML would not be perpendicular (Fig. 11.178).
- Have the patient *slowly open the mouth wide open* while holding the position.
- Immobilize the head.
- *Respiration:* Suspend.

Fig. 11.178 Parietoacanthial sinuses: open-mouth Waters method.

Central ray

- *Horizontal* to the IR and exiting the acanthion.

Collimation

- Adjust the radiation field to extend 1 inch (2.5 cm) beyond the lateral skin shadows, superiorly to include just the shadow of the top of the head, and inferiorly to the occlusal plane. The exposure field should be no larger than 8 × 10 inches (18 × 24 cm). Place the side marker in the collimated exposure field.

Structures shown

The sphenoidal sinuses projected through the open mouth along with the maxillary sinuses (Fig. 11.179).

The following should be clearly seen:
- Evidence of proper collimation and presence of the side marker placed clear of anatomy of interest
- Sphenoidal sinuses projected through the open mouth
- Maxillary sinuses
- OML in proper position (sufficient neck extension), as demonstrated by:
  □ Petrous pyramids lying immediately *inferior* to the floor of the maxillary sinuses
- No rotation or tilt, demonstrated by:
  □ Equal distance between the lateral border of the skull and the lateral border of the orbit on both sides
  □ Orbits and maxillary sinuses symmetric on each side
  □ MSP of head aligned with long axis of collimated field
- Soft tissue, bony trabecular detail, and air-fluid levels, if present

Maxillary sinus
Upper teeth

Sphenoidal sinuses

Lower teeth

Fig. 11.179 Open-mouth Waters modification shows sphenoidal sinuses projected through open mouth along with maxillary sinuses.

Fig. 11.180 SMV sinuses.

Fig. 11.181 Upright radiography diagram: SMV sinuses.

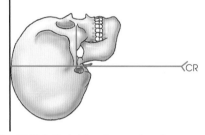
Fig. 11.182 Upright radiography diagram: SMV sinuses, preferred position of skull.

⚕ SUBMENTOVERTICAL PROJECTION

Image receptor + grid: Positioned by manufacturer or department protocol for proper anatomy display orientation; CR plate: 10 × 12 inches (24 × 30 cm), lengthwise.

Position of patient

The success of the SMV projection depends on placing the IOML as nearly parallel as possible with the plane of the IR and directing the central ray perpendicular to the IOML. The upright position is recommended for all paranasal sinus images and is more comfortable for the patient. The following steps are observed:

- Use a chair that supports the patient's back to obtain greater freedom in positioning the patient's body to place the IOML parallel with the IR.
- Seat the patient far enough away from the vertical grid device that the head can be fully extended (Fig. 11.180).
- If necessary to examine short-necked or hypersthenic patients, angle the vertical grid device downward to achieve a parallel relationship between the grid and the IOML (Fig. 11.181). The disadvantage of angling the vertical grid device is that the central ray is not horizontal, and air-fluid levels may not be shown as easily as when the central ray is truly horizontal.

Position of part

- Hyperextend the patient's neck as far as possible, and rest the head on its vertex. If the patient's mouth opens during hyperextension, ask the patient to keep the mouth closed to move the mandibular symphysis anteriorly.
- Adjust the patient's head so that the MSP is perpendicular to the midline of the IR.
- Adjust the tube so that the central ray is perpendicular to the IOML (Fig. 11.182; also see Figs. 11.180 and 11.181).
- Immobilize the patient's head. In the absence of a head clamp, place a suitably backed strip of adhesive tape across the tip of the chin and anchor it to the sides of the radiographic unit. Do not put the adhesive surface directly on the patient's skin.
- *Respiration:* Suspend.

Central ray

- *Horizontal* and perpendicular to the IOML through the sella turcica. The central ray enters on the MSP approximately ¾ inch (1.9 cm) anterior to the level of the EAM.

Collimation

- Adjust the radiation field to extend 1 inch (2.5 cm) beyond the tip of the nose and on the lateral sides. The exposure field should be no larger than 8 × 10 inches (18 × 24 cm). Place the side marker in the collimated exposure field.

Structures shown

A symmetric image of the anterior portion of the base of the skull. The sphenoidal sinus and ethmoidal air cells are shown (Fig. 11.183).

EVALUATION CRITERIA

The following should be clearly seen:
- Evidence of proper collimation and presence of the side marker placed clear of anatomy of interest
- Sphenoid and ethmoid sinuses

- No tilt (MSP positioned perpendicular to IR), demonstrated by:
  - Equal distance from the lateral border of the skull to the mandibular condyles on both sides
- IOML positioned parallel to IR (sufficient neck extension), demonstrated by:
  - Superimposition of anterior frontal bone by mental protuberance
  - Insufficient neck extension will cause mandible to superimpose ethmoid sinuses.
- Mandibular condyles anterior to petrous pyramids
- Soft tissue, bony trabecular detail, and air-fluid levels, if present

Maxillary sinus
Ethmoidal sinuses
Mandible
Vomer
Sphenoidal sinus
Pharynx
Petrosa

Fig. 11.183 SMV sinuses.

References

1. HEW 76-8013, Handbook of Selected Organ Doses.
2. Schüller A. Die schädelbasis im rontgenbild. *Fortschr Röntgenstr.* 1905;11:215.
3. Towne EB. Erosion of the petrous bone by acoustic nerve tumor. *Arch Otolaryngol.* 1926;4:515.
4. Grashey R. Atlas typischer röntgenbilder vom normalen menschen. In *Lehmann's medizinische atlanten.* vol 5. ed 2. Munich: JF Lehmann; 1912.
5. Altschul W. Beiträg zur röntgenologie des gehörorganes. *Z Hals Nas Ohr.* 1926;14:335.
6. Haas L. Verfahren zur sagittalen aufnahme der sellagegend. *Fortschr Röntgenstr.* 1927;36:1198.
7. Schüller A. Die schädelbasis im rontgenbild. *Fortschr Röntgenstr.* 1905;11:215.
8. Pfeiffer W. Beitrag zum wert des axialen schädelskiagrammes. *Arch Laryngol Rhinol.* 1916;30(1).
9. Waters CA. Modification of the occipitofrontal position in roentgenography of the accessory nasal sinuses. *Arch Radiol Electrother.* 1915;20(15).
10. Zanelli A. Le proiezioni radiografiche dell'articolazione temporomandibolare. *Radiol Med.* 1929;16:495.
11. Cross KS. Radiography of the nasal accessory sinuses. *Med J Aust.* 1927;14:569.
12. Flecker H. Roentgenograms of the antrum. *AJR Am J Roentgenol.* 1928;20:56 (letter).
13. Waters CA. A modification of the occipitofrontal position in the roentgen examination of the accessory nasal sinuses. *Arch Radiol Ther.* 1915;20(15).
14. Mahoney HO. Head and sinus positions. *Xray Techn.* 1930;1:89.

12

TRAUMA RADIOGRAPHY

SUMMARY OF PROJECTIONS

PROJECTIONS, POSITIONS, AND METHODS

Page	Essential	Anatomy	Projection	Position	Method
124	🐦	Cervical vertebrae	Lateral	Dorsal decubitus	
125	🐦	Cervicothoracic vertebrae	Lateral	Dorsal decubitus	
126		Cervical vertebrae	AP axial	Supine	
137		Cervical intervertebral foramina	AP axial oblique	Supine	
128		Thoracic vertebrae	Lateral	Dorsal decubitus	
128		Lumbar vertebrae	Lateral	Dorsal decubitus	
129	🐦	Chest: *Lungs and heart*	AP	Supine	
131	🐦	Abdomen	AP	Supine	
133	🐦	Abdomen	AP or PA	R or L lateral decubitus	
134	🐦	Abdomen	Lateral	Dorsal decubitus	
135		Pelvis	AP	Supine	
136	🐦	Hip	Lateral	Supine	Danelius-Miller
137	🐦	Hip	Modified axiolateral	Supine	Clements-Nakayama
138	🐦	Skull	Lateral	Dorsal decubitus	
140	🐦	Skull	AP	Supine	
140	🐦	Skull	AP axial	Supine	Reverse Caldwell
140	🐦	Skull	AP axial	Supine	Reverse Towne
142		Facial bones	Acanthioparietal	Supine	Reverse Waters
143		Upper extremity	AP	Variable	
143		Upper extremity	Lateral	Variable	
146		Lower extremity	AP	Variable	
146		Lower extremity	Lateral	Variable	

Icons in the Essential column indicate projections frequently performed in the United States and Canada. Students should be competent in these projections.

AP, Anteroposterior; *L,* left; *LAO,* left anterior oblique; *PA,* posteroanterior; *R,* right; *RAO,* right anterior oblique.

Introduction

Trauma is defined as severe injury or damage to the body caused by an accident or violence. Victims of trauma require immediate and specialized care, which is commonly provided in larger hospitals within a specialized unit termed the *emergency department* (ED). Physicians and many nurses specialize in trauma care. Imaging professionals are essential to the diagnosis of injuries sustained during traumatic events, so extra study in this area of imaging is necessary. Trauma radiography can be an exciting and challenging environment for a properly prepared imaging professional. These procedures can be intimidating and stressful for individuals unprepared for the innumerable injuries seen in the ED. The essential key to quality imaging procedures for trauma patients is proper study and preparation for imaging professionals.

Preparation for the trauma environment requires an understanding of the following: the most common traumatic injuries, the most commonly affected populations, types of trauma care facilities, specialized imaging equipment designed for imaging of trauma patients, the role of the imaging technologist as part of the ED team, and imaging procedures commonly performed on trauma patients. This chapter provides the information necessary to improve the skills and confidence of all imaging professionals caring for trauma patients.

Trauma Statistics

Trauma-related injuries affect persons in all age ranges. Fig. 12.1 shows trauma incidence by age and gender, as reported in the 2016 annual report of the American College of Surgeons' National Trauma Data Bank (NTDB). The database contains more than 7 million records from 747 hospitals and is the largest collection of data on US/Canadian trauma. These data show that trauma patients most commonly are male and range in age from teenagers to early adults. Fig. 12.2 shows the distribution of trauma injuries by cause; the most common are falls, followed by motor vehicle–traffic accidents (MVTAs). Firearms rank last as a cause of injury, however, the 2016 NTDB report also shows

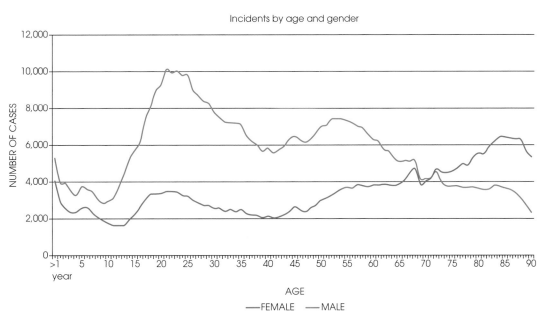

Fig. 12.1 NTDB annual report, 2016, table showing number of trauma incidents by age and gender. *NTDB*, National Trauma Data Bank.

(Reprinted by permission of the American College of Surgeons.)

that firearms have the highest fatality rate. The data show the most common trauma patients and mechanisms of injury, but the imaging professional who chooses to work in the ED must be prepared to care for patients of every age exhibiting a vast array of injuries.

Many types of facilities provide emergency medical care, ranging from major medical centers to small outpatient clinics in rural areas. The term *trauma center* denotes a specific level of emergency medical care as defined by the American College of Surgeons Commission on Trauma (ACS COT). Four levels of care are defined. Level I is the most comprehensive, and Level IV is the most basic. A *Level I* trauma center is usually a university-based center, research facility, or large medical center. It provides the most comprehensive emergency medical care available with complete imaging capabilities and all types of specialty physicians available on site 24 hours/day. Imaging professionals are also available 24 hours/day. A *Level II* trauma center probably has all of the same specialized care available but is not a research or teaching hospital, and some specialty physicians may not be available on site. *Level III* trauma centers are usually located in smaller communities where Level I or Level II care is unavailable. Level III centers generally do not have all specialists available but can resuscitate, stabilize, assess, and prepare a patient for transfer to a larger trauma center. A *Level IV* trauma center may not be a hospital at all, but rather a clinic or other outpatient setting. These facilities usually provide care for minor injuries and offer stabilization, as well as transfer arrangements to a larger trauma center for patients with more serious injuries.

Trauma injuries can occur by several types of forces, including *blunt, penetrating, explosive,* and *heat*. Examples of blunt trauma are MVTAs, which include motorcycle accidents, collisions with pedestrians, falls, and aggravated assaults. Penetrating trauma events include gunshot wounds (GSWs), stab wounds, impalement injuries, and foreign body ingestion or aspiration. Explosive trauma causes injury by several mechanisms, including pressure shock waves, high-velocity projectiles, and burns. Heat trauma includes burn injuries, which may be caused by numerous agents, including fire, steam, hot water, chemicals, electricity, and frostbite.

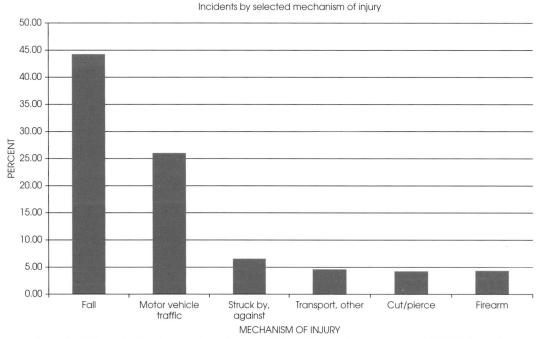

Fig. 12.2 NTDB annual report, 2016, table showing number of patients injured by each mechanism. *NTDB,* National Trauma Data Bank.

(Reprinted by permission of the American College of Surgeons.)

Preliminary Considerations

SPECIALIZED EQUIPMENT

Time is a crucial element in the care of a trauma patient. To minimize the time needed to acquire diagnostic x-ray images, many EDs have dedicated radiographic equipment located in the department or immediately adjacent to the department. Trauma radiographs must be taken with minimal patient movement, requiring more maneuvering of the tube and image receptor (IR). Specialized trauma radiographic systems are available and are designed to provide greater flexibility in x-ray tube and IR maneuverability (Fig. 12.3). These specialized systems help minimize movement of the injured patient while imaging procedures are performed. In addition, some EDs are equipped with specialized beds or stretchers that have a movable tray to hold the IR. This type of stretcher allows for the use of a mobile radiographic unit and eliminates both the requirement and risk for transferring an injured patient to the radiographic table.

Computed tomography (CT) is widely used for imaging of trauma patients. In many cases, CT is the first imaging modality used, now that image acquisition has become almost instantaneous. (Refer to Chapter 25 in Volume 3 for a detailed explanation and description of CT.) The only major concern with CT imaging compared with radiography is the radiation dose. The debate centers on the exclusive use of CT, when lower-dose radiographs may be sufficient for a diagnosis. Patients who are at high risk and who are not good candidates for quality radiographs based on their injuries may be referred to CT first.

Mobile radiography is often a necessity in the ED. Many patients have injuries that prohibit transfer to a radiographic table, or their condition may be too critical to interrupt treatment. Trauma radiographers must be competent in performing mobile radiography on almost any part of the body and must be able to use accessory devices (e.g., grids, air-gap technique) to produce quality mobile images.

Mobile fluoroscopic units, usually referred to as *C-arms* because of their shape, are becoming more commonplace in EDs. C-arms are used for fracture reduction procedures, foreign body localization in extremities, and reduction of joint dislocations (Fig. 12.4).

An emerging imaging technology has the potential to have a significant effect on trauma radiography. The Statscan Critical Imaging System (Lodox Systems [Pty.], Ltd., Johannesburg, South Africa) is a relatively new imaging device that produces full-body imaging scans in approximately 13 seconds without the need to move the patient (Figs. 12.5 to 12.7). At present, approximately 17 of these systems are available worldwide. At a cost of approximately $450,000, this technology is an expensive addition to a trauma-imaging department.

Positioning aids are essential for quality imaging in trauma radiography. Sponges, sandbags, and tape used creatively are often the trauma radiographer's most useful tools. Most patients who are injured cannot hold the required positions because of pain or impaired consciousness. Other patients cannot be moved into the proper position because to do so would exacerbate their injury. Proper use of positioning aids assists in quick adaptation of procedures to accommodate the patient's condition.

Grids and IR holders are also an important part of trauma radiography because many projections require the use of a horizontal central ray. Grids should be inspected regularly because a damaged grid often causes image artifacts. IR holders enable the radiographer to perform cross-table lateral projections (dorsal decubitus position) on numerous body parts with minimal distortion. To prevent unnecessary exposure, ED personnel should not hold the IR.

Fig. 12.3 Dedicated C-arm-type trauma radiographic room with patient on the table.

(Courtesy Siemens Healthcare.)

Fig. 12.4 Mobile fluoroscopic C-arm.

(Courtesy GE Healthcare.)

A   B

Fig. 12.5 (A) Statscan system configured for AP projection. (B) Statscan system configured for lateral projection.

(Courtesy Lodox Systems (Pty.), Ltd.)

Fig. 12.6 Statscan of patient with multiple GSWs. (A) AP full-body scan—13 seconds required for acquisition. Shrapnel and projectile pathways identified by zooming in on areas of full-body scan. (B) Skull. (C) Diaphragm area. (D) Pelvis.

(Courtesy Lodox Systems (Pty.), Ltd.)

Fig. 12.7 Statscan of motor vehicle-traffic accident victim with blunt trauma. (A) AP full-body scan. Tension pneumothorax shown without additional processing. (B) Zoomed lower pelvis showing multiple fractures *(arrows)*. (C) Zoomed bony thorax showing rib fractures *(arrows)*.

(Courtesy Lodox Systems (Pty.), Ltd.)

EXPOSURE FACTORS

Patient motion is always a consideration in trauma radiography. The shortest possible exposure time that can be set should be used in all procedures, except when a breathing technique is desired. Unconscious patients cannot suspend respiration for the exposure. Conscious patients are often in extreme pain and unable to cooperate for the procedure.

Radiographic exposure factor compensation may be required when exposures are made through immobilization devices such as a spine board or backboard. Most trauma patients arrive at the hospital with some type of immobilization device (Fig. 12.8). Pathologic changes should also be considered when technical factors are set. Internal bleeding in the abdominal cavity would absorb a greater amount of radiation than a bowel obstruction.

Fig. 12.8 (A) Typical backboard and neck brace used for trauma patients. (B) Backboard, brace, and other restraints are used on the patient throughout transport. (C) All restraints remain with and on the patient until all x-ray examinations are completed.

POSITIONING OF THE PATIENT

The primary challenge of the trauma radiographer is to obtain a high-quality, diagnostic image on the first attempt when the patient is unable to move into the desired position. Many methods are available to adapt a routine projection and obtain the desired image of the anatomic part. To minimize the risk of aggravating the patient's condition, the x-ray tube and IR should be positioned, rather than the patient or the part. The stretcher can be positioned adjacent to the vertical Bucky or upright table as the patient's condition allows (Fig. 12.9). This location enables accurate positioning with minimal patient movement for cross-table lateral images (dorsal decubitus positions) on numerous parts of the body. In addition, the grid in the table or vertical Bucky is usually of a higher ratio than grids used for mobile radiography, so image contrast is improved. Another technique to increase efficiency while minimizing patient movement is to obtain all anteroposterior (AP) projections of the requested examinations while moving superiorly to inferiorly. All lateral projections of the requested examinations are then performed while moving inferiorly to superiorly. This method moves the x-ray tube in the most expeditious manner.

When radiographs are taken to localize a penetrating foreign object, such as metal, glass fragments, or bullets, entrance and exit wounds should be marked with a radiopaque marker that is visible on all projections (Fig. 12.10). Two exposures at right angles to each other will demonstrate the depth and path of the projectile.

Fig. 12.9 Stretcher positioned adjacent to vertical Bucky to expedite positioning. Note x-ray tube in position for lateral projections.

Fig. 12.10 Proper placement of radiopaque markers *(inside red circles)* on each side of bullet entrance wound. Red circles are "stickies" that contain radiopaque marker.

Radiographer's Role as Part of the Trauma Team

The role of the radiographer within the ED ultimately depends on the department protocol and staffing and the extent of emergency care provided at the facility. Regardless of the size of the facility, the primary responsibilities of a radiographer in an emergency situation include the following:

- Perform quality diagnostic imaging procedures as requested.
- Practice ethical radiation protection for self, patient, and other personnel.
- Provide competent patient care.

Ranking these responsibilities is impossible because they occur simultaneously, and all are vital to quality care in the ED.

DIAGNOSTIC IMAGING PROCEDURES

Producing a high-quality diagnostic image is an obvious role of any radiographer; a radiographer in the trauma environment has the added responsibility to perform that task efficiently. Efficiency and productivity are common and practical goals for the radiology department. In the ED, efficiency is often crucial to saving the patient's life. Diagnostic imaging in the ED is paramount to an accurate, timely, and often lifesaving diagnosis.

RADIATION PROTECTION

One of the most important duties and ethical responsibilities of the trauma radiographer is radiation protection of the patient, members of the trauma team, and the radiographer himself or herself. In critical care situations, members of the trauma team cannot leave the patient while imaging procedures are being performed. The trauma radiographer must ensure that the other team members are protected from unnecessary radiation exposure. Common practices should minimally include the following:

- Close collimation to the anatomy of interest to reduce scatter
- Gonadal shielding for patients of child-bearing age (when doing so does not interfere with the anatomy of interest)
- Lead aprons for all personnel who remain in the room during the procedure
- Exposure factors that minimize patient dose and scattered radiation
- Announcement of impending exposure to allow unnecessary personnel to exit the room

Consideration must also be given to patients on nearby stretchers. If these patients are less than 6 feet away from the x-ray tube, appropriate shielding should be provided. Some of the greatest exposures to patients and medical personnel result from fluoroscopic procedures. If the C-arm fluoroscopic unit is used in the ED, special precautions should be in place to ensure that fluoroscopic exposure time is kept to a minimum and that all personnel are wearing protective aprons.

PATIENT CARE

As with all imaging procedures, trauma procedures require a patient history. The patient may provide this history, if he or she is conscious, or the attending physician may inform the radiographer of the injury and the patient's status. If the patient is conscious, the radiographer should explain what he or she is doing in detail and in terms the patient can understand. The radiographer should listen to the patient's rate and manner of speech, which may provide insight into the patient's mental and emotional status. The radiographer should make eye contact with the patient to provide comfort and reassurance. A trip to the ED is an emotionally stressful event, regardless of the severity of injury or illness.

Radiographers are often responsible for the total care of the trauma patient while performing diagnostic imaging procedures. It is crucial that the radiographer constantly assess the patient's condition, recognize any signs of deterioration or distress, and report any change in the status of the patient's condition to the attending physician. The trauma radiographer must be knowledgeable in taking vital signs, as well as in knowing normal ranges, and must be competent in performing cardiopulmonary resuscitation (CPR), administering oxygen, and dealing with all types of medical emergencies. The radiographer must be prepared to perform these procedures when covered by a standing physician's order or as departmental policy allows. The radiographer should also be familiar with the location and contents of the adult and pediatric crash carts and should understand how to use the suctioning devices.

The CAB (*compressions, airway, and breathing*) of basic life support techniques must be constantly assessed during radiographic procedures. Visual inspection and verbal questioning enable the radiographer to determine whether the status of the patient changes during the procedure. Table 12.1 provides a guide for the trauma radiographer regarding changes in status that should be reported immediately to the attending physician. Table 12.1 also includes only the *common* injuries in which the radiographer may be the sole health care professional with the patient during the imaging procedure. Patients with multiple trauma injuries and those in respiratory or cardiac arrest usually are imaged with a mobile radiographic unit while ED personnel are present in the room. In these situations, the primary responsibility of the trauma radiographer is to produce quality images in an efficient manner while practicing ethical radiation protection measures.

TABLE 12.1

Guide for reporting patient status change

Noted symptom	Possible cause	When to report to physician immediately
Cool, clammy skin	Shock[a] Vasovagal reaction[b]	Other symptoms of shock present
Excessive sweating (diaphoresis)	Shock[a]	Other symptoms of shock present
Slurred speech	Head injury Stroke (cerebrovascular accident)[c] Drug or ethanol influence[d]	Accompanied by vomiting, especially if vomiting stops when patient is moved to different position
Agitation or confusion	Head injury Drug or ethanol influence[d]	Accompanied by vomiting, especially if vomiting stops when patient is moved to different position
Vomiting (without abdominal complaints) (hyperemesis)	Head injury Hyperglycemia[e] Drug or ethanol overdose	Position of patient abruptly stimulates vomiting or abruptly stops vomiting
Increased drowsiness (lethargy)	Shock[a] Head injury Hyperglycemia[e]	Other symptoms of shock present or accompanied by vomiting
Loss of consciousness (unresponsive to voice or touch)	Shock[a] Head injury Hyperglycemia[e]	Immediately
Pale or bluish skin pallor (cyanosis)	Airway compromise Hypovolemic shock	Immediately
Bluish nail beds	Circulatory compromise	Immediately
Patient complains of thirst	Shock[a] Hyperglycemia[e] Hypoglycemia	Other symptoms of shock present
Patient complains of tingling or numbness (paresthesia) or inability to move a limb	Spinal cord injury Peripheral nerve impairment	Accompanied by any symptoms of shock or altered consciousness
Seizures	Head injury	Immediately
Patient states that he or she cannot feel your touch (paralysis)	Spinal cord injury Peripheral nerve impairment	Accompanied by any symptoms of shock or altered consciousness
Extreme eversion of foot	Fracture of proximal femur or hip joint	Report only if x-ray request specifies "frog leg" lateral projection of hip. This movement would exacerbate patient's injury and cause intense pain. Surgical lateral position should be substituted. Watch for changes in abdominal size and firmness.
Increasing abdominal distention and firmness to palpation	Internal bleeding from pelvic fracture[f] or organ laceration	Immediately

[a]*Hypovolemic* or *hemorrhagic shock* is a medical condition in which levels of blood plasma in the body are abnormally low, such that the body cannot properly maintain blood pressure, cardiac output of blood, and normal amounts of fluid in the tissues. It is the most common type of shock in trauma patients. Symptoms include diaphoresis, cool and clammy skin, decrease in venous pressure, decrease in urine output, thirst, and altered state of consciousness.

[b]*Vasovagal reaction* is also called a vasovagal attack, situational syncope, and vasovagal syncope. It is a reflex of the involuntary nervous system or a normal physiologic response to emotional stress. Patients may complain of nausea, feeling flushed (warm), and feeling lightheaded. They may appear pale before they lose consciousness for several seconds.

[c]*Cerebrovascular accident* is commonly called a stroke and may be caused by thrombosis, embolism, or hemorrhage in the vessels of the brain.

[d]*Drugs or alcohol.* Patients under the influence of drugs, alcohol or both commonly present in the ED. In this situation, the usual symptoms of shock and head injury are unreliable. Be on guard for aggressive physical behaviors and abusive language.

[e]*Hyperglycemia* is also known as diabetic ketoacidosis. The cause is increased blood glucose levels. The patient may exhibit any combination of symptoms noted and has fruity-smelling breath.

[f]*Pelvic fractures* have a high mortality rate (mortality with open fractures may be 50%). Hemorrhage and shock are often associated with this type of injury.

Best Practices in Trauma Radiography

Radiography of the trauma patient seldom allows for the use of "routine" positions and projections. In addition, the trauma patient requires special attention to patient care techniques while difficult imaging procedures are performed. The following best practices provide some universal guidelines for the trauma radiographer.

1. **Speed:** Trauma radiographers must produce quality images in the shortest amount of time. Speed in performing a diagnostic examination is crucial to saving the patient's life. Many practical methods that increase examination efficiency without sacrificing image quality are introduced in this chapter.

2. **Accuracy:** Trauma radiographers must provide accurate images with a minimal amount of distortion and with the maximum amount of recorded detail. Alignment of the central ray, the part, and the IR is imperative in trauma radiography. Using the shortest exposure time minimizes the possibility of involuntary and uncontrollable patient motion on the image.

3. **Quality:** Quality does not have to be sacrificed to produce an image quickly. The patient's condition should not be used as an excuse for careless positioning and accepting less than high-quality images.

4. **Positioning:** Careful precautions must be taken to ensure that performance of the imaging procedure does not worsen the patient's injuries. The "golden rule" of two projections at right angles from one another still applies. As often as possible, the radiographer should position the tube and the IR, rather than the patient, to obtain the desired projections.

5. **Practice standard precautions:** Exposure to blood and body fluids should be expected in trauma radiography. The radiographer should wear gloves, mask, eye shields, and gown when appropriate. IR and sponges should be placed in nonporous plastic to protect them from body fluids. Hand hygiene should be performed frequently, especially between patients. All equipment and accessory devices should be kept clean and ready for use.

6. **Immobilization:** The radiographer should *never* remove any immobilization device without a physician's orders. The radiographer should provide proper immobilization and support to increase patient comfort and to minimize risk for motion.

7. **Anticipation:** Anticipating required special projections or diagnostic procedures for certain injuries makes the radiographer a vital part of the ED team. Patients requiring surgery generally require an x-ray of the chest. In facilities where CT is not readily available for emergency patients, fractures of the pelvis may require a cystogram to determine the status of the urinary bladder. The radiographer should know which procedures are often referred to CT first or for additional images. Being prepared for and understanding the necessity of these additional procedures and images instills confidence in and creates an appreciation for the role of the radiographer in the emergency setting.

8. **Attention to detail:** The radiographer should *never* leave a trauma patient (or any patient) unattended during imaging procedures. The patient's condition may change at any time, and it is the radiographer's responsibility to note these changes and report them immediately to the attending physician. If the radiographer cannot process images while maintaining eye contact with the patient, he or she should call for help. Someone must be with the injured patient at all times.

9. **Attention to department protocol and scope of practice:** The radiographer should know department protocols and practice only within his or her own competence and abilities. The scope of practice for radiographers varies from state to state and from country to country. The radiographer should study and understand the scope of his or her role in the emergency setting. The radiographer should not provide or offer a patient anything by mouth. The radiographer should always ask the attending physician before giving the patient anything to eat or drink, no matter how persistent the patient may be.

10. **Professionalism:** Ethical conduct and professionalism in all situations and with every person is a requirement of all health care professionals, but the conditions encountered in the ED can be particularly complicated. The radiographer should adhere to the Code of Ethics for radiologic technologists (see Chapter 1) and the radiography practice standards. The radiographer should be aware of the people present or nearby at all times when discussing a patient's care. The ED radiographer is exposed to countless tragic conditions. Emotional reactions are common and expected but must be controlled until emergency care of the patient is complete.

Radiographic Procedures in Trauma

The projections included in this chapter address the trauma-related positions and projections listed in the American Registry of Radiologic Technologists (ARRT) radiography examination content specifications and align with the American Society of Radiologic Technologists (ASRT) radiography curriculum.

Most Level I trauma centers have replaced conventional trauma skull and facial bone radiographs (e.g., AP, cross-lateral, reverse Caldwell and Towne, and reverse Waters) with CT scan of the head and/or facial bones (Fig. 12.11). Research articles continue to delineate the advantages of CT over radiography. The American College of Radiology (ACR) Appropriateness Criteria state that CT head without IV contrast is usually appropriate in closed head trauma on patients who meet the most widely accepted patient evaluation criteria scales—the Glasgow Coma Scale (GCS), the New Orleans Head CT Criteria, and the Canadian CT Head Rule. Many smaller facilities may not have CT readily available, thus, trauma skull positioning remains valuable knowledge for the radiographer.

PATIENT PREPARATION

Remembering that the patient has endured an emotionally disturbing and distressing event, in addition to the physical injuries he or she may have sustained, is important. If the patient is conscious, speak calmly and look directly into the patient's eyes while explaining the procedures that have been ordered. Assume that the patient can hear you, even if he or she does not respond. Check the patient thoroughly for items that might cause an artifact on the images. Explain what you are removing from the patient and why. Place all removed personal effects, especially valuables, in the proper container used by the facility (i.e., plastic bag) or in the designated secure area. Each facility has a procedure regarding proper storage of a patient's personal belongings. Know the procedure and follow it carefully.

Fig. 12.11 CT scan of skull showing displaced fracture *(white arrow)*. Intracranial air is present *(black open arrow)*.

(Courtesy Sunie Grossman, RT(R), St. Bernard's Medical Center, Jonesboro, AR.)

BREATHING INSTRUCTIONS

Most injured patients have difficulty following the recommended breathing instructions for routine projections. For these patients, exposure factors should be set using the shortest possible exposure time to minimize motion on the radiograph, necessitating use of the large focal spot. The decrease in resolution from using a large focal spot is minimal compared with the significant loss of resolution due to patient motion. If a breathing technique is desired, this can be explained to a conscious trauma patient in the usual manner. If the patient is unconscious or unresponsive, careful attention should be paid to the rate and degree of chest wall movement. If inspiration is desired on the image, the exposure should be timed to correspond to the highest point of chest expansion. Conversely, if the routine projection calls for exposure on expiration, the exposure should be made when the patient's chest wall falls to its lowest point.

IMMOBILIZATION DEVICES

A wide variety of immobilization devices are used to stabilize injured patients. Standard protocol is to perform radiographic images without removing immobilization devices. After injuries have been diagnosed or ruled out, the attending physician gives the order for immobilization devices to be removed or changed, or to remain in place.

Many procedures necessitate the use of some sort of immobilization to prevent involuntary and voluntary motion. Many patient care textbooks discuss prudent usage of such immobilization devices. The key issues in the use of immobilization in trauma are to avoid exacerbating the patient's injury and to avoid increasing his or her discomfort.

IMAGE RECEPTOR SIZE AND COLLIMATED FIELD

The orientation of the IR, image plate sizes, and recommended collimated field sizes are the same in trauma procedures as those specified for the routine projection of the anatomy of interest. Occasionally, the physician may request that more of a part be included, and then a larger IR or exposure field size is acceptable. When using flat panel digital radiography (DR) detectors, be sure to collimate to the anatomy of interest to provide optimal quality images and ethical radiation protection for the patient and other personnel who may be required to be in the room during the imaging procedures. Exposure of unnecessary tissue generates excessive scatter, which is a primary source of radiation exposure for radiographers and other health care professionals.

CENTRAL RAY, PART, AND IMAGE RECEPTOR ALIGNMENT

Unless otherwise indicated for the procedure, the central ray should be directed perpendicular to the midpoint of the grid, IR, or both. Tips for minimizing distortion are detailed in the procedures in which distortion is a potential threat to image quality.

IMAGE EVALUATION

Ideally, trauma images should be of optimal quality to ensure prompt and accurate diagnosis of the patient's injuries. Evaluate images for proper positioning and technique as indicated in the routine projections. Allowances can be made when true right-angle projections (AP, posteroanterior [PA], and lateral) must be altered as a result of the patient's condition.

DOCUMENTATION

Deviation from routine projections is necessary in many instances. Documenting the alterations in routine projections for the attending physician and radiologist is important, so that they can interpret the images properly. In addition, the radiographer often has to determine whether the anatomy of interest has been adequately shown and must perform additional projections (within the scope of the ordered examination) on an injured part to aid in proper diagnosis. Notations concerning additional projections are extremely helpful for the interpreting physicians.

ABBREVIATIONS USED IN CHAPTER 12

CPR	Cardiopulmonary resuscitation
CR	Central ray
CVA	Cerebrovascular accident
EAM	External acoustic meatus
ED	Emergency department
GSW	Gunshot wound
IOML	Infraorbitomeatal line
IVU	Intravenous urography
KUB	Kidneys, ureters, and bladder
MCP	Midcoronal plane
MML	Mentomeatal line
MSP	Midsagittal plane
MVTA	Motor vehicle-traffic accident
OML	Orbitomeatal line
SID	Source-to-image receptor distance

See Addendum B for a summary of all abbreviations used in Volume 2.

Trauma Radiography

⚜ LATERAL PROJECTION[a]
Dorsal decubitus position
Trauma positioning tips

- *Always* perform this projection first, before any other projections. Level I centers may refer patients with indications for cervical spine imaging to CT first, depending on concomitant injuries.
- The *attending physician* or radiologist must review this image to rule out vertebral fracture or dislocation before other projections are performed.
- Use a 72-inch (183-cm) SID whenever attainable.
- Move the patient's head and neck as little as possible.
- *Shield gonads and other personnel in the room.*

Patient position considerations

- The patient is generally immobilized on a backboard and in a cervical collar.
- The patient should relax the shoulders as much as possible.
- The patient should look straight ahead without any rotation of the head or neck.
- Place IR in a holder at the top of the shoulder (Fig. 12.12).
- Check that the IR is perfectly vertical.

---

[a]See Mobile Lateral Projection in Vol. 3, Chapter 20, pp. 24–25.

Central ray

- *Horizontal* and perpendicular to the IR. Centered to MCP at the level of C4.

Collimation

- Adjust the radiation field to include the sella turcica (located 2 inches [5 cm] anterior and superior to the external acoustic meatus [EAM]) to T1 (located 2 inches [5 cm] above the jugular notch). The AP field margins should extend 1 inch (2.5 cm) beyond the skin shadow. Place the side marker in the collimated exposure field.

Structures shown

The entire cervical spine, from sella turcica to the top of T1, must be shown in profile with minimal rotation and distortion (Fig. 12.13). Evidence of proper collimation should be visible. Cross-table lateral images of the cervical vertebrae demonstrate the height and alignment of the vertebral bodies and intervertebral disk spaces, as well as the zygapophyseal joints.

NOTE: If all seven cervical vertebrae, including the spinous process of C7 and the C7-T1 interspace, are not clearly visible, a lateral projection of the cervicothoracic region must be performed.

Horizontal CR to C4

Fig. 12.12 Patient and image receptor positioned for trauma lateral projection of cervical spine using dorsal decubitus position. The X marks the central ray entrance point.

Fig. 12.13 Dorsal decubitus position lateral projection of cervical spine performed on a trauma patient. (A) Dislocation of C3 and C4 articular processes *(arrow)*. C7 is not well shown, so lateral projection of cervicothoracic vertebrae should also be performed. (B) Fracture of pedicles with dislocation of C5 and C6. Note superior portion of C7 shown on this image.

✦ LATERAL PROJECTION[b]
Dorsal decubitus position

This projection is often called the *swimmer's technique*.

Trauma positioning tips

- This projection should be performed if the entire cervical spine, including C7 and the interspace between C7 and T1, is not shown on the dorsal decubitus lateral projection. The patient must be able to move both arms. Do not move the patient's arms without permission from the attending physician and review of the lateral projection.
- If required and the patient is in stable condition, position the stretcher adjacent to a vertical Bucky to increase efficiency and obtain optimal image quality.
- *Shield gonads and other personnel in the room.*

---

[b]See Chapter 9, Vol. 1, pp. 460–461, for a complete description.

Patient position considerations

- Position the patient supine, usually on a backboard and in a cervical collar.
- Have the patient depress the shoulder closest to the tube as much as possible. *Do not push on the patient's shoulder.*
- Instruct the patient to raise the arm closest to the grid IR over the head. Assist the patient as needed, but *do not use force or move the limb too quickly* (Fig. 12.14).
- Ensure that the patient is looking straight ahead without any rotation of the head or neck.
- Ensure that the grid IR is exactly vertical in the holder to prevent distortion.
- Instruct the patient to breathe normally, if he or she is conscious, and use a long exposure time technique to blur the overlying ribs.

Central ray

- *Horizontal* and perpendicular to the IR entering MCP at the level of the C7-T1 interspace, which is about 2 inches (5 cm) above the jugular notch.
- If the shoulders are aligned in the same horizontal plane, angle 3 to 5 degrees cephalic, enter the patient at MCP at the level of the C7-T1 interspace.

Collimation

- Adjust the radiation field to extend from the level of the mastoid tip to 1 inch (2.5 cm) below the jugular notch and no larger than 10 × 12 inches (24 × 30 cm). The entire soft tissues of the neck should also be included. Place the side marker in the collimated exposure field.

Structures shown

The lower cervical and upper thoracic vertebral bodies and spinous processes should be seen in profile between the shoulders. Exposure should be sufficient to demonstrate bony cortical margins and trabeculation, as well as soft tissues in the neck (Fig. 12.15). Evidence of proper collimation should be visible.

◤ COMPENSATING FILTER

The use of a compensating filter can improve image quality, owing to the extreme difference in thickness between the upper thorax and the lower cervical spine.

NOTE: A grid is required to improve image contrast. If a breathing technique cannot be used, make the exposure with respiration suspended.

Horizontal CR to C7-T1

Fig. 12.14 Patient and image receptor positioned for trauma lateral projection of cervicothoracic vertebrae using dorsal decubitus position.

Fig. 12.15 Dorsal decubitus position lateral projection of cervicothoracic region performed on a trauma patient. Negative examination. Note excellent image of C7-T1 joint with use of Ferlic swimmer's filter *(arrow)*.

AP AXIAL PROJECTION[c]

Trauma positioning tips

- *Do not perform this projection until the attending physician has reviewed the lateral projection.*
- This projection is usually performed after the lateral projection.
- If the patient is on a backboard and gurney, obtain proper assistance to safely lift the backboard and place the grid IR in position centered to MSP at the level of C4.
- Move the patient's head and neck as little as possible.
- *Shield gonads and other personnel in the room.*

---

[c]See Standard Projection in Vol. 1, Chapter 9, pp. 445–446.

Patient position considerations

- Position the patient supine, usually on a backboard and in a cervical collar.
- Have the patient relax the shoulders as much as possible.
- Ensure that the patient is looking straight ahead without any rotation of the head or neck.

Central ray

- The central ray is directed 15 to 20 degrees cephalad to the center of the IR and enters MSP at slightly inferior to the thyroid cartilage. Exits at the level of C4 (Fig. 12.16).

Collimation

- Adjust the radiation field to 10 inches (25 cm) in length and 1 inch (2.5 cm) beyond the skin shadow on both sides. Place the side marker in the collimated exposure field.

Structures shown

C3 through T1 or T2, including interspaces and surrounding soft tissues, should be shown with minimal rotation and distortion. Exposure technique should show cortical margins and soft tissue shadows (Fig. 12.17). Evidence of proper collimation should be visible.

NOTE: If the patient is not on a backboard or an x-ray table, preferably the attending physician should lift the patient's head and neck while the radiographer positions the IR under the patient.

Fig. 12.16 Patient and image receptor positioned for trauma AP axial projection of cervical vertebrae. *CR,* Central ray.

Fig. 12.17 AP axial projection of cervical vertebrae performed on an 11-year-old trauma patient. Cervical spine is completely dislocated between C2 and C3 *(arrow).* The patient died on the x-ray table after x-ray examinations were performed.

AP AXIAL OBLIQUE PROJECTION

Trauma positioning tips

- *Do not perform this projection until the attending physician has reviewed the lateral projection.*
- If the patient is on a backboard, obtain appropriate help to safely lift the board and place the IR in position centered at the level of C4 and to adjacent mastoid process (about 3 inches [7.6 cm] lateral to MSP).
- Move the patient's head and neck as little as possible.
- Do not use a grid IR because the compound central ray angle results in grid cutoff. Some equipment does not allow the x-ray tube head to move in a compound angle. On these machines, only the 45-degree angle is used and a grid IR may be used to improve contrast.
- *Shield gonads and other personnel in the room.*

Patient position considerations

- Position the patient supine, usually on a backboard and in a cervical collar.
- Have the patient relax the shoulders as much as possible.
- Ensure that the patient is looking straight ahead without any rotation of the head or neck.

Central ray

- Angled 45 degrees lateromedially. When a double angle is used, also angle 15 to 20 degrees cephalad.
- Enters slightly lateral to MSP at the level of the thyroid cartilage and passing through C4 (Fig. 12.18).

Collimation

- Adjust the radiation field to 12 inches (30 cm) in length and 1 inch (2.5 cm) beyond the skin shadow on both sides. Place the side marker in the collimated exposure field.

Structures shown

Cervical and upper thoracic vertebral bodies, pedicles, open intervertebral disk spaces, and open intervertebral foramina of the side that the central ray enters are shown. This projection provides excellent detail of the facet joints, and it is important in detecting subluxations and dislocations (Fig. 12.19). If the 15-degree cephalic angle is not used, the intervertebral foramina are foreshortened. Evidence of proper collimation should be visible.

NOTE: If the patient is not on a backboard or an x-ray table, preferably the attending physician should lift the patient's head and neck while the radiographer positions the IR under the patient.

Fig. 12.18 Patient and IR positioned for trauma AP axial oblique projection of cervical vertebrae. Central ray *(CR)* is positioned 45 degrees mediolaterally and, if possible, 15 to 20 degrees cephalad.

Fig. 12.19 AP axial oblique projection of cervical vertebrae performed on a trauma patient using 45-degree angle. Radiograph was made using non-grid exposure technique. Negative image. Note excellent alignment of vertebral bodies and intervertebral foramen.

LATERAL PROJECTIONS
Dorsal decubitus positions
Trauma positioning tips

- *Always* perform dorsal decubitus positions before AP projections of the spine because the attending physician should review the dorsal decubitus lateral projections to rule out vertebral fracture or dislocation *before* other projections are performed.
- Move the patient as little as possible.
- Use of a grid is necessary to improve image contrast. Use a vertical Bucky, if not working with a C-arm configured unit, to maximize positioning and for optimal image quality.
- *Shield gonads and other personnel in the room.*

Patient position considerations

- The patient is generally immobilized and on a backboard.
- Have the patient cross the arms over the chest to remove them from the anatomy of interest.
- *Thoracic spine:* Place the top of the IR 1.5 to 2 inches (3.8 to 5 cm) above the patient's relaxed shoulders. DR field projected size is from the jugular notch to the inferior costal margin and 7 inches (18 cm) in AP width, centered at the level of MCP.
- *Lumbar spine:* Center the IR at the level of the iliac crests (Fig. 12.20).

DR field projected size extends from the xiphoid to the midsacrum and 8 inches (20 cm) in AP width, centered at the level of MCP.
- Ensure that the grid IR is perfectly vertical.

Central ray

- *Horizontal* and perpendicular to the longitudinal center of the IR and going through the spine.

Collimation

- Adjust the radiation field to 17 inches (43 cm) in length and 7 to 8 inches (18 to 20 cm) in the AP dimension. Place the side marker in the collimated exposure field.

Structures shown

For the thoracic spine, the image should include T3/T4 through L1. The lumbar spine image should, at a minimum, include T12 to the sacrum. The vertebral bodies should be seen in profile, with minimal rotation and distortion. Exposure should be sufficient to show cortical margins and bony trabeculation, as well as surrounding soft tissues (Fig. 12.21). Evidence of proper collimation should be visible.

NOTE: A lateral projection of the cervicothoracic spine must be performed to allow for visualization of the upper thoracic vertebrae in profile.

Horizontal CR to top of iliac crest

Fig. 12.20 Patient and image receptor positioned for trauma lateral projection of lumbar spine using dorsal decubitus position and vertical Bucky device.

Fig. 12.21 Dorsal decubitus position lateral projection of lumbar spine performed on a trauma patient. (A) Fracture and dislocation of L2 *(black arrow)*. Note backboard *(white arrow)*. (B) Compression fracture of body of L2 *(arrow)*. This coned-down image provides better detail of fracture area.

☀ AP PROJECTION[d,e]

Trauma positioning tips

- Most trauma patients must be imaged in the supine position. If it is necessary to see air-fluid levels, a cross-table lateral x-ray beam (dorsal decubitus position) can be performed. (*Note:* Patients with chest trauma with suspected vascular injury may be referred to CT first.)
- Obtain help in lifting the patient to position the IR if the stretcher is not equipped with an IR tray or a C-arm configured trauma unit is not being used.
- Check for signs of respiratory distress or changes in level of consciousness during radiographic examination. *Report any changes to the attending physician immediately.*
- Assess the patient's ability to follow breathing instructions.

[d]See Standard Projection in Vol. 1, Chapter 3, pp. 119–120.
[e]See Mobile Projection in Vol. 3, Chapter 20, pp. 10–11.

- Use the maximum SID possible to minimize magnification of the heart shadow.
- Use universal precautions if wounds, bleeding, or both are present, and protect the IR with plastic covering.
- Mark entrance and exit wounds with radiopaque indicators if evaluating a penetrating injury.
- Use of a grid improves image contrast.
- *Shield gonads and other personnel in the room.*

Patient position considerations

- Position the top of the IR 1.5 to 2 inches (3.8 to 5 cm) above the patient's shoulders.
- Move the patient's arms away from the thorax and out of the collimated field.

- Ensure that the patient is looking straight ahead, with the chin extended out of the collimated field.
- Check for rotation by determining whether the shoulders are equidistant to the IR or stretcher. This position places MCP parallel to the IR, minimizing image distortion.
- The exposure should be made at the end of deep inhalation. Breathing instructions are provided to the conscious patient, if possible, or to the medical personnel assisting with breathing for an unconscious patient.

Central ray

- Perpendicular to the center of the IR at MSP and at a level 3 inches (7.6 cm) below the jugular notch (Fig. 12.22).

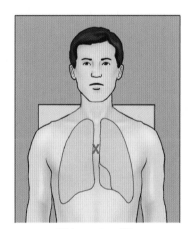

CR to center of IR

Fig. 12.22 Patient and image receptor *(IR)* positioned for trauma AP projection of chest. *CR,* Central ray.

Collimation

- Adjust the radiation field to no larger than 14 × 17 inches (35 × 43 cm), oriented to accommodate the patient's body habitus. On smaller patients, the exposure field should extend 1 inch (2.5 cm) beyond the skin shadows. Place the side marker in the collimated exposure field.

Structures shown

AP projection of the thorax is shown. The lung fields should be included in their entirety, with minimal rotation and distortion present. Adequate aeration of the lungs must be imaged to show the lung parenchyma (Fig. 12.23). Evidence of proper collimation should be visible.

NOTE: Fractured ribs are often incidentally diagnosed on AP chest images in the ED. Use of a grid and an adjustment in breathing instructions can improve rib visibility, if needed.

Fig. 12.23 AP upright projection of chest performed on a trauma patient. (A) Multiple buckshot in chest caused hemopneumothorax. *Arrows* show margin of collapsed lung with free air laterally. Arrowhead shows fluid level at costophrenic angle, left lung. (B) Open safety pin lodged in esophagus of a 13-month-old infant.

⚕ AP PROJECTION[f,g]

Trauma positioning tips

- *Note:* Sonography is often used to evaluate abdominal trauma.
- Use of a grid provides optimal image quality. If not working with a C-arm configured unit, verify transfer to a standard x-ray table with the attending physician before moving the patient.
- Determine the possibility of fluid accumulation within the abdominal cavity to establish appropriate exposure factors.
- For patients with blunt force or projectile injuries, check for signs of internal bleeding during radiographic examination and *report any changes to the attending physician immediately.*
- Mark entrance and exit wounds with radiopaque markers if evaluating projectile injuries.

---

[f]See Standard Projection in Vol. 1, Chapter 4, pp. 138–139.
[g]See Mobile Projection in Vol. 3, Chapter 20, pp. 14–15.

- Assess the ability of the patient to follow breathing instructions.
- Use standard precautions if wounds, bleeding, or both are present, and protect the IR with plastic covering if it is to come in contact with the patient.
- *Shield gonads, if possible, and other personnel in the room.*

Patient position considerations

- Ask ED personnel to assist in transferring the patient to the radiographic table, if possible.
- If not working with a C-arm-configured trauma unit and transfer is not advisable, obtain assistance to lift the patient carefully to position the grid IR under the patient, centered to the level of iliac crest (Fig. 12.24). (On patients with a long torso, a second AP projection of the upper abdomen may be required to show the diaphragm and lower ribs.)
- If the patient is on a stretcher, check that the grid IR is parallel with MCP. Correct tilting with sponges, sandbags, or

rolled towels. The grid IR must be perfectly horizontal to prevent grid cutoff and image distortion. If you are unable to correct tilt on grid IR, angle the central ray to maintain part-IR-central ray alignment.

- Instruct the conscious patient to exhale and hold his or her breath for the exposure. Inform medical personnel assisting with breathing for an unconscious patient to suspend respiration for the exposure.

Central ray

- Perpendicular to the center of the IR entering the patient at MSP at the level of the iliac crests.

Collimation

- Adjust the radiation field to 17 inches (43 cm) in length on adult sthenic patients, and the width should be approximately 1 inch (2.5 cm) beyond the skin margin but no larger than the IR. Place the side marker in the collimated exposure field.

Fig. 12.24 Patient and image receptor positioned for trauma AP projection of abdomen. *CR,* Central ray.

Structures shown

AP projection of the abdomen is shown. The entire abdomen, including the pubic symphysis and/or diaphragm (depending upon the injury), should be included without distortion or rotation. Exposure should be adequate to show tissue interfaces, such as the lower margin of the liver, kidney shadows, psoas muscles, and transverse processes of lumbar vertebrae (Fig. 12.25). Evidence of proper collimation should be visible.

Fig. 12.25 AP projection of abdomen performed on a trauma patient. (A) Table knife in stomach along with other small metallic foreign bodies swallowed by the patient. (B) Coin in stomach swallowed by the patient.

⚕ AP PROJECTION[h,i]

Left lateral decubitus position

Trauma positioning tips

- If not using a C-arm-configured unit, a vertical Bucky provides optimal image quality. If the patient must be imaged using a mobile radiographic unit, a grid IR is required.
- Verify with the attending physician that patient movement is possible and whether the image is necessary to assess fluid accumulation or free air in the abdominal cavity.
- The left lateral decubitus position shows free air in the abdominal cavity because the density of the liver provides good contrast for visualization of any free air.
- If fluid accumulation is of primary interest, the side down, or dependent side, must be elevated off the stretcher or table to be completely shown.
- Check for signs of internal bleeding during the radiographic examination and *report any changes to the attending physician immediately.*

---

[h]See Standard Projection in Vol. 1, Chapter 4, pp. 140–141.
[i]See Mobile Projection in Vol. 3, Chapter 20, pp. 16–17.

- Use universal precautions if wounds, bleeding, or both are present, and protect the IR with plastic covering. Mark all entrance and exit wounds with radiopaque markers when imaging for penetrating injuries.
- *Shield gonads, if possible, and personnel in the room.*

Patient position considerations

- Carefully and slowly turn the patient into the recumbent left lateral position. Flex the knees to provide stability.
- If the image is being taken for visualization of fluid, carefully place a block under the length of the abdomen to ensure that the entire right side is visualized.
- Ensure that MCP is vertical to prevent image distortion.
- Center the IR 2 inches (5 cm) above the iliac crests to include the diaphragm (Fig. 12.26).
- The patient should be in the lateral position at least 5 minutes before the exposure to allow any free air to rise and be visualized.
- Instruct the patient to exhale and hold their breath for the exposure.

Central ray

- *Horizontal* and perpendicular to the IR, entering the patient at MSP at a level 2 inches (5 cm) above the iliac crests to include the diaphragm.

Collimation

- Adjust the radiation field to approximately 14 × 17 inches (35 × 43 cm). Collimate to 1 inch beyond the skin shadows on thinner adults and pediatric patients. Place the side marker in the collimated exposure field.

Structures shown

Air and fluid levels within the abdominal cavity are shown. This projection is especially helpful in assessing free air in the abdomen when an upright position cannot be used. Exposure should be adequate to show tissue interfaces, such as the lower margin of the liver, kidney shadows, psoas muscles, and the transverse processes of the lumbar vertebrae (Fig. 12.27). Evidence of proper collimation should be visible.

Horizontal CR to center of IR

Fig. 12.26 Patient and image receptor positioned for trauma AP projection of abdomen using left lateral decubitus position and using vertical Bucky device.

Fig. 12.27 Left lateral decubitus position AP projection of abdomen performed on a trauma patient. Free intraperitoneal air is seen on upper right side of abdomen *(arrow)*. Radiograph is slightly underexposed to show free air more easily.

♠ LATERAL PROJECTION[j]
Dorsal decubitus position
Trauma positioning tips

- *Note:* This position is substituted for the lateral decubitus position in patients too injured or too ill to be turned onto their side.
- Verify whether the image is necessary to assess fluid accumulation or free air in the abdominal cavity. Exposure factors are often decreased for free air since the air must be visualized against the anterior tissues of the abdomen.
- If fluid accumulation is of primary interest, ensure that the IR is centered to the level of MCP.
- Check for signs of internal bleeding during the radiographic examination and *report any changes to the attending physician immediately.*
- Use universal precautions if wounds, bleeding, or both are present, and protect the IR with plastic covering. Mark all entrance and exit wounds with radiopaque markers when imaging for penetrating injuries.
- *Shield gonads, if possible, and personnel in the room.*

[j]See Standard Projection in Vol. 1, Chapter 4, p. 143.

Patient position considerations

- Position the gurney with either side of the patient adjacent to the vertical Bucky device, with wheels locked. If mobile radiography is required, be sure that the grid IR is exactly vertical to avoid distortion.
- Center the IR 2 inches (5 cm) above the iliac crests to include the diaphragm (Fig. 12.28).
- Carefully position the patient's arms over his or her head or across the upper chest to remove them from the image.
- Ensure that MSP is perpendicular to avoid rotation.
- Instruct the patient to exhale and hold his or her breath for the exposure.

Central ray

- *Horizontal* and perpendicular to the IR, entering the patient at MCP at a level 2 inches (5 cm) above the iliac crests to include the diaphragm.

Collimation

- Adjust the radiation field to approximately 14 × 17 inches (35 × 43 cm). Collimate to 1 inch (2.5 cm) beyond the skin shadows on thinner adults and pediatric patients. Place the side marker in the collimated exposure field.

Structures shown

Air and fluid levels within the abdominal cavity are shown. This projection is especially helpful in assessing free air in the abdomen when an upright position cannot be used. Exposure should be adequate to show tissue interfaces and the prevertebral space (Fig. 12.29). Evidence of proper collimation should be visible.

Horizontal CR 2 inches above iliac crests

Fig. 12.28 Patient and image receptor positioned for trauma dorsal decubitus position, lateral projection of the abdomen. *CR,* Central ray.

Fig. 12.29 Dorsal decubitus, lateral projection of the abdomen. *Arrows* mark calcifications in the abdominal aorta.

AP PROJECTION[k,l]

Trauma positioning tips

- *Note:* Level I centers often refer patients with pelvic trauma to CT first because research has shown that CT is superior in showing fracture extent and associated visceral and vascular damage.
- Up to 50% of pelvic fractures are fatal due to vascular damage and shock. The mortality risk increases with the energy of the force and according to the health of the victim.
- Pelvic fractures have a high incidence of internal hemorrhage. Alert the attending physician immediately if the abdomen becomes distended and firm.

[k]See Standard Projection in Vol. 1, Chapter 8, pp. 393–394.
[l]See Mobile Projection in Vol. 3, Chapter 20, pp. 18–19.

- Hemorrhagic shock is common with pelvic and abdominal injuries. Reassess the patient's level of consciousness repeatedly while performing radiographic examinations.
- *Do not* attempt internal rotation of the limbs for true AP projection of proximal femora on this projection.
- Collimate closely to reduce scatter radiation.
- Shield gonads, if possible, and other personnel in the room.

Patient position considerations

- The patient is supine, possibly on a backboard and with external immobilization.
- Obtain appropriate assistance to safely transfer the patient to the radiographic table to allow the use of a Bucky, if not working with a C-arm-configured unit.

- If unable to transfer the patient, use a grid IR positioned under the immobilization device or patient. Ensure that the grid IR is horizontal and parallel to MCP to minimize distortion and rotation.
- Position the grid IR centered at MSP at a level 2 inches (5 cm) inferior to the anterior superior iliac spine or 2 inches (5 cm) superior to the pubic symphysis.
- Instruct the patient to suspend respiration for the exposure, if possible.

Central ray

- Directed perpendicular to the center of the IR (Fig. 12.30). Carefully align to avoid distortion and grid cutoff.

Collimation

- Adjust the radiation field to approximately 14 × 17 inches (35 × 43 cm), and no larger than the IR. Adjust to 1 inch (2.5 cm) beyond the skin shadows on both sides on thinner adults or pediatric patients. Place the side marker in the collimated exposure field.

Structures shown

The pelvis and proximal femora should be shown in their entirety, with minimal rotation and distortion. Femoral necks are foreshortened, and lesser trochanters are seen. Exposure technique should show cortical margins, bony trabeculation, and soft tissue (Fig. 12.31). Evidence of proper collimation should be visible.

Fig. 12.30 Patient and image receptor positioned for trauma AP projection of pelvis. *CR,* Central ray.

Fig. 12.31 AP projection of pelvis performed on a trauma patient. (A) Entire right limb torn off after being hit by a car. Pelvic bone was disarticulated at pubic symphysis and sacroiliac joint. The patient survived. (B) Separation of pubic bones *(arrowheads)* anteriorly and associated fracture of left ilium *(arrow).*

⚕ AXIOLATERAL PROJECTION[m]
DANELIUS-MILLER METHOD

Trauma positioning tips
- This projection is often referred to as a "cross-table lateral" or "surgical lateral" hip.
- Use care and appropriate assistance to safely elevate the unaffected limb out of the collimated field.
- Do *not* attempt to internally rotate the affected limb.
- *Shield gonads, if possible, and other personnel in the room.*

Patient position considerations
- The patient is supine, possibly on a backboard and with external immobilization.

[m]See Standard Projection in Vol. 1, Chapter 8, pp. 406–407.

- Position a grid IR parallel with the femoral neck, centered to the most prominent portion of the greater trochanter and at a level to place the midline of the hip in the midline of the IR.
- Obtain appropriate assistance to safely elevate the unaffected limb, flex the knee, and position the thigh vertical, if possible.
- Support and immobilize the elevated limb. *Do not* rest on the collimator or tube housing, as this may cause injury to the patient or affect the central ray/IR relationship.
- If the patient is conscious, instruct them to suspend respiration for the exposure.

Central ray
- *Horizontal* and perpendicular to the center of the IR (Fig. 12.32). Carefully align to avoid distortion and grid cutoff.

Collimation
- Adjust the radiation field to approximately 10 × 12 inches (24 × 30 cm), and no larger than the IR. Adjust to 1 inch (2.5 cm) beyond the skin shadows on the anterior and posterior sides on thinner adults or pediatric patients. Place the side marker in the collimated exposure field.

Structures shown
The acetabulum, head, neck, and trochanters of the femur. Exposure technique should show cortical margins, bony trabeculation, and soft tissue (Fig. 12.33). Any orthopedic appliance should be seen in its entirety. Evidence of proper collimation should be visible.

Fig. 12.32 Patient and image receptor positioned for cross-table lateral hip, axiolateral projection (Danelius-Miller method).

Fig. 12.33 Axiolateral projection of the hip (Danelius-Miller method).

⚜ MODIFIED AXIOLATERAL PROJECTION[n]

CLEMENTS-NAKAYAMA MODIFICATION

Trauma positioning tips

- *Note:* This modification is used on patients with suspected bilateral hip fractures, bilateral hip arthroplasty, or limited movement of the unaffected limb.
- Position a grid IR aligned parallel to the femoral neck at a height to place the center of the hip on the IR.

---

[n]See Standard Projection in Vol. 1, Chapter 8, pp. 408–409.

- Tilt the top of the grid IR back (away from the hip) 15 degrees.
- *Shield gonads, if possible, and other personnel in the room.*

Patient position considerations

- The patient is supine, possibly on a backboard and with external immobilization.
- *Do not* attempt internal rotation of the limb.

Central ray

- Directed 15 degrees posteriorly and aligned perpendicular to the femoral neck and grid IR (Fig. 12.34).

Collimation

- Adjust the radiation field to approximately 10 × 12 inches (24 × 30 cm), and no larger than the IR. Adjust to 1 inch (2.5 cm) beyond the skin shadows on both sides on thinner adults or pediatric patients. Place the side marker in the collimated exposure field.

Structures shown

The acetabulum and the head, neck, and trochanters of the femur in lateral profile. Exposure technique should show cortical margins, bony trabeculation, and soft tissue (Fig. 12.35). Any orthopedic appliance should be seen in its entirety. Evidence of proper collimation should be visible.

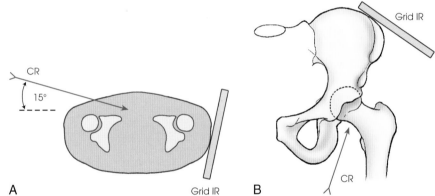

Fig. 12.34 Central ray (CR) and image receptor *(IR)* angles for Clements-Nakayama method for trauma hip. (A) CR angles 15 degrees posteriorly with grid top tilted 15 degrees away from the patient. (B) CR enters at femoral neck.

Fig. 12.35 Clements-Nakayama method with 15-degree central ray angulation.

✦ LATERAL PROJECTION°
Dorsal decubitus position
Trauma positioning tips

- *Note:* Patients with head injuries are often referred to CT imaging first because of its superiority in showing associated soft tissue and vascular damage.
- Robinson et al.[1] recommended using the dorsal decubitus lateral projection to show traumatic sphenoid sinus effusion (Fig. 12.36). The group stated that this finding may be the only clue to the presence of a basal skull fracture.
- Because the scalp and face are vascular, these areas tend to bleed profusely. Protect IRs with plastic covering and practice universal precautions.
- A grid IR is used for this projection. Elevate the patient's head on a

°See Standard Projection in Vol. 2, Chapter 11, pp. 34–37.

radiolucent sponge *only after cervical injury, such as fracture or dislocation, has been ruled out.*
- Vomiting is a symptom of intracranial injury. *If a patient begins to vomit, log-roll him or her to a lateral position to prevent aspiration, and alert the attending physician immediately.*
- *Alert the attending physician immediately if there is any change in the patient's level of consciousness or if the pupils are unequal.*
- Collimate closely to reduce scatter radiation. Recommend visualizing 1 inch of light beyond skin line. Check vertex, anterior, posterior, and base of skull to ensure entire anatomy of interest is included.
- Correctly place the side marker in light field.
- *Shield gonads and other personnel in the room. Shield thyroid and thymus glands on children.*

Patient position considerations
- Have the patient relax the shoulders.
- After cervical spine injury has been ruled out, the patient's head may be positioned to align the interpupillary line perpendicular to the IR and MSP vertical.
- If the patient is wearing a cervical collar, carefully minimize rotation and tilt of the cranium.
- Ensure that the grid IR is vertical.

Central ray
- *Horizontal* and perpendicular to a point 2 inches (5 cm) above the EAM (Fig. 12.37).

Collimation
- Adjust the radiation field to 12 inches (30 cm) in the AP dimension and 10 inches (24 cm) in the superoinferior dimension. Place the side marker in the collimated exposure field.

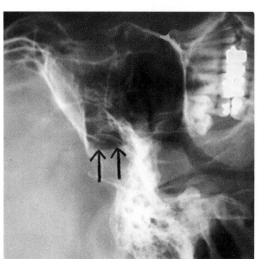

Fig. 12.36 Dorsal decubitus, lateral skull showing sphenoid sinus effusion *(arrows).*

Horizontal CR
2 inches above EAM

Fig. 12.37 Patient and image receptor positioned for trauma lateral projection of cranium using dorsal decubitus position. Note sponge in place to raise head to show posterior cranium (after checking lateral cervical spine radiograph). *CR,* Central ray; *EAM,* external acoustic meatus.

Structures shown

A profile image of the superimposed halves of the cranium is seen with detail of the side closer to the IR shown (Fig. 12.38). With some injuries, air-fluid levels can be shown in the sphenoid sinuses. Evidence of proper collimation should be visible.

Fig. 12.38 Dorsal decubitus position lateral projection of cranium performed on a trauma patient. (A) Two gunshot wounds entering at level of C1 and traveling forward to face and lodging in area of zygomas. Note bullet fragments in external acoustic meatus area. (B) Multiple frontal skull fractures *(arrows)* caused by hitting windshield during a motor vehicle accident (MVA).

Trauma Radiography

⚕ AP AND AP AXIAL PROJECTIONS[1]

REVERSE CALDWELL METHOD AND TOWNE METHOD[p]

Trauma positioning tips

- Profuse bleeding should be anticipated with head and facial injuries. Use universal precautions and protect IRs and sponges with plastic.
- Cervical spine injury should be ruled out before attempting to position the head.
- AP and reverse Caldwell demonstrate the anterior cranium. The AP axial projection, Towne method, shows the posterior cranium.
- Vomiting is a symptom of an intracranial injury. If a patient begins to vomit, logroll him or her to a lateral position to prevent aspiration and alert the attending physician immediately.

[p]See Standard Projection in Vol. 2, Chapter 11, pp. 38–49.

- Alert the attending physician if the patient's level of consciousness decreases or if pupils are unequal.
- A grid IR or Bucky should be used to ensure proper image contrast.
- *Shield gonads and other personnel in the room.*

Patient position considerations

- If not using a C-arm–configured unit, and if the patient's condition allows, obtain appropriate assistance to safely transfer the patient to the x-ray table using the immobilization device and proper transfer techniques. Transfer allows the use of the Bucky and minimizes risk of injury to the patient when positioning the IR.
- If the patient is not transferred to the radiographic table, the grid IR should be placed under the immobilization device. If no such device is present, the *attending physician* should carefully lift the patient's head and neck while the radiographer positions the grid IR under the patient.

- *AP and AP axial (reverse Caldwell):* Position the patient's head to place the orbitomeatal line (OML) and MSP perpendicular to the IR.
- *AP axial (Towne method):* Position the patient's head to place OML or infraorbitomeatal line (IOML) and MSP perpendicular to the IR. If the patient is wearing a cervical collar, the OML or IOML cannot be positioned perpendicularly, thus, the central ray angle may have to be increased to 60 degrees caudad to maintain a 30-degree angle to OML maintained.

Central ray

- *AP projection:* Perpendicular to MSP at the nasion (Fig. 12.39).
- *AP axial projection (reverse Caldwell):* Angled 15 degrees cephalad entering MSP at the nasion (Fig. 12.40).
- *AP axial projection (Towne method):* Angled 30 degrees caudad to the OML or 37 degrees to the IOML (Fig. 12.41). The central ray passes through the EAM and exits the foramen magnum.

Fig. 12.39 Patient and image receptor positioned for trauma AP projection of cranium. *CR,* Central ray.

Fig. 12.40 Patient, image receptor, and central ray (CR) angled 15 degrees cephalad for trauma AP axial, reverse Caldwell of the cranium.

Fig. 12.41 Patient and image receptor positioned for trauma AP axial projection, Towne method, of cranium using 30-degree central ray *(CR)* angulation.

Collimation

- Adjust the radiation field to 10 × 12 inches (24 × 30 cm). Check for light extending approximately 1 inch beyond the skin shadows surrounding the cranium. Place the side marker in the collimated exposure field.

Structures shown

AP and reverse Caldwell demonstrate the anterior cranium (Fig. 12.42). The reverse Caldwell demonstrates the petrous ridges in the lower third of the magnified orbits (Fig. 12.43). AP axial projection, Towne method, shows the posterior cranium and foramen magnum (Fig. 12.44). Cranium should be demonstrated without tilt or rotation. Exposure should demonstrate penetration of cranial bones and surrounding soft tissues. Evidence of proper collimation should be visible.

Fig. 12.43 AP axial, reverse Caldwell of cranium. Note screws (anterior and lateral surfaces) from recent surgery. Petrous ridges are slightly too low in the orbits, most likely due to misalignment of orbitomeatal line with image receptor plane. Slight rotation and tilt also present.

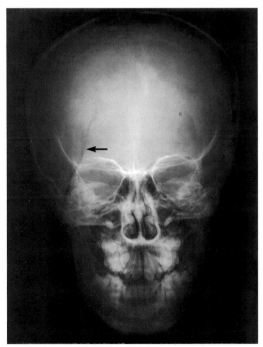

Fig. 12.42 AP projection of cranium performed on a trauma patient. Fracture of occipital bone *(arrow)*.

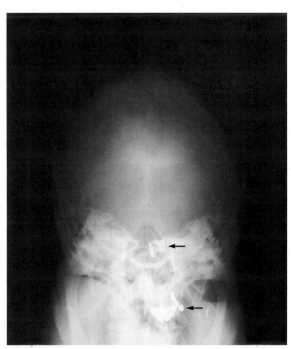

Fig. 12.44 AP axial projection, Towne method, performed on a trauma patient with gunshot wound to the head. Metal clip *(upper arrow)* indicates entrance of bullet on anterior cranium. Flattened bullet and fragments *(lower arrow)* are lodged in area of C2.

ACANTHIOPARIETAL PROJECTION[q]

REVERSE WATERS METHOD

Trauma positioning tips

- Anticipate profuse bleeding with facial trauma. Protect IRs with plastic covering and practice universal precautions.
- Cervical spine injury should be ruled out before positioning of the head is attempted.
- *Alert the attending physician if the patient's level of consciousness decreases or if pupils are unequal.*
- A grid IR or Bucky is used to ensure proper image contrast.
- *Shield gonads and other personnel in the room.*

Patient position considerations

- If required and if the patient's condition allows, carefully and slowly transfer the patient to the x-ray table using the immobilization device and proper transfer techniques. Transfer allows use of the Bucky and minimizes risk for injury to the patient when the IR is positioned.
- If mobile radiography must be used, the grid IR should be placed under

[q]See Standard Projection in Vol. 2, Chapter 11, pp. 65–66.

the immobilization device. If no such device is present, the *attending physician* should carefully lift the patient's head and neck while the radiographer positions the grid IR under the patient.
- Trauma patients are often unable to hyperextend the neck far enough to allow placement of the OML 37 degrees to the IR and the MML perpendicular to the plane of the IR. In these patients, the acanthioparietal projection, or the reverse Waters projection, can be achieved by adjusting the central ray so that it enters the acanthion while remaining parallel with the MML.
- MSP should be perpendicular to prevent rotation.

Central ray

- Angled cephalad until it is parallel with MML. Enters at the acanthion (Fig. 12.45).

Collimation

- Adjust the radiation field to 10 × 12 inches (24 × 30 cm). Check that the light field extends 1 inch (2.5 cm) beyond the lateral sides of the face and 1 inch (2.5 cm) above the superior orbital margins and inferiorly to the tip of the chin. Place the side marker in the collimated exposure field.

Structures shown

The superior facial bones are shown (Fig. 12.46). The image should be similar to the parietoacanthial projection or routine Waters method and should show symmetry of the face. Evidence of proper collimation should be visible.

Fig. 12.45 Central ray *(CR)* aligned parallel to mentomeatal line for trauma acanthioparietal projection, reverse Waters method, of cranium.

Fig. 12.46 Acanthioparietal projections, reverse Waters method, performed on trauma patients to show facial bones. (A) Fracture of right orbital floor *(arrow)* with blood-filled maxillary sinus (note no air is in sinus). The patient hit face on steering wheel during MVA. (B) Blowout fracture of left orbital floor *(arrow)* with blood-filled maxillary sinus (note no air is in sinus). Patient was hit with a fist.

Trauma positioning tips

- Use standard precautions, and cover IRs and positioning aids in plastic if wounds are present.
- When lifting an injured limb, support it at both joints and lift slowly. Lift only enough to place the IR under the part—sometimes only 1 to 2 inches (2.5 to 5 cm). Always obtain help in lifting injured limbs and positioning the IRs to minimize patient discomfort.
- If the limb is severely injured, *do not* attempt to position for true AP or lateral projections. Expose the two projections, 90 degrees apart, while moving the injured limb as little as possible.

- Check the patient's status during radiographic examination. Shock can occur from crushing injuries to extremities.
- Long bone radiographs must include both joints on the image.
- Separate examinations of the adjacent joints *may be required* if injury indicates. Do not attempt to "short cut" by performing only one projection of the long bone.
- *Shield gonads and other personnel in the room.*

Patient position considerations

- If possible, demonstrate the desired position for a conscious patient. Assist the patient in attempting to assume the position, rather than moving the injured limb.
- If the patient is unable to position the limb close to that required, move the IR and x-ray tube to obtain the desired projection (Figs. 12.47 to 12.50).

CR to center of IR

Fig. 12.47 Patient and image receptor *(IR)* positioned for trauma AP projection of forearm. *CR,* Central ray.

2-inch block   Horizontal CR to center of IR

Fig. 12.48 Patient and image receptor *(IR)* positioned for trauma cross-table lateral projection of forearm. *CR,* Central ray.

Trauma Radiography

Fig. 12.49 AP projection of forearm performed on a trauma patient. Fracture of midportion of radius and ulna *(arrows)*.

- Shoulder injuries should be initially imaged "as is" without rotating the limb. The "reverse" PA oblique projection of the scapular Y (an AP oblique) is useful in showing dislocation of the glenohumeral joint with minimal patient movement. The patient's affected side is elevated 45 degrees and supported in position (Figs. 12.51 and 12.52).
- If imaging while the patient is still on a stretcher, check to ensure that the IR is perfectly horizontal to minimize image distortion.
- The central ray must be directed perpendicular to the IR to minimize distortion.
- Immobilization techniques for the IR and upper limb are useful in obtaining an optimal image with minimal patient discomfort.

Fig. 12.50 Cross-table lateral projection of forearm performed on a trauma patient. Gunshot wound to forearm with fracture of radius and ulna and extensive soft tissue damage.

Fig. 12.51 Patient and image receptor positioned for trauma AP oblique projection of shoulder to show scapular Y. (Reverse of PA oblique, scapular Y—see Chapter 6.) *CR,* Central ray.

Structures shown

Images of the anatomy of interest, 90 degrees from one another, should be shown. Exposure technique should be sufficient to visualize cortical margins, bony trabeculation, and surrounding soft tissues. Both joints should be included in projections of long bones. Projections of adjacent joints must be centered to the joint to show the articular ends properly (Figs. 12.53 and 12.54). Evidence of proper collimation should be visible.

CR to center of IR

Fig. 12.53 Patient and image receptor *(IR)* positioned for trauma AP projection of humerus. *CR*, Central ray.

Fig. 12.52 AP oblique projection of shoulder (reverse of PA oblique, scapular Y) performed on a trauma patient. Several fractures of scapula *(arrows)* with significant displacement.

Fig. 12.54 AP projection of humerus performed on a trauma patient. Fracture of midshaft of humerus.

Trauma positioning tips

- Use standard precautions, and cover IRs and positioning aids in plastic if open wounds are present.
- Immobilization devices are often present with injuries to the lower extremities, especially in cases with suspected femoral fractures. *Perform image procedures with immobilization in place, unless directed to remove them by the attending physician.*
- When lifting an injured extremity, support at both joints and lift slowly. Lift only enough to place the IR under the part—sometimes only 1 to 2 inches (2.5 to 5 cm). Always obtain help in lifting injured extremities and in positioning IRs to minimize patient discomfort (Fig. 12.55).

- If the extremity is severely injured, *do not* attempt to position it for true AP and lateral projections. Take two projections, 90 degrees apart, moving the injured extremity as little as possible.
- Long bone examinations must include both joints. Separate images may be required.
- Examinations of adjacent joints may be required if the condition indicates. The central ray and IR must be properly centered to the joint of interest to show the anatomy properly.
- Check on patient status during radiographic examination. Shock can occur with severe injuries to the lower extremities.
- A grid IR should be used on thicker anatomic parts, such as the femur.
- *Shield gonads and other personnel in the room.*

Patient position considerations

- Demonstrate or describe the desired position for the patient and allow him or her to attempt to assume the position, rather than moving the injured extremity. Assist the patient as needed.
- If the patient is unable to position the extremity close to the required true position, move the IR and x-ray tube to obtain projection (Figs. 12.56 and 12.57).
- If imaging while the patient is still on a stretcher, check to ensure that the IR is perfectly horizontal to minimize image distortion.
- The central ray must be directed perpendicular to the IR to minimize distortion.
- Immobilization techniques for the IR and lower extremity are extremely useful in obtaining optimal quality with minimal patient discomfort.

Fig. 12.55 Proper method of lifting lower extremity for placement of image receptor (for AP projection) or placement of elevation blocks (for cross-table lateral). Lift only high enough to place IR or blocks underneath. Note that two hands are used to lift this patient with a broken leg gently.

2-inch block   Horizontal CR to center of IR

Fig. 12.56 Patient and image receptor *(IR)* positioned for trauma cross-table lateral projection of lower leg. IR and central ray *(CR)* may be moved superiorly or inferiorly to center for other portions of lower extremity. Note positioning blocks placed under extremity to elevate it so that all anatomy of interest is seen.

Fig. 12.57 Cross-table lateral projection of lower extremity performed on a trauma patient. (A) Dislocation of tibia from talus *(double arrows)* and fracture of fibula *(arrow)*. (B) Complete fracture and displacement of femur. Proximal femur is seen in AP projection, and distal femur is rotated 90 degrees at fracture point, resulting in lateral projection. Note artifacts caused by immobilization devices.

Trauma Radiography

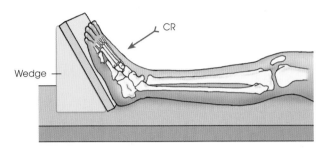

Fig. 12.58 Patient and image receptor *(IR)* positioned for trauma AP projection of foot or toes. IR is supported with sandbags for positioning against foot. *CR,* Central ray.

Structures shown

Images of the anatomy of interest, 90 degrees from each other, should be shown. Exposure technique should be sufficient to visualize cortical margins, bony trabeculation, and surrounding soft tissues. Both joints should be included in examinations of long bones. Images of articulations must be properly centered to show anatomy properly (Figs. 12.58 and 12.59). Evidence of proper collimation should be visible.

Fig. 12.59 AP projection of foot performed on a trauma patient. (A) Fracture and dislocation of tarsal bones with exposure technique adjusted for optimal image of this area. (B) Gunshot wounds to great toe.

Follow-up imaging procedures by other modalities are often warranted when radiography reveals a traumatic injury. In many instances, however, radiography is *not* the modality used first for detection of injuries sustained in a trauma. Because of this fact, most trauma centers have CT readily available or a dedicated unit for trauma cases (Figs. 12.60 to 12.63). The role of sonography in trauma imaging has increased significantly, and it provides the advantage of yielding a great deal of diagnostic information without radiation exposure. Magnetic resonance imaging (MRI) has also increased in its utility in trauma imaging, primarily owing to decreased scan times provided by newer scan protocols and techniques.

Computed Tomography

In many major trauma centers, CT is readily available for emergency imaging. This fact has influenced the decision-making policies associated with diagnostic imaging of trauma. CT is the first imaging modality used for trauma to the following parts of the body:

- Head and brain
- Cervical spine
- Thorax
- Pelvis

Fig. 12.60 CT scan of C5 showing multiple fractures *(arrows)* resulting from a fall from a tree.

(Courtesy Sunie Grossman, RT(R), St. Bernard's Medical Center, Jonesboro, AR.)

Fig. 12.61 CT scan of pelvis showing fracture of left ilium *(arrow)* with fragment displacement. Clothing and backboard artifacts are evident.

(Courtesy St. Bernard's Medical Center, Jonesboro, AR.)

Fig. 12.62 Three-dimensional reconstruction of pelvis from the patient in Fig. 12.52. Multiple pelvic fractures are well visualized *(arrows)*.

(Courtesy St. Bernard's Medical Center, Jonesboro, AR.)

Fig. 12.63 (A) AP and lateral computer tomography (CT) scout images of cranium. Note knife placement in cranium. Conventional cranium radiographs were not obtained on this trauma patient. The patient was sent directly to CT scanner for these images and sectional images before going to surgery. The patient recovered and returned home. (B) Axial and coronal CT sectional images of cranium at level of the eye. The patient was shot in the left eye with a BB gun. Note BB *(arrow).* Adjacent black area is air. The patient now has monocular vision.

(A, Courtesy Tony Hofmann, RT(R)(CT), Shands Hospital School of Radiologic Technology, Jacksonville, FL; B, courtesy Mark H. Layne, RT(R).)

The GCS is often the diagnostic indicator for the necessity of a head CT scan. The GCS is used to provide an objective and consistent neurologic evaluation. The highest possible score is 15, and the lowest possible score is 3. The GCS score and other head injury signs and symptoms, such as headache, loss of consciousness, posttraumatic amnesia, and seizure, are used to determine whether a head CT scan is required. Patients with cervical spine injuries are often referred to CT first—especially patients with multiple injuries and associated symptoms of cord injury. CT of the thorax is often the first imaging modality used in cases of suspected aortic dissection. Chest radiography is still the gold standard for many emergency cases involving the thorax, but because of time factors, patients with certain types of force trauma are sent directly to the CT scanner. CT of the pelvis is often performed in place of radiography because CT shows the extent of pelvic fractures better than radiography and offers the advantage of showing injuries to the pelvic organs and vasculature simultaneously.

Diagnostic Medical Sonography

The role of sonography in emergency imaging is evolving and increasing rapidly. Focused abdominal sonography in trauma (FAST) has been recognized as a valuable trauma diagnostic imaging tool. Research continues to assess the role of sonography in trauma imaging, and a wide variety of procedures have been studied so far, such as pediatric fracture reduction; chest and thoracic trauma, specifically pneumothorax and hemorrhage in the abdomen and pelvis; cranial trauma in infants; and superficial musculoskeletal sprains and tears. Advantages of sonography in trauma include lack of radiation exposure and improved efficiency of image access. The disadvantage is that sonography image quality is critically operator-dependent, and the ED physician may be uncomfortable with image interpretation, requiring the presence of a radiologist.

Reference

1. Robinson AE, et al. Traumatic sphenoid sinus effusion. *AJR Am J Roentgenol.* 1967;101:795.

Bibliography

ACR Appropriateness Criteria®. *Head trauma*, revised 2015. Available at: https://acsearch.acr.org/list. (Accessed August 25, 2017.)

American College of Emergency Physicians. Policy statement: emergency ultrasound guidelines. *Ann Emerg Med.* 2009;53:550.

American College of Surgeons. *National Trauma Databank annual report.* Available at: http://www.facs.org/trauma/ntdb/docpub.html; 2016. (Accessed August 24, 2017.)

Bagley L. Imaging of spinal trauma. *Radiol Clin North Am.* 2006;44(1).

Centers for Disease Control and Prevention. Guidelines for field triage of injured patients: recommendations of the national expert panel on field triage. *MMWR Morb Mortal Wkly Rep.* 2009. Available at: http://www.cdc.gov/mmwr/preview/mmwrhtml/rr5801a1.htm. (Accessed August 4, 2009.)

Jagoda A, et al. Clinical policy: neuroimaging and decision making in adult mild traumatic brain injury in the acute setting. *Ann Emerg Med.* 2008;52:714.

Kool D, Blickman J. Advanced trauma life support. ABCDE from a radiological point of view. *Emerg Radiol.* 2007;14:135.

Shanmuganathan K, Matsumoto J. Imaging of penetrating chest trauma. *Radiol Clin North Am.* 2006;44:225.

13

CONTRAST ARTHROGRAPHY

Overview

Contrast computed tomography (CT), shoulder magnetic resonance imaging (MRI) with and without contrast, and ultrasound (US) have drastically reduced the need for radiographic contrast arthrography (Fig. 13.1). Radiography of joints is still recommended as the initial imaging for many of the joints once imaged using contrast arthrography, yet the most recent recommendations by the American College of Radiology (ACR) rank radiographic contrast arthrography from very low to not at all as an appropriate diagnostic tool. Exceptions include the following:

- Contraindications for administration of gadolinium or lack of expertise for US exams[1]
- Aspiration in suspected septic or inflammatory arthropathies of the shoulder[1]
- After knee arthroplasty as a routine follow-up or for complications[2]
- To rule out the hip as the referred pain source after other negative imaging[3]

Arthrography (Greek *arthron,* meaning "joint") is radiography of a joint or joints. *Pneumoarthrography, opaque arthrography,* and *double-contrast arthrography* are terms used to denote radiologic examinations of the soft tissue structures of joints (menisci, ligaments, articular cartilage, bursae) after injection of one or two contrast agents into the capsular space. A gaseous medium is used in pneumoarthrography, a water-soluble iodinated medium is used in opaque arthrography (Fig. 13.2), and a combination of gaseous

Fig. 13.1 (A) Non–contrast-enhanced MRI of shoulder. (B) Non–contrast-enhanced MRI of knee, showing torn medial meniscus *(arrow).*

Fig. 13.2 Bilateral opaque arthrogram of bilateral congenital hip dislocations.

and a water-soluble iodinated medium is used in double-contrast arthrography. Although contrast studies may be performed on any encapsulated joint, the shoulder is the most frequent site of investigation. The joints discussed in this chapter—shoulder, knee, and hip—are the ones most likely to be imaged using radiographic contrast arthrography. Other joints may be imaged occasionally with arthrography. As noted previously, MRI, CT, and US are the modalities most likely to be used to demonstrate pathologies of the joints and associated soft tissues.

Arthrogram examinations are usually performed with a local anesthetic. The injection is made under careful aseptic conditions, usually in a combination fluoroscopic-radiographic examining room that has been carefully prepared in advance. The sterile items required, particularly the length and gauge of the needles, vary according to the part being examined. The sterile tray and the non-sterile items should be set up on a conveniently placed instrument cart or a small two-shelf table (Fig. 13.3).

After aspirating any effusion, the radiologist injects the contrast agent or agents and manipulates the joint to ensure proper distribution of the contrast material. The examination is usually performed by fluoroscopy and spot images. Conventional radiographic images may be obtained when special images, such as an axial projection of the shoulder or an intercondyloid fossa position of the knee, are desired.

Fig. 13.3 Sterile arthrogram tray.

SUMMARY OF PATHOLOGY

Condition	Definition
Developmental dysplasia of the hip	Denotes a wide spectrum of congenital hip abnormalities, ranging from acetabular dysplasia, joint laxity, and subluxation to complete dislocation
Dislocation	Displacement of a bone from a joint
Joint capsule tear	Rupture of the joint capsule
Ligament tear	Rupture of the ligament
Meniscus tear	Rupture of the meniscus
Rotator cuff tear	Rupture of any muscle of the rotator cuff

ABBREVIATIONS USED IN CHAPTER 13

ACR	American College of Radiology
DDH	Developmental dysplasia of the hip
MRI	Magnetic resonance imaging
PA	Posteroanterior

See Addendum B for a summary of all abbreviations used in Volume 2.

Shoulder Arthrography

Arthrography of the shoulder is performed primarily for the evaluation of partial or complete tears in the rotator cuff or glenoid labrum, persistent pain or weakness, and frozen shoulder. A single-contrast technique (Fig. 13.4) or a double-contrast technique (Fig. 13.5) may be used.

The usual injection site is approximately ½ inch (1.3 cm) inferior and lateral to the coracoid process. Because the joint capsule is usually deep, use of a spinal needle is recommended.

For a single-contrast arthrogram (Fig. 13.6), approximately 10 to 12 mL of positive contrast medium is injected into the shoulder. For double-contrast examinations, approximately 3 to 4 mL of positive contrast medium and 10 to 12 mL of air are injected into the shoulder.

Fig. 13.4 Normal AP single-contrast shoulder arthrogram with contrast medium surrounding the biceps tendon sleeve and lying in the intertubercular (bicipital) groove *(arrows)*. The axillary recess is filled but has normal medial filling defect *(arrowheads)*, created by the glenoid labrum.

Fig. 13.5 Normal AP double-contrast shoulder arthrogram.

Fig. 13.6 Single-contrast arthrogram showing a rotator cuff tear *(arrowheads)*.

The projections most often used are the anteroposterior (AP) (internal and external rotation), 30-degree AP oblique, axillary (Figs. 13.7 and 13.8), and tangential. (See Volume 1, Chapter 6, for a description of patient and part positioning).

After double-contrast shoulder arthrography is performed, CT may be used to examine some patients. CT images may be obtained at approximately 5-mm intervals through the shoulder joint. In shoulder arthrography, CT has been found to be sensitive and reliable in diagnosis. Radiographs and CT scans of the same patient are presented in Figs. 13.5 and 13.9. Shoulder arthrography is increasingly performed with MRI, with injection of gadolinium contrast medium into the joint capsule (see Fig. 13.9B).

Clavicle

Humeral head

Contrast medium in glenoid cavity

Scapula

Fig. 13.7 Normal axillary single-contrast shoulder arthrogram.

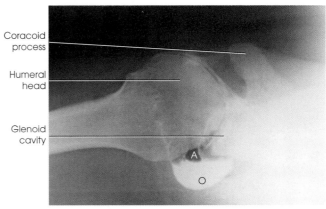

Coracoid process

Humeral head

Glenoid cavity

Fig. 13.8 Normal axillary double-contrast shoulder arthrogram projection of patient in supine position. Opaque medium *(O)* and air-created *(A)* density are seen anteriorly.

Fig. 13.9 (A) CT shoulder arthrogram. Radiographic arthrogram in this patient was normal (see Fig. 13.5). CT shoulder arthrogram shows small chip fracture *(arrow)* on the anterior surface of the glenoid cavity. Head of humerus *(H)*, air surrounding biceps tendon *(arrowhead)*, air contrast medium *(A)*, opaque contrast medium *(O)*, and glenoid portion of scapula *(G)* are evident. (B) MRI arthrogram of shoulder with injection of gadolinium contrast medium.

Contrast Arthrography of the Knee

VERTICAL RAY METHOD

Contrast arthrography of the knee by the vertical ray method requires the use of a stress device. The following steps are taken:

- Place the limb in the frame to widen or "open up" the side of the joint space under investigation. This widening, or spreading, of the intrastructural spaces permits better distribution of the contrast material around the meniscus.

- After the contrast material is injected, place the limb into the stress device (Fig. 13.10). To delineate the medial side of the joint, place the stress device just above the knee, and then laterally stress the lower leg.

- When contrast arthrograms are to be made by conventional radiography, turn the patient to the prone position and fluoroscopically localize the centering point for each side of the joint. The mark ensures accurate centering for closely collimated studies of each side of the joint. The images obtained of each side of the joint usually consist of an AP projection and a 20-degree right and left AP oblique projection.

- Obtain the oblique position by leg rotation or by central ray angulation (Fig. 13.11).

- On completion of these studies, remove the frame and perform lateral and intercondyloid fossa projections.

NOTE: Anderson and Maslin[4] recommended that tomography be used in knee arthrography. In addition, the technique can frequently be used for other contrast-filled joint capsules.

Fig. 13.10 Patient lying on lead rubber for gonad shielding and positioned in stress device on fluoroscopic table.

Femoral condyle

Meniscus

Tibia

Fig. 13.11 Vertical ray double-contrast knee arthrogram.

Double-Contrast Arthrography of the Knee

HORIZONTAL RAY METHOD

The horizontal central ray method of performing double-contrast arthrography of the knee was first described by Andrén and Wehlin[5] and later by Freiberger et al.[6] These investigators found that using a horizontal x-ray beam position and a comparatively small amount of each of the two contrast agents (gaseous medium and water-soluble iodinated medium) improved double-contrast delineation of the knee joint structures. With this technique, the excess of the heavier iodinated solution drains into the dependent part of the joint, leaving only the desired thin opaque coating on the gas-enveloped uppermost part—the part under investigation.

Medial meniscus

- Adjust the patient into a semiprone position that places the posterior aspect of the medial meniscus uppermost (Fig. 13.12).
- To widen the joint space, manually stress the knee.
- Draw a line on the medial side of the knee and direct the central ray along the line and centered to the meniscus.
- With rotation toward the supine position, turn the leg 30 degrees for each of the succeeding five exposures.
- Direct the central ray along the localization line for each exposure, ensuring that it is centered to the meniscus.

Lateral meniscus

- Adjust the patient into a semiprone position that places the posterior aspect of the lateral meniscus uppermost (Fig. 13.13).
- To widen the joint space, manually stress the knee.
- As with the medial meniscus, make six images on one image receptor (IR).
- With movement toward the supine position, rotate the leg 30 degrees for each of the consecutive exposures, from the initial prone oblique position to the supine oblique position.
- Adjust the central ray angulation as required to direct it along the localization line and center it to the meniscus.

NOTE: To show the cruciate ligaments after imaging of the menisci is completed,[7] the patient sits with the knee flexed 90 degrees over the side of the radiographic table. A firm cotton pillow is placed under the knee and is adjusted so that some forward pressure can be applied to the leg. With the patient holding a grid IR in position, a closely collimated lateral projection is made.

Fig. 13.12 Image showing a tear *(arrow)* in the medial meniscus.

Fig. 13.13 Normal lateral meniscus *(arrows)*.

Hip Arthrography

Hip arthrography is most often performed on children in a surgery suite by an orthopedic surgeon. Arthrography is used to evaluate lateral femoral head displacement and after closed reduction to ensure that there is no folding or impingement of soft tissues (see Fig. 13.2, pretreatment, and Figs. 13.14 and 13.15, posttreatment). In adults, the primary use of hip arthrography is to detect a loose hip prosthesis or to confirm the presence of infection.

The cement used to fasten hip prosthesis components has barium sulfate added to make the cement and the cement-bone interface radiographically visible (Fig. 13.16). Although the addition of barium sulfate to cement is helpful in confirming proper seating of the prosthesis, it makes evaluation of the same joint by arthrography difficult.

Because cement and contrast material may appear similar in radiographic images (Figs. 13.17 and 13.18), subtraction images are recommended (Fig. 13.19). Chapter 27 in Volume 3 explains subtraction techniques. A common puncture site for hip arthrography is ¼ inch (0.6 cm) distal to the inguinal crease and ¼ inch (0.6 cm) lateral to the palpated femoral pulse. A spinal needle is useful for reaching the joint capsule.

Fig. 13.14 AP opaque arthrogram showing treated congenital right hip dislocation in the same patient as in Fig. 13.2.

Fig. 13.15 Axiolateral "frog" right hip of a patient treated for congenital dislocation of the hip.

Fig. 13.16 AP hip radiograph showing radiopaque cement *(arrows)* used to secure a hip prosthesis.

Fig. 13.17 AP hip arthrogram showing hip prosthesis in proper position. Cement with radiopaque additive is difficult to distinguish from contrast medium used to perform arthrography *(arrows)*.

Fig. 13.18 AP hip radiograph after injection of contrast medium.

Fig. 13.19 Digital subtraction hip arthrogram in the same patient as in Fig. 13.18. Contrast medium around a prosthesis in the proximal lateral femoral shaft *(arrows)* indicates that the prosthesis is loose. Lines on the medial and lateral aspects of the femur *(arrowheads)* are subtraction registration artifacts caused by slight patient movement during injection of contrast medium. (See Chapter 27 for a description of subtraction technique.)

Other Joints

Essentially, any joint can be evaluated by arthrography. A wrist arthrogram is included here as an example (Fig. 13.20).

Fig. 13.20 Opaque arthrogram of wrist, showing rheumatoid arthritis.

References

1. ACR Appropriateness Criteria®. *Acute shoulder pain*; 2010.
2. ACR Appropriateness Criteria®. *Imaging after total knee arthroplasty*; 2011.
3. ACR Appropriateness Criteria®. *Chronic hip pain*; 2011.
4. Anderson PW, Maslin P. Tomography applied to knee arthrography. *Radiology*. 1974;110:271.
5. Andrén L, Wehlin L. Double-contrast arthrography of knee with horizontal roentgen ray beam. *Acta Orthop Scand*. 1960;29:307.
6. Freiberger RH, et al. Arthrography of the knee by double contrast method. *AJR Am J Roentgenol*. 1966;97:736.
7. Mittler S, et al. A method of improving cruciate ligament visualization in double-contrast arthrography. *Radiology*. 1972;102:441.

14

MYELOGRAPHY AND OTHER CENTRAL NERVOUS SYSTEM IMAGING

REBECCA H. KEITH

For descriptive purposes, the central nervous system (CNS) is divided into two parts: (1) the *brain,*[a] which occupies the cranial cavity, and (2) the *spinal cord,* which is suspended within the vertebral canal.

[a]Many italicized words are defined at the end of the chapter.

Brain

The brain is composed of an outer portion of gray matter called the *cortex* and an inner portion of *white matter.* The brain consists of the *cerebrum, cerebellum,* and *brain stem,* which is continuous with the spinal cord after leaving the cranial cavity (Fig. 14.1). The brain stem consists of the *midbrain, pons,* and *medulla oblongata.*

The cerebrum is the largest part of the brain and is referred to as the *forebrain.* Its surface is convoluted by shallow sulci and deeper grooves (*fissures*) that divide it into lobes and lobules. There are four lobes of the cerebrum, each named for its location within the cranium: the frontal lobe, parietal lobe, occipital lobe, and temporal lobe. The stemlike portion that connects the cerebrum to the pons and cerebellum is termed the *midbrain.* The cerebellum, pons, and medulla oblongata make up the *hindbrain.*

A deep cleft, called the *longitudinal sulcus* (interhemispheric fissure), separates the cerebrum into *right* and *left hemispheres,* which are closely connected by bands of nerve fibers, or commissures. The largest commissure between the cerebral hemispheres is the *corpus callosum.* The corpus callosum is a midline structure inferior to the longitudinal sulcus. Each cerebral hemisphere contains a fluid-filled cavity called a *lateral ventricle.* At the diencephalon, or second portion of the brain, the pair of oval-shaped gray matter masses of the thalamus surround the *third ventricle.* Inferior to the diencephalon is the *pituitary gland,* the master endocrine gland of the body. The pituitary gland resides in the hypophyseal fossa of the sella turcica.

The cerebellum, the largest part of the hindbrain, is separated from the cerebrum by a deep transverse cleft. The hemispheres of the cerebellum are connected by a median constricted area called the *vermis.* The surface of the cerebellum contains numerous transverse sulci that account for its cauliflower-like appearance. The tissues between the curved sulci are called *folia.* The pons, which forms the upper part of the hindbrain, is the commissure, or bridge, between the cerebrum, cerebellum, and medulla oblongata. The medulla oblongata, which extends between the pons and spinal cord, forms the lower portion of the hindbrain. All the fiber tracts between the brain and spinal cord pass through the medulla.

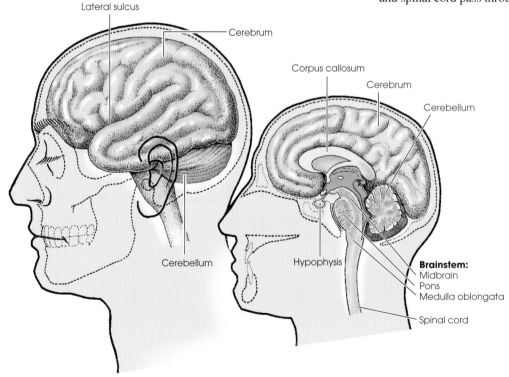

Fig. 14.1 Lateral surface and midsection of brain.

Spinal Cord

The spinal cord is a slender, elongated structure consisting of an inner gray, cellular substance, which has a butterfly shape on the transverse section and an outer white, fibrous substance (Figs. 14.2 and 14.3). The cord extends from the brain, where it is connected to the medulla oblongata at the level of the foramen magnum, to the approximate level of the space between the first and second lumbar vertebrae. The spinal cord ends in a pointed extremity called the *conus medullaris* (see Fig. 14.3). The *filum terminale* is a delicate fibrous strand that extends from the terminal tip and attaches the cord to the upper coccygeal segment.

In an adult, the spinal cord is 18 to 20 inches (46 to 50 cm) long and is connected to 31 pairs of spinal nerves. Each pair of spinal nerves arises from two roots (dorsal and ventral) at the sides of the spinal cord. The nerves are transmitted through the intervertebral and sacral foramina. Spinal nerves below the termination of the spinal cord extend inferiorly through the vertebral canal. These nerves resemble a horse's tail and are referred to as the *cauda equina.* The spinal cord and nerves work together to transmit and receive sensory, motor, and reflex messages to and from the brain.

Meninges

The brain and spinal cord are enclosed in three continuous protective membranes called *meninges.* The inner sheath, called the *pia mater* (Latin, meaning "tender mother"), is highly vascular and closely adherent to the underlying brain and cord structure.

The delicate central sheath is called the *arachnoid.* This membrane is separated from the pia mater by a comparatively wide space called the *subarachnoid space,* which is widened in certain areas. These areas of increased width are called *subarachnoid cisterns.* The widest area is the cisterna magna (cisterna cerebellomedullaris). This triangular cavity is situated in the lower posterior fossa between the base of the cerebellum and the dorsal surface of the medulla oblongata. The subarachnoid space is continuous with the ventricular system of the brain and communicates with it through the foramina of the fourth ventricle. The ventricles of the brain and the subarachnoid space contain *cerebrospinal fluid* (CSF). CSF is the tissue fluid of the brain and spinal cord; it surrounds and cushions the structures of the CNS.

The outermost sheath, called the *dura mater* (Latin, meaning "tough mother"), forms the strong fibrous covering of the brain and spinal cord. The dura is separated from the arachnoid by the *subdural space* and from the vertebral periosteum by the *epidural space.* These spaces do not communicate with the ventricular system. The dura mater is composed of two layers throughout its cranial portion. The outer layer lines the cranial bones, serving as periosteum to their inner surface. The inner layer protects the brain and supports the blood vessels. The inner layer also has four partitions that provide support and protection for the various parts of the brain. One of these partitions, the *falx cerebri,* runs through the longitudinal fissure and provides support for the cerebral hemispheres. The *tentorium cerebelli* is a tent-shaped fold of dura that separates the cerebrum and cerebellum. Changes in the normal positions of these structures often indicate pathology. The dura mater extends below the spinal cord (to the level of the second sacral segment) to enclose the spinal nerves, which are prolonged inferiorly from the cord to their respective exits. The lower portion of the dura mater is called the *dural sac.* The dural sac encloses the cauda equina.

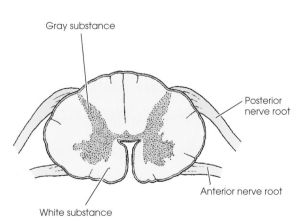

Fig. 14.2 Transverse section of spinal cord.

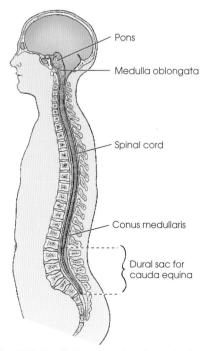

Fig. 14.3 Sagittal section showing spinal cord.

Ventricular System

The ventricular system of the brain consists of four irregular, fluid-containing cavities that communicate with one another through connecting channels (Figs. 14.4 through 14.6). The two upper cavities are an identical pair and are called the *right* and *left lateral ventricles.* They are situated, one on each side of the midsagittal plane, in the inferior medial part of the corresponding hemisphere of the cerebrum.

Each lateral ventricle consists of a central portion called the *body* of the cavity. The body is prolonged anteriorly, posteriorly, and inferiorly into horn-like portions that give the ventricle an approximate U shape. The prolonged portions are known as the *anterior, posterior, or occipital,* and *inferior or temporal horns.* Each lateral ventricle is connected to the third ventricle by a channel called the *interventricular foramen*, or foramen of Monro, through which it communicates directly with the third ventricle and indirectly with the opposite lateral ventricle.

The *third ventricle* is a slit-like cavity with a quadrilateral shape. It is situated in the midsagittal plane just inferior to the level of the bodies of the lateral ventricles. This cavity extends anteroinferiorly from the pineal gland, which produces a recess in its posterior wall, to the optic chiasm, which produces a recess in its anteroinferior wall.

The interventricular foramina, one from each lateral ventricle, open into the anterosuperior portion of the third ventricle. The cavity is continuous posteroinferiorly with the fourth ventricle by a passage known as the *cerebral aqueduct,* or aqueduct of sylvius.

The *fourth ventricle* is diamond-shaped and located in the area of the hindbrain. The fourth ventricle is anterior to the cerebellum and posterior to the pons and the upper portion of the medulla oblongata. The distal, pointed end of the fourth ventricle is continuous with the central canal of the medulla oblongata. CSF exits the fourth ventricle into the subarachnoid space via the *median aperture* (foramen of Magendie) and the *lateral apertures* (foramen of Luschka). The central canal continues inferiorly to the conus medullaris and functions to carry CSF and nutrients throughout the spinal cord (Fig. 14.7).

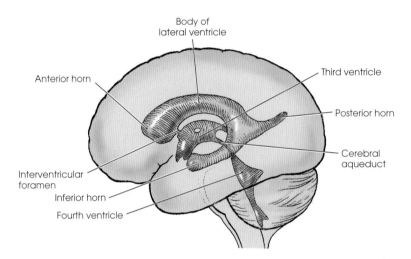

Fig. 14.4 Lateral aspect of cerebral ventricles in relation to surface of brain.

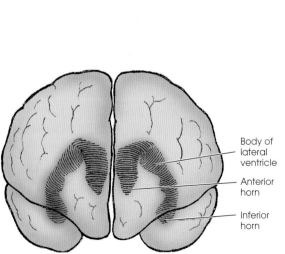

Fig. 14.5 Anterior aspect of lateral cerebral ventricles in relation to surface of brain.

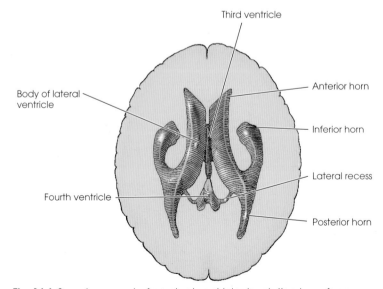

Fig. 14.6 Superior aspect of cerebral ventricles in relation to surface of brain.

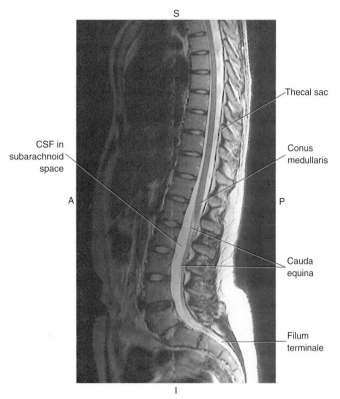

S

Thecal sac

CSF in
subarachnoid
space

Conus
medullaris

A

P

Cauda
equina

Filum
terminale

I

Fig. 14.7 Mid-sagittal T2-weighted magnetic resonance image demonstrating spinal cord within the vertebral canal, along with thecal sac and *cerebrospinal fluid (CSF)* flowing in the subarachnoid space.

Plain Radiographic Examination

Neuroradiologic assessment should begin with noninvasive imaging procedures. Radiographs of the cerebral and visceral cranium and the vertebral column may be obtained to show bony anatomy. In traumatized patients (see Chapters 9 and 12), radiographs are obtained to detect bone injury, subluxation, or dislocation of the vertebral column and to determine the extent and stability of the bone injury. Computed tomography (CT) is often employed first in a trauma setting due to its speed and ability to demonstrate both soft tissue and bony anatomy (see Chapter 25).

For a traumatized patient with possible CNS involvement, a cross-table lateral cervical spine radiograph may be obtained to rule out fracture or misalignment of the cervical spine. Approximately two-thirds of significant pathologic conditions affecting the spine can be detected on this initial image. Care must be taken to image the entire cervical spine adequately, including the C7–T1 articulation. Employing the Swimmer's technique (see Chapter 9) may be necessary to show this anatomic region radiographically.

After the cross-table lateral radiograph has been checked and cleared by a physician or advanced practitioner, the following cervical spine projections should be obtained: AP, bilateral AP oblique (trauma technique may be necessary), and AP to show the dens. A vertebral arch, or pillar image, of the cervical spine may provide additional information about the posterior portions of the cervical vertebrae (see Chapter 9). An upright lateral cervical spine radiograph may also be requested to show alignment of the vertebrae better and to assess the normal lordotic curvature of the spine.

Radiographs of the spine should always be obtained before myelography. Routine images of the vertebral column are helpful in assessing narrowed disk spaces because of degeneration of the disk, osteoarthritis, postoperative changes in the spine, and other pathologies of the vertebral column. Because the contrast agents used in myelography may obscure some anomalies, noncontrast spinal images complement the myelographic examination and often provide additional information.

Routine skull images may be obtained when the possibility of a skull fracture exists. In trauma patients, a cross-table lateral or upright lateral skull radiograph may be obtained to show air-fluid levels in the sphenoid sinus. In many instances, these air-fluid levels may be the initial indication of a basilar skull fracture. A noncontrast head CT is indicated in head trauma patients who experience a loss of consciousness or other neurologic symptoms. In addition, skull images are helpful in diagnosing reactive bone formation and general alterations in the skull resulting from various pathologic conditions, including Paget disease, fibrous dysplasia, hemangiomas, and changes in the sella turcica.

Myelography

Myelography (Greek, *myelos,* "marrow; the spinal cord") is the general term applied to radiologic examination of the CNS structures situated within the vertebral canal. This examination is performed by introducing a nonionic, water-soluble contrast medium into the subarachnoid space by spinal puncture, most commonly at the L2–L3 or L3–L4 interspace or into the thecal sac via a lateral C1–C2 puncture. Injections into the subarachnoid space are termed *intrathecal injections.* A tilting table facilitates the positioning of the contrast medium to the desired region.

Most myelograms are performed on an outpatient basis, with patients recovering for approximately 4 to 8 hours after the procedure before being released to return home. In many parts of the United States, magnetic resonance imaging (MRI) (see Chapter 26) has largely replaced myelography. Myelography continues to be the preferred examination method for assessing disk disease in patients with contraindications to MRI, such as pacemakers or metallic posterior spinal fusion rods.

Myelography is employed to show extrinsic spinal cord compression caused by a herniated disk, bone fragments, or tumors and spinal cord swelling resulting from traumatic injury. These encroachments appear radiographically as a deformity in the subarachnoid space or an obstruction of the passage of the column of contrast medium within the subarachnoid space. Myelography is also useful for identifying a narrowing of the subarachnoid space by evaluating the dynamic flow patterns of the CSF. Myelography may also demonstrate CSF leak and be used for surgical planning.

CONTRAST MEDIA

A non–water-soluble iodinated ester (iophendylate [Pantopaque]) was introduced in 1942. Because the body could not absorb it, this lipid-based contrast medium required removal after the procedure. Frequently, some contrast remained in the canal and could be seen on noncontrast radiographs of patients who had the myelography procedure before the introduction of the newer medium. Iophendylate was used in myelography for many years but is no longer commercially available. The first water-soluble nonionic iodinated contrast agent, metrizamide, was introduced in the late 1970s. Thereafter, water-soluble contrast media quickly became the agents of choice. Nonionic water-soluble contrast media provides good visualization of nerve roots (Fig. 14.8) and allows for good enhancement for follow-up CT of the spine, often immediately following the radiographic myelogram. In addition, the body readily absorbs these agents. Over the past two decades, nonionic water-soluble agents, including iopamidol (Isovue) and iohexol (Omnipaque), have become the most commonly used agents for myelography. To reduce the chance of infection, single-dose vials are recommended. Improvements in nonionic contrast agents have resulted in fewer side effects.

Fig. 14.8 Myelogram using nonionic water-soluble contrast medium (iopamidol) on a postsurgical patient.

Technologists who perform myelography should be educated regarding the use of contrast media. Intrathecal administration of ionic contrast media may cause severe and fatal neurotoxic reactions. Because vials of ionic and nonionic agents may look similar, radiology departments are encouraged to store contrast media for myelography separately from other agents. Proper medication guidelines must be followed when intrathecal agents are administered. Contrast vials should be checked three times and checked with the physician or advanced practitioner performing the examination. They should be kept until the procedure has been completed. All appropriate documentation must be completed.

PREPARATION OF THE EXAMINING ROOM

One of the radiographer's responsibilities is to prepare the examination room before the patient's arrival. The radiographic equipment should be checked. Because the procedure involves aseptic technique, the table and overhead equipment must be cleaned. The footboard should be attached to the table, and the padded shoulder supports should be placed and ready for adjustment to the patient's height. The fluoroscopy tower should be locked so that it cannot accidentally come in contact with the spinal needle, sterile field, or both (Fig. 14.9).

The spinal puncture and injection of contrast medium are performed in the radiology department utilizing sterile technique. The Centers for Disease Control and Prevention (CDC) requires that surgical masks be worn when a catheter is being placed or material injected into the spinal canal or subdural space. Subcutaneous and intramuscular local anesthetic is administered. Under fluoroscopic observation, placement of the 20- to 25-gauge spinal needle in the subarachnoid space is verified and the nonionic iodinated contrast medium injected. The sterile tray and the nonsterile items required for this initial procedure should be ready for convenient placement.

EXAMINATION PROCEDURE

Premedication of the patient for myelography may be necessary, depending on the patient. The patient should be well hydrated, however, because a nonionic water-soluble contrast medium is used. To reduce apprehension and prevent alarm at unexpected maneuvers during the procedure, the radiographer should explain the details of myelography to the patient before the examination begins. The patient should be informed that the angulation of the examining table will change repeatedly and acutely. The patient should also be told why their head must be maintained in a fully extended position when the table is tilted to the Trendelenburg position. The radiographer must ensure that the patient will be safe when the table is acutely angled and that everything possible is being done to avoid causing unnecessary discomfort. Most facilities require an informed consent form to be completed and signed by the patient and physician. The risks and benefits of the procedure and of possible alternatives should be addressed.

Scout images, including a cross-table lateral lumbar spine prone (Fig. 14.10), are often requested. Some physicians/practitioners prefer to have the patient placed on the table in the prone position for the spinal puncture. Alternately, some physicians/practitioners have the patient adjusted in the lateral position, with the spine flexed to widen the interspinous spaces for easier introduction of the needle.

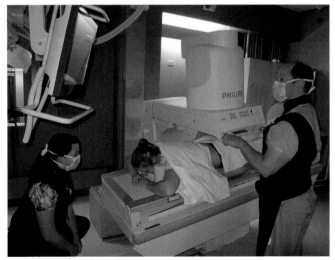

Fig. 14.9 Patient set up with shoulder supports and fluoroscopy tower in locked position.

Fig. 14.10 Lateral scout projection of cross-table lumbar spine myelogram.

The physician/practitioner may withdraw CSF for laboratory analysis. Approximately 9 to 12 mL of nonionic contrast medium is slowly injected under intermittent imaging. After completing the injection, the physician removes the spinal needle. Travel of the column of contrast medium is observed and controlled fluoroscopically. Angulation of the table allows gravity to direct the contrast medium to the area of interest. Spot images are taken throughout the procedure. The radiographer obtains images at the level of any blockage or distortion in the outline of the contrast column. Conventional radiographic studies, with the central ray directed vertically or horizontally, may be performed as requested by the radiologist. The *conus projection* is used to show the *conus medullaris*. For this projection, the patient is placed in the AP position with the central ray centered to T12–L1. A 10 × 12-inch (24 × 30-cm) exposure field is used. Cross-table lateral radiographs are obtained using a crosswise image receptor with a grid and close collimation (Figs. 14.11 through 14.15).

The position of the patient's head must be guarded as the contrast medium column nears the cervical area to prevent the medium from passing into the cerebral ventricles. Acute extension of the head compresses the cisterna magna and prevents further ascent of the contrast medium. Because the cisterna magna is situated posteriorly, neither forward nor lateral flexion of the head will compress the cisternal cavity. The technologist should employ proper radiation protection practices, including wearing lead gloves if support of the patient's head during fluoroscopy is deemed necessary.

After completion of the procedure, the patient must be monitored in an appropriate recovery area. Most physicians/practitioners recommend that the patient's head and shoulders be elevated 30 to 45 degrees during recovery. Bed rest for several hours is recommended, and fluids are encouraged. The puncture site must be examined before the patient is released from the recovery area. If the myelogram is performed on an outpatient basis, the patient should be instructed regarding limitations, including no driving, and warning signs of adverse reactions.

Fig. 14.11 (A) Lumbar myelogram. Cross-table lateral showing needle tip in the subarachnoid space. (B) Lumbar myelogram. Cross-table lateral showing contrast enhancement.

Fig. 14.12 Cervical myelogram. AP projection showing symmetric nerve roots *(arrows)* and axillary pouches *(a)* on both sides and spinal cord.

Fig. 14.13 Myelogram. Prone cross-table lateral projection showing dentate ligament and posterior nerve roots *(arrow)*.

Fig. 14.14 Myelogram. Prone, cross-table lateral projection showing contrast medium passing through the foramen magnum and lying against the lower clivus *(arrows)*.

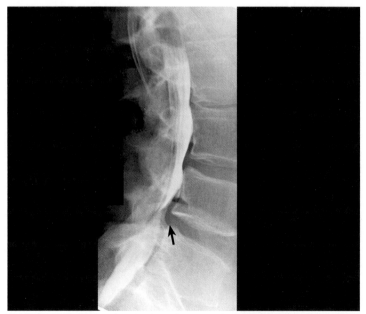

Fig. 14.15 Myelogram. Lateral projection showing narrowing of the subarachnoid space *(arrow)*.

LUMBAR PUNCTURE

For some diagnoses, a *lumbar puncture* is performed under fluoroscopic guidance. This procedure involves a similar setup to myelography, but without the contrast administration steps. In this procedure, the spinal needle is inserted, and CSF is withdrawn for laboratory analysis, or medication may be given intrathecally. Lumbar puncture exams may be performed for diagnostic means, such as in infections (meningitis), demyelinating diseases (multiple sclerosis), bleeding (subarachnoid hemorrhage), in situations when the pressure around the brain and spinal cord must be measured (increased intracranial pressure), and to inject medications. Alternately, lumbar punctures may be performed for treatment purposes, such as to relieve increased spinal pressure, to give anesthesia, or during a blood patch (CSF leak) (Fig. 14.16).

Vertebral Augmentation

Vertebral augmentation includes several percutaneous techniques aimed at stabilizing weakened vertebral bodies. Vertebroplasty, kyphoplasty, and mesh-container-plasty are interventional radiology procedures used to treat spinal osteoporotic compression fractures and other pathologies, such as bone weakened by neoplasia of the vertebral bodies that do not respond to conservative treatment. Vertebral compression fractures (VCFs) are common, especially in older patients with a history of osteoporosis. Estimates indicate that osteoporosis causes more than 700,000 vertebral fractures per year in the United States. About half of these fractures occur silently without any pain. Some fractures are extremely painful, however, and severely limit the patient's quality of life. The morbidity of symptomatic VCFs is significant, causing chronic pain, sleep loss, depression, and a loss of the ability to perform activities of daily living. Vertebral augmentation is used in cases of severe pain that does not improve over many weeks of conservative treatment.

Percutaneous vertebroplasty is defined as the injection of a radiopaque bone cement (e.g., polymethyl methacrylate) into a painful compression fracture under fluoroscopic guidance. This procedure is typically performed in the special procedures suite or the operating room with the patient sedated but awake. A specialized trocar needle is advanced into the fractured vertebral body under fluoroscopy (Fig. 14.17). Intraosseous venography using nonionic contrast media is performed to confirm needle placement. When the physician is satisfied with the needle placement, the cement is injected (Fig. 14.18). The cement stabilizes fracture fragments and leads to reduction in pain. Postprocedural imaging includes AP and lateral projections of the spine to confirm cement position (Fig. 14.19). A CT scan may also be performed.

Fig. 14.16 Prone position for lumbar puncture and myelography. Fluoroscopic image demonstrating spinal needle localization.

Fig. 14.17 Lateral projection of a compressed vertebral body with bone needle in place.

Fig. 14.18 Bone cement injected during vertebroplasty under image guidance.

Percutaneous kyphoplasty differs from vertebroplasty in that a balloon catheter is used to expand the compressed vertebral body to near its original height before injection of the bone cement. Inflation of the balloon creates a pocket for the placement of the cement. Kyphoplasty can help restore the spine to a more normal curvature and reduce hunchback deformities.

Percutaneous mesh-container-plasty utilizes a bone expansion brace to cut the bone tissues. After the brace is withdrawn, a mesh container is advanced into the cavity and the cement is injected into the container. This technique restores vertebral body height and strengthens bony trabeculae.

The success of these procedures is measured by significant reduction of pain, reduced disability, and improved quality of life reported by the patient. With proper patient selection and technique, success rates of 80% to 90% have been reported. Vertebral augmentation procedures have risks of serious complications, however.

Major complications occur in less than 1% of patients treated for compression fractures. The most common complication is leakage of the cement before it hardens. Pulmonary embolism and death, although rare, have been reported. Patients should be encouraged to discuss risks, benefits, and alternatives with their physicians. Technologists who perform these procedures need to be properly educated and ensure that informed consent has been documented.

Fig. 14.19 (A) and (B) AP and lateral projections show bone cement in L1.

Other Neuroradiographic Procedures

PROVOCATIVE DISKOGRAPHY

Diskography is a procedure performed under fluoroscopic guidance to determine whether the disc is the source of a patient's chronic back pain. The examination is performed with a small quantity of water-soluble nonionic iodinated medium injected into the center of the disk. Diskography is used in the investigation of internal disk lesions, such as rupture of the nucleus pulposus, which cannot be shown by other imaging procedures (Fig. 14.20). Patients are given only a local anesthetic so that they remain fully conscious and able to inform the physician about pain when the needles are inserted and the injection is made. Attempts are made to replicate the patient's chronic pain during the injection. CT is usually performed after diskography to look for clefts or tears. Spinal fusion is often recommended based on a positive provocation of pain. The need for this procedure should be carefully evaluated because there is controversy regarding the sensitivity and specificity of the examination. Some authors have suggested that diskography may increase the chance of later disk disruption. MRI and CT have largely replaced diskography.

INTERVENTIONAL PAIN MANAGEMENT

Image-guided interventional pain management is becoming a common treatment for chronic back pain that does not respond to conservative treatment. Pretreatment assessment of the patient's pain and a thorough history are necessary. Fluoroscopy, CT, and ultrasonography are often used to confirm needle placement. Interventional pain management physicians perform a variety of injections using corticosteroids and local anesthetics to reduce inflammation and improve symptoms. Procedures can be performed at all levels of the spine and include facet injections, nerve root blocks, and epidural steroid injections. Various needle types can be used, but needles with a stylet are most common to prevent tissue from being trapped in the lumen. Size and tip configuration are determined by the physician. Patients are placed in the prone position (Fig. 14.21). A pillow placed under the pelvis may help with patient comfort. C-arm fluoroscopy is commonly used to determine needle placement. The C-arm may have to be rotated several times to identify the needle path. Images are taken to document the procedure, needle position, and contrast distribution. PA and lateral projections are needed to confirm needle depth. The tip of the needle and an identifiable bony landmark must be included in the images. The precise nature of the injections is thought to improve patient outcomes compared with blind injections. The success of the treatment is based on the patient's self-report of pain reduction.

Fig. 14.20 Lumbar diskogram showing normal nucleus pulposus of round contour type.

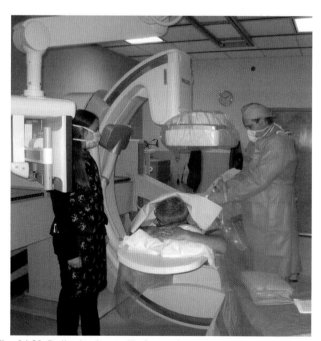

Fig. 14.21 Patient set up with C-arm for pain management injection.

Definition of Terms

arachnoid: Thin delicate membrane surrounding the brain and spinal cord.

brain: Portion of the CNS contained within the cranium.

cauda equina: Collection of nerves located in the spinal canal inferior to the spinal cord.

cerebellum: Part of the brain located in the posterior cranial fossa behind the brain stem.

cerebral aqueduct: Opening between the third and fourth ventricles.

cerebrum: Largest uppermost portion of the brain.

conus medullaris: Most inferior portion of the spinal cord.

cortex: Outer surface layer of the brain.

CSF: Cerebrospinal fluid—the fluid that flows through and protects the ventricles, subarachnoid space, brain, and spinal cord.

dura mater: Tough outer layer of the meninges, which lines the cranial cavity and spinal canal.

epidural space: Outside or above the dura mater.

falx cerebri: Fold of dura mater that separates the cerebral hemispheres.

filum terminale: Threadlike structure that extends from the distal end of the spinal cord.

hindbrain: Portion of the brain within the posterior fossa; it includes the pons, medulla oblongata, and cerebellum.

intrathecal injection: Injection into the subarachnoid space of the spinal canal.

kyphoplasty: Interventional radiology procedure used to treat vertebral body compression fractures using a specialized balloon and bone cement.

lumbar puncture: Procedure involving the insertion of a spinal needle into the subdural space to remove CSF for laboratory analysis, relieve pressure, or to inject medication (also known as spinal tap).

pons: Oval-shaped area of the brain anterior to the medulla oblongata.

spinal cord: Extension of the medulla oblongata that runs through the spinal canal to the upper lumbar vertebrae.

tentorium cerebelli: Layer of dura that separates the cerebrum and cerebellum.

vermis: Wormlike structure that connects the two cerebellar hemispheres.

vertebroplasty: Interventional radiology procedure used to treat vertebral body compression fractures by stabilizing bone fragments with cement.

Bibliography

Bontrager KL, Lampignano J. *Textbook of radiographic positioning and related anatomy.* ed 8. St Louis: Elsevier; 2014.

Boyajian SS. Interventional pain management: an overview for primary care physicians. *J Am Osteopath Assoc.* 2005;105(9 suppl 4):S1.

Brown DB, et al. Treatment of chronic symptomatic vertebral compression fractures with percutaneous vertebroplasty. *AJR Am J Roentgenol.* 2004;182:319.

Carragee EJ, et al. A gold standard evaluation of the discogenic pain diagnosis as determined by provocative discography. *Spine.* 2006;31:18.

Centers for Disease Control and Prevention. Safe injection practices to prevent transmission of infections to patients; 2007. Available at: http://www.cdc.gov/injectionsafety/ip07.

Chandra RV, et al. Vertebroplasty and kyphoplasty for osteoporotic vertebral fractures: what are the latest data? *Am J Neuroradiol.* 2018;39(5):798–806.

Chen C, et al. Safety and efficacy studies of vertebroplasty, kyphoplasty, and mesh-container-plasty for the treatment of vertebral compression fractures: preliminary report. *PLoS ONE.* 2016;11(3):e0151492. Available at: https://doi.org/10.1371/journal.pone.0151492.

Furlow B. Pain management imaging. *Radiol Technol.* 2009;80:447.

Hirsch JA, et al. American College of Radiology Practice parameter for the performance of vertebral augmentation; 2017. Available at: https://www.acr.org/-/media/ACR/Files/Practice-Parameters/myelog-cisternog.pdf. (Accessed September 2021.)

Hudgins AJ, et al. Difficult lumbar puncture: Pitfalls and tips from the trenches. *Am J Neuroradiol.* 2017;38(7):1276–1283. https://doi.org/10.3174/ajnr.A5128.

Kelley LL, Petersen C. *Sectional anatomy for imaging professionals.* ed 4. St Louis: Elsevier; 2018.

Kieffer SA, et al. American College of Radiology practice parameter for the performance of myelography and cisternography; 2013. Available at: https://www.acr.org/-/media/ACR/Files/Practice-Parameters/myelog-cisternog.pdf. (Accessed September 2021.)

Landers MH. Indications for spinal injections in the chronic pain patient. *Pain Med.* 2008;V9:S1.

Linger L. Percutaneous polymethacrylate vertebroplasty. *Radiol Technol.* 2004;76:109.

Manchikanti L, et al. The role of fluoroscopic interlaminar epidural injections in managing chronic pain of lumbar disc herniation or radiculitis: a randomized, double-blind trial. *Pain Pract.* 2013;13(7):547–558. Available at: https://onlinelibrary.wiley.com/doi/abs/10.1111/papr.12023. (Accessed September 2018.)

Marcia S, et al. What is the role of vertebral augmentation for osteoporotic fractures? A review of the recent literature. *Neuroradiology.* 2018;60:777.

McCormick Z, et al. Diagnostic value, prognostic value, and safety of provocation discography. *Pain Med.* 2018;19(1):3–8. Available at: https://academic.oup.com/painmedicine/article/19/1/3/3074755. (Accessed September 2018.)

McDonald RJ, et al. Percutaneous vertebroplasty: overview, clinical applications and current state. *Appl Radiol.* 2017;46(1):24–30.

Palmer WE. Spinal injections for pain management. *Radiology.* 2016;V281(3).

Thiyagarajah AR, et al. Discography: overview; 2016. Available at: https://emedicine.medscape.com/article/1145703-overview. (Accessed August 2017.)

Wheeler AH. Therapeutic injections for pain management. Available at: http://emedicine.medscape.com. (Accessed September 2009.)

15

DIGESTIVE SYSTEM: SALIVARY GLANDS, ALIMENTARY CANAL, AND BILIARY SYSTEM

SUMMARY OF PROJECTIONS

PROJECTIONS, POSITIONS, AND METHODS

Page	Essential	Anatomy	Projection	Position	Method
201		Parotid gland	Tangential		
203		Parotid and submandibular glands	Lateral	R or L	
207	⚜	Soft palate, pharynx, larynx, and cervical esophagus	Lateral	Upright/seated R or L	
208	⚜	Soft palate, pharynx, larynx, and cervical esophagus	AP	Upright/seated	
218	⚜	Esophagus	AP or PA		
218	⚜	Esophagus	AP or PA oblique	RAO or LPO	
218	⚜	Esophagus	Lateral	R or L	
223	⚜	Stomach and duodenum	PA		
225		Stomach and duodenum	PA axial		
226	⚜	Stomach and duodenum	PA oblique	RAO	
228	⚜	Stomach and duodenum	AP oblique	LPO	
230	⚜	Stomach and duodenum	Lateral	R only	
232	⚜	Stomach and duodenum	AP		
234		Superior stomach and distal esophagus	PA oblique	RAO	WOLF
237	⚜	Small intestine	PA or AP		
250	⚜	Large intestine	PA		
251	⚜	Large intestine	PA axial		
253	⚜	Large intestine	PA oblique	RAO	
254	⚜	Large intestine	PA oblique	LAO	
255	⚜	Large intestine	Lateral	R or L	
256	⚜	Large intestine	AP		
257	⚜	Large intestine	AP axial		
258	⚜	Large intestine	AP oblique	LPO	
259	⚜	Large intestine	AP oblique	RPO	
261	⚜	Large intestine	AP or PA	R lateral decubitus	
263	⚜	Large intestine	PA or AP	L lateral decubitus	
265		Large intestine	Lateral	R or L ventral decubitus	
266		Large intestine	AP, PA, oblique, lateral	Upright	
272		Percutaneous transhepatic cholangiography	AP/AP oblique	Supine/RPO	
274		Postoperative (T-tube) cholangiography	AP/AP oblique	Supine/RPO	
276		Endoscopic retrograde cholangiopancreatography	AP/AP oblique	Supine/RPO	

Icons in the Essential column indicate projections frequently performed in the United States and Canada. Students should be competent in these projections.

AP, Anteroposterior; *L,* left; *LAO,* left anterior oblique; *LPO,* left posterior oblique; *PA,* posteroanterior; *R,* right; *RAO,* right anterior oblique; *RPO,* right posterior oblique.

Digestive System

The *digestive system* consists of two parts: the *accessory glands* and the *alimentary canal*. The accessory glands, which include the *salivary glands, liver, gallbladder,* and *pancreas,* secrete digestive enzymes into the alimentary canal. The alimentary canal is a musculomembranous tube that extends from the mouth to the anus. The regions of the alimentary canal vary in diameter according to functional requirements. The greater part of the canal, which is about 29 to 30 ft (8.6 to 8.9 m) long, lies in the abdominal cavity. The component parts of the alimentary canal (Fig. 15.1) are the *mouth,* in which food is masticated and converted into a bolus by insalivation; the *pharynx* and *esophagus,* which are the organs of swallowing; the *stomach,* in which the digestive process begins; the *small intestine,* in which the digestive process is completed; and the *large intestine,* which is an organ of egestion and water absorption that terminates at the *anus.*

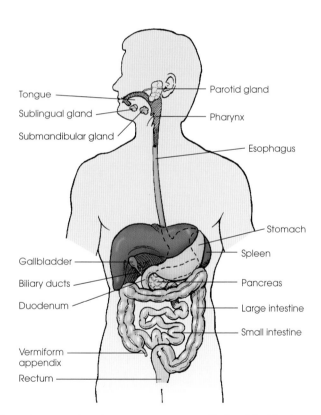

Tongue

Sublingual gland

Submandibular gland

Parotid gland

Pharynx

Esophagus

Stomach

Spleen

Gallbladder

Biliary ducts

Duodenum

Pancreas

Large intestine

Small intestine

Vermiform appendix

Rectum

Fig. 15.1 Alimentary canal and accessory organs, with liver lifted to show gallbladder.

Mouth

The *mouth,* or *oral cavity,* is the first division of the digestive system (Fig. 15.2). It encloses the dental arches and receives the saliva secreted by the salivary glands. The cavity of the mouth is divided into (1) the *oral vestibule,* the space between the teeth and the cheeks, and (2) the *oral cavity,* or mouth proper, the space within the dental arches. The roof of the oral cavity is formed by the hard and soft palates. The floor is formed principally by the tongue, and it communicates with the pharynx posteriorly via the *oropharynx.*

The *hard palate* is the anteriormost portion of the roof of the oral cavity. The hard palate is formed by the horizontal plates of the maxillae and palatine bones. The anterior and lateral boundaries are formed by the inner wall of the maxillary alveolar processes, which extend superiorly and medially to blend with the horizontal processes. The height of the hard palate varies considerably, and it determines the angulation of the inner surface of the alveolar process. The angle is less when the palate is high and is greater when the palate is low.

The *soft palate* begins behind the last molar and is suspended from the posterior border of the hard palate. Highly sensitive to touch, the soft palate is a movable musculomembranous structure that functions chiefly as a partial septum between the mouth and the pharynx. At the center of the inferior border, the soft palate is prolonged into a small, pendulous process called the *uvula.* On each side of the uvula, two arched folds extend laterally and inferiorly. The *anterior arches* project forward to the sides of the base of the tongue. The *posterior arches* project posteriorly to blend with the posterolateral walls of the pharynx. The triangular space between the anterior and posterior arches is occupied by the palatine *tonsil.*

The *tongue* is situated in the floor of the oral cavity, with its base directed posteriorly and its *apex* directed anteriorly (Fig. 15.3; see Fig. 15.2). The tongue is freely movable. The tongue is composed of numerous muscles and is covered with a mucous membrane that varies in complexity in the different regions of the organ. The extrinsic muscles of the tongue form the greater part of the oral floor. The

mucous membrane covering the undersurface of the tongue is reflected laterally over the remainder of the floor to the gums. This part of the floor lies under the free anterior and lateral portions of the tongue and is called the *sublingual space.* Posterior movement of the free anterior part of the tongue is restricted by a median vertical band, or fold, of mucous membrane called the *frenulum of the tongue,* which extends between the undersurface of the tongue and the sublingual space. On each side of the frenulum, extending around the outer limits of the sublingual space and over the underlying salivary glands, the mucous membrane is elevated into a crest-like ridge called the *sublingual fold.* In the relaxed state, the two folds are quite prominent and are in contact with the gums.

The *teeth* serve the function of *mastication,* the process of chewing and grinding food into small pieces. During mastication, the teeth cut, grind, and tear food, which is then mixed with saliva and swallowed, and later digested. The saliva softens the food, keeps the mouth moist, and contributes digestive enzymes.

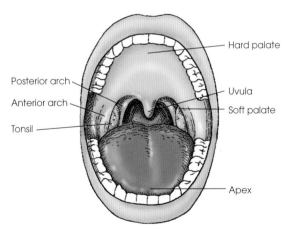

Fig. 15.2 Anterior view of oral cavity.

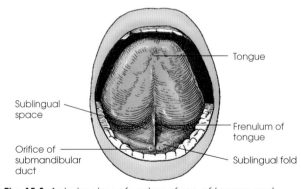

Fig. 15.3 Anterior view of undersurface of tongue and floor of mouth.

Salivary Glands

The three pairs of salivary glands produce approximately 1 L of saliva each day. The glands are named the *parotid, submandibular,* and *sublingual* (Fig. 15.4). Each gland is composed of numerous lobes, and each lobe contains small lobules. The whole gland is held together by connective tissue and a fine network of blood vessels and ducts. The minute ducts of the lobules merge into larger tributaries, which unite and form the large efferent duct that conveys the saliva from the gland to the mouth.

Each of the *parotid glands,* the largest of the salivary glands, consists of a flattened superficial portion and a wedge-shaped deep portion (Fig. 15.5). The superficial part lies immediately anterior to the external ear and extends inferiorly to the mandibular ramus and posteriorly to the mastoid process. The deep, or retromandibular, portion extends medially toward the pharynx. The *parotid duct* runs anteriorly and medially to open into the oral vestibule opposite the second upper molar.

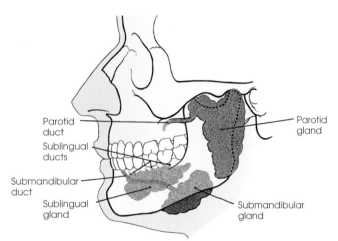

Fig. 15.4 Salivary glands from left lateral aspect.

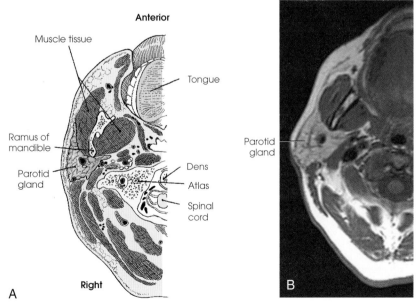

Fig. 15.5 (A) Horizontal section of face, showing relationship of parotid gland to mandibular ramus. Auricle is not shown. (B) Axial MRI of parotid gland.

(B, Courtesy J. Louis Rankin, BS, RT(R)(MR).)

The *submandibular glands* are large, irregularly shaped glands. On each side, a submandibular gland extends posteriorly from a point below the first molar almost to the angle of the mandible (Fig. 15.6). Although the upper part of the gland rests against the inner surface of the mandibular body, its greater portion projects below the mandible. The *submandibular duct* extends anteriorly and superiorly to open into the mouth on a small papilla at the side of the frenulum of the tongue.

The *sublingual glands,* the smallest pair, are narrow and elongated in form (see Fig. 15.6). These glands are located in the floor of the mouth beneath the sublingual fold. Each is in contact with the mandible laterally and extends posteriorly from the side of the frenulum of the tongue to the submandibular gland. Numerous small *sublingual ducts* exist. Some of these ducts open into the floor of the mouth along the crest of the sublingual fold, and others open into the submandibular duct. The main sublingual duct opens beside the orifice of the submandibular duct.

Pharynx

The *pharynx* serves as a passage for air and food and is common to the respiratory and digestive systems (Figs. 15.7 and 15.8). The pharynx is a musculomembranous, tubular structure situated in front of the vertebrae and behind the nose, mouth, and larynx. Approximately 5 inches (13 cm) in length, the pharynx extends from the undersurface of the body of the sphenoid bone and the basilar part of the occipital bone inferiorly to the level of the disk between the sixth and seventh cervical vertebrae, where it becomes continuous with the esophagus. The pharyngeal cavity is subdivided into nasal, oral, and laryngeal portions.

The *nasopharynx* lies posteriorly above the *soft* and *hard* palates. (The upper part of the hard palate forms the floor of the nasopharynx.) Anteriorly, the nasopharynx communicates with the posterior apertures of the nose. Hanging from the posterior aspect of the soft palate is a small conical process, the *uvula*. On the roof and posterior wall of the nasopharynx, between the orifices of the auditory tubes,

the mucosa contains a mass of lymphoid tissue known as the *pharyngeal tonsil* (or *adenoids* when enlarged). Hypertrophy of this tissue interferes with nasal breathing and is common in children. This condition is well shown in a lateral radiographic image of the nasopharynx.

The *oropharynx* is the portion extending from the soft palate to the level of the *hyoid bone*. The base, or root, of the tongue forms the anterior wall of the oropharynx. The *laryngeal pharynx* lies posterior to the larynx, its anterior wall being formed by the posterior surface of the larynx. The laryngeal pharynx extends inferiorly and is continuous with the esophagus.

The air-containing nasal and oral pharynges are well visualized in lateral images except during the act of phonation, when the soft palate contracts and tends to obscure the nasal pharynx. An opaque medium is required to show the lumen of the laryngeal pharynx, although it can be distended with air during the *Valsalva maneuver* (an increase in intrathoracic pressure produced by forcible expiration effort against the closed glottis).

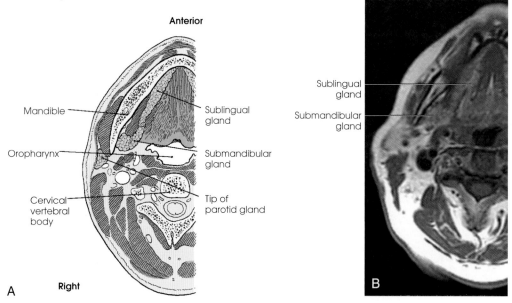

Fig. 15.6 (A) Horizontal section of face, showing relationship of submandibular and sublingual glands to surrounding structures. Auricle is not shown. (B) Axial MRI of submandibular and sublingual glands.

(B, Courtesy J. Louis Rankin, BS, RT(R)(MR).)

Fig. 15.7 (A) Interior posterior view of neck. (B) Coronal MRI of neck.

(B, Courtesy J. Louis Rankin, BS, RT(R)(MR).)

Fig. 15.8 (A) Sagittal section of face and neck. (B) Sagittal MRI of neck.

(B, Courtesy J. Louis Rankin, BS, RT(R)(MR).)

Larynx

The larynx is the organ of voice (Figs. 15.9 and 15.10; see Figs. 15.7 through 15.10). Serving as the air passage between the pharynx and the trachea, the larynx is also one of the divisions of the respiratory system.

The larynx is a movable, tubular structure; is broader above than below; and is approximately 1½ inches (3.8 cm) in length. Situated below the root of the tongue and in front of the laryngeal pharynx, the larynx is suspended from the hyoid bone and extends from the level of the superior margin of the fourth cervical vertebra to its junction with the trachea at the level of the inferior margin of the sixth cervical vertebra. The thin, leaf-shaped *epiglottis* is situated behind the root of the tongue and the hyoid bone and above the laryngeal entrance. It has been stated that the epiglottis serves as a trap to prevent leakage into the larynx between acts of swallowing. The *thyroid cartilage* forms the laryngeal prominence, or *Adam's apple.*

The inlet of the larynx is oblique, slanting posteriorly as it descends. A pouch-like fossa called the *piriform recess* is located on each side of the larynx and external to its orifice. The piriform recesses are well shown as triangular areas on frontal projections when insufflated with air (Valsalva maneuver) or when filled with an opaque medium.

The entrance of the larynx is guarded superiorly and anteriorly by the epiglottis and laterally and posteriorly by folds of mucous membrane. These folds, which extend around the margin of the laryngeal inlet from their junction with the epiglottis, function as a sphincter during swallowing. The *laryngeal cavity* is subdivided into three compartments by two pairs of mucosal folds that extend anteroposteriorly from its lateral walls. The superior pairs of folds are the *vestibular folds,* or false vocal cords. The space above them is called the *laryngeal vestibule.* The lower two folds are separated from each other by a median fissure called the *rima glottidis.* They are known as the *vocal folds,* or true vocal folds (see Fig. 15.10). The vocal cords are vocal ligaments that are covered by the vocal folds. The ligaments and the rima glottidis constitute the vocal apparatus of the larynx and are collectively referred to as the *glottis.*

Esophagus

The *esophagus* is a long, muscular tube that carries food and saliva from the laryngopharynx to the stomach (see Fig. 15.1). The adult esophagus is approximately 10 inches (24 cm) long and ¾ inch (1.9 cm) in diameter. The esophagus begins at the inferior border of the cricoid cartilage, which is approximately at the level of the sixth cervical vertebra (C6). The esophagus terminates at the cardiac opening of the stomach, at about the level of the eleventh thoracic vertebra (T11) (Fig. 15.11).

Similar to the rest of the alimentary canal, the esophagus has a wall composed of four layers. Beginning with the outermost layer and moving in, the layers are as follows:
- Fibrous layer
- Muscular layer
- Submucosal layer
- Mucosal layer

The *esophagus* lies in the midsagittal plane (MSP) and is divided into three major sections with four natural narrowed areas or constrictions (Fig. 15.12A and B). The *cervical esophagus* begins at its first natural constriction, the *pharyngoesophageal constriction* occurs at the junction to the pharynx. The cervical portion of the esophagus is about 1.2 to 2 inches (3 to 5 cm) long, stretching from C6 to T1. The middle portion is the *thoracic esophagus,* which measures about 7 to 8.7 inches (18 to 22 cm) in length. The thoracic esophagus features two constrictions. The first occurs where the aortic arch and left main stem bronchus cross the esophagus, the *aortobronchial constriction,* and the second is where the left atrium of the heart compresses the esophagus. The *abdominal esophagus* measures about 1.2 to 2.4 inches (3 to 6 cm) long and begins at the final natural narrowing, the *diaphragmatic constriction.*

The esophagus descends the thorax parallel and anterior to the thoracic vertebrae and posterior to the trachea and heart (see Fig. 15.11). As the esophagus nears the diaphragm, it shifts anteriorly and to the left, crossing from the right side of the thoracic aorta to lie anterior to it. The esophagus then passes through the diaphragm at the *esophageal hiatus,* at the approximate level of T10. Finally, the esophagus curves sharply left, increases in diameter, and joins the stomach at the *esophagogastric junction,* which is at the level of the T11. The expanded portion of the terminal esophagus, which lies in the abdomen, is called the *cardiac antrum.*

The proximal and distal ends of the esophagus are bordered by sphincters that regulate the passage of materials. The *upper esophageal sphincter (UES)* is at its junction with the pharynx and functions to prevent air from entering the esophagus during respiration. Relaxation of the UES allows trapped air to escape the esophagus and stomach, commonly termed belching or burping. The distal sphincter is explained with the stomach anatomy.

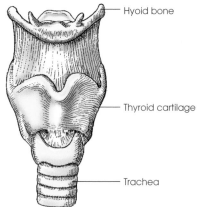

Fig. 15.9 Anterior aspect of larynx.

Hyoid bone

Thyroid cartilage

Trachea

Base of tongue

Epiglottis

Vestibular fold (false vocal cord)

Vocal fold (true vocal cord)

Rima glottidis open

Rima glottidis closed

Fig. 15.10 Superior aspect of larynx (open and closed true vocal folds).

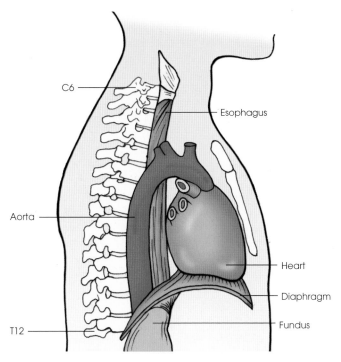

Fig. 15.11 Lateral view of thorax shows esophagus positioned anterior to vertebral bodies and posterior to trachea and heart.

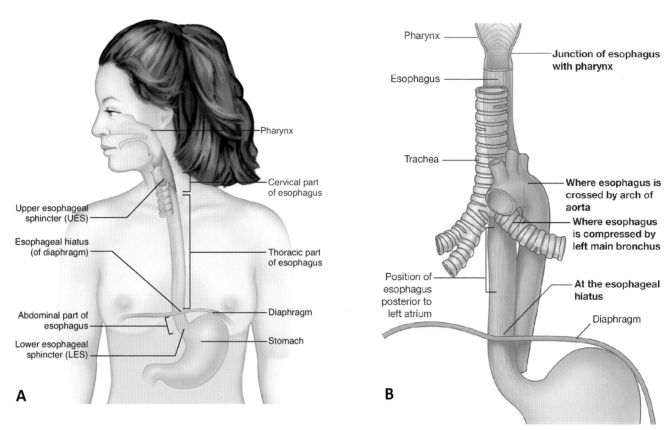

Fig. 15.12 (A) Anterior view of esophageal divisions. (B) Locations of natural constrictions of the esophagus.

(A, Modified from Patton K, Thibodeau G. *Anatomy and Physiology.* 8th ed. St. Louis: Mosby; 2013. B, From Drake R, Vogl W, Mitchell AWM. *Gray's Anatomy for Students.* 2nd ed. Philadelphia: Churchill Livingstone; 2010.)

Stomach

The *stomach* is the dilated, sac-like portion of the digestive tract extending between the esophagus and the small intestine (Fig. 15.13). Its wall is composed of the same four layers as the esophagus.

The stomach is divided into the following four parts:
- Cardia
- Fundus
- Body
- Pyloric portion

The *cardia* of the stomach is the section immediately surrounding the esophageal opening. The *fundus* is the superior portion of the stomach that expands superiorly and fills the dome of the left hemidiaphragm. When the patient is in the upright position, the fundus is usually filled with gas; in radiography, this is referred to as the *gas bubble*. Descending from the fundus and beginning at the level of the cardiac notch is the *body* of the stomach. The inner mucosal layer of the body of the stomach contains numerous longitudinal folds called *rugae*. When the stomach is full, the rugae are smooth. The body of the stomach ends at a vertical plane passing through the *angular notch*. Distal to this plane is the *pyloric portion* of the stomach, which consists of the *pyloric antrum*, to the immediate right of the angular notch, and the narrow *pyloric canal*, which communicates with the duodenal bulb.

The stomach has anterior and posterior surfaces. The right border of the stomach is marked by the *lesser curvature*. The lesser curvature begins at the esophagogastric junction, is continuous with the right border of the esophagus, and is a concave curve ending at the pylorus. The left and inferior borders of the stomach are marked by the *greater curvature*. The greater curvature begins at the sharp angle at the esophagogastric junction, the *cardiac notch,* and follows the superior curvature of the fundus and then the convex curvature of the body down to the pylorus. The greater curvature is four to five times longer than the lesser curvature.

Fig. 15.13 (A) Anterior surface of stomach. (B) Interior view. (C) Axial CT image of upper abdomen showing position of stomach in relation to surrounding organs. Note contrast media *(white)* and air *(black)* in stomach. (D) Axial CT image showing stomach without contrast media. Note air *(arrow)* and empty stomach.

(D, Courtesy Heath Yarbrough, RT(R)(MR)(CT), NEA Baptist Memorial Hospital, Jonesboro, AR.)

The entrance to and the exit from the stomach are controlled by muscular sphincters. The esophagus joins the stomach at the esophagogastric junction through an opening termed the *cardiac orifice*. The muscle controlling the cardiac orifice is called the *cardiac sphincter* or the *lower esophageal sphincter (LES)*. The opening between the stomach and the small intestine is the *pyloric orifice*, and the muscle controlling the pyloric orifice is called the *pyloric sphincter*.

The size, shape, and position of the stomach depend on body habitus and vary with posture and the amount of stomach contents (Fig. 15.14). In persons with a hypersthenic habitus, the stomach is almost horizontal and is high, with its most dependent portion well above the umbilicus. In persons with an asthenic habitus, the stomach is vertical and occupies a low position, with its most dependent portion extending well below the transpyloric, or interspinous, line. Between these two extremes are the intermediate types of bodily habitus with corresponding variations in shape and position of the stomach. The habitus of 85% of the population is either sthenic or hyposthenic. Radiographers should become familiar with the various positions of the stomach in the different types of body habitus so that accurate positioning of the stomach is ensured.

The stomach has several functions in the digestive process. The stomach serves as a storage area for food until it can be digested further. It is also where food is broken down. Acids, enzymes, and other chemicals are secreted to break food down chemically. Food is also mechanically broken down through churning and peristalsis. Food that has been mechanically and chemically altered in the stomach is transported to the duodenum as a material called *chyme*.

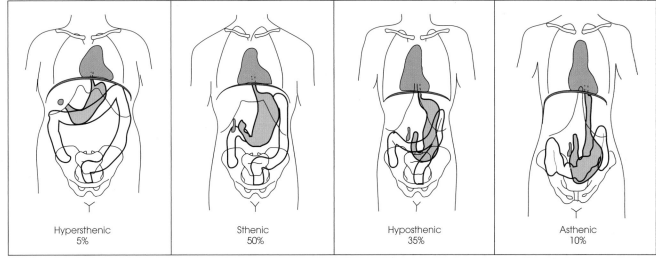

| Hypersthenic 5% | Sthenic 50% | Hyposthenic 35% | Asthenic 10% |

Fig. 15.14 Size, shape, and position of stomach and large intestine for the four different types of body habitus. Note extreme difference between hypersthenic and asthenic types.

Small Intestine

The *small intestine* extends from the pyloric sphincter of the stomach to the ileocecal valve, where it joins the large intestine at a right angle. Digestion and absorption of food occur in this portion of the alimentary canal. The length of the adult small intestine averages about 22 ft (6.5 m), and its diameter gradually diminishes from approximately 1½ inches (3.8 cm) in the proximal part to approximately 1 inch (2.5 cm) in the distal part. The wall of the small intestine contains the same four layers as the walls of the esophagus and stomach. The mucosa of the small intestine contains a series of finger-like projections called *villi,* which assist the processes of digestion and absorption.

The small intestine is divided into the following three portions:

• Duodenum
• Jejunum
• Ileum

The *duodenum* is 8 to 10 inches (20 to 24 cm) long and is the widest portion of the small intestine (Fig. 15.15). It is retroperitoneal and is relatively fixed in position. Beginning at the pylorus, the duodenum follows a C-shaped course. Its four regions are described as the *first* (superior), *second* (descending), *third* (horizontal or inferior), and *fourth* (ascending) portions. The segment of the first portion is called the *duodenal bulb* because of its radiographic appearance when it is filled with an opaque contrast medium. The second portion is about 3 or 4 inches (7.6 to 10 cm) long. This segment passes inferiorly along the head of the pancreas and in close relation to the undersurface of the liver. The common bile duct and the pancreatic duct usually unite to form the *hepatopancreatic ampulla,* which opens on the summit of the *greater duodenal papilla* in the duodenum. The third portion passes toward the left at a slight superior inclination for a distance of about 2½ inches (6 cm) and continues as the fourth portion on the left side of the vertebrae. This portion joins the jejunum at a sharp curve called the *duodenojejunal flexure* and is supported by the *suspensory muscle of the duodenum* (ligament of Treitz). The duodenal loop, which lies in the second portion, is the most fixed part of the small intestine and normally lies in the upper part of the umbilical region of the abdomen; however, its position varies with body habitus and with the amount of gastric and intestinal contents.

The remainder of the small intestine is arbitrarily divided into two portions, with the upper two fifths referred to as the *jejunum* and the lower three fifths referred to as the *ileum.* The jejunum and the ileum are gathered into freely movable loops, or gyri, and are attached to the posterior wall of the abdomen by the mesentery. The loops lie in the central and lower part of the abdominal cavity within the arch of the large intestine.

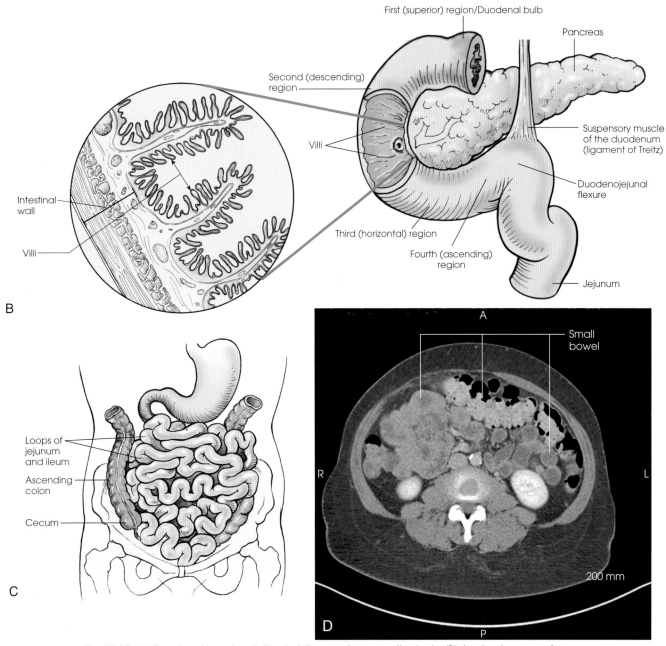

Fig. 15.15 (A) Duodenal loop in relation to biliary and pancreatic ducts. (B) Anatomic areas of duodenum. *Inset:* Cross-section of duodenum, showing villi. (C) Loops of small intestine lying in central and lower abdominal cavity. (D) CT axial image of small bowel loops with contrast media.

(D, Courtesy Kacey Higgins, RT(R)(CT), NEA Baptist Memorial Hospital, Jonesboro, AR.)

Large Intestine

The *large intestine* begins in the right iliac region, where it joins the ileum of the small intestine, forms an arch surrounding the loops of the small intestine, and ends at the anus (Fig. 15.16). The large intestine has four main parts, as follows:

- Cecum
- Colon
- Rectum
- Anal canal

The large intestine is about 5 ft (1.5 m) long and is greater in diameter than the small intestine. The wall of the large intestine contains the same four layers as the walls of the esophagus, stomach, and small intestine. The muscular portion of the intestinal wall contains an external band of longitudinal muscle that forms into three thickened bands called *taeniae coli*. One band is positioned anteriorly, and two are positioned posteriorly. These bands create a pulling muscle tone that forms a series of pouches called the *haustra*. The main functions of the large intestine are reabsorption of fluids and elimination of waste products.

The *cecum* is the pouch-like portion of the large intestine that is below the junction of the ileum and the colon. The cecum is approximately 2½ inches (6 cm) long and 3 inches (7.6 cm) in diameter. The *vermiform appendix* is attached to the posteromedial side of the cecum. The appendix is a narrow, worm-like tube that is about 3 inches (7.6 cm) long. The *ileocecal valve* is just below the junction of the ascending colon and the cecum. The valve projects into the lumen of the cecum and guards the opening between the ileum and the cecum.

A

B

C

Fig. 15.16 (A) Anterior aspect of large intestine positioned in abdomen. (B) Anterior aspect of large intestine. (C) Axial CT image of upper abdomen showing actual image of transverse colon positioned in anterior abdomen.

The *colon* is subdivided into ascending, transverse, descending, and sigmoid portions. The *ascending colon* passes superiorly from its junction with the cecum to the undersurface of the liver, where it joins the transverse portion at an angle called the *right colic flexure* (formerly hepatic flexure). The *transverse colon,* which is the longest and most movable part of the colon, crosses the abdomen to the undersurface of the spleen. The transverse portion makes a sharp curve, called the *left colic flexure* (formerly splenic flexure), and ends in the descending portion. The *descending colon* passes inferiorly and medially to its junction with the *sigmoid portion* at the superior aperture of the lesser pelvis. The sigmoid colon curves to form an S-shaped loop and ends in the rectum at the level of the third sacral segment.

The *rectum* extends from the sigmoid colon to the anal canal. The *anal canal* terminates at the *anus,* which is the external aperture of the large intestine (Fig. 15.17). The rectum is approximately 6 inches (15 cm) long. The distal portion, which is about 1 inch (2.5 cm) long, is constricted to form the anal canal. Just above the anal canal is a dilatation called the *rectal ampulla*. Following the sacrococcygeal curve, the rectum passes inferiorly and posteriorly to the level of the pelvic floor and bends sharply anteriorly and inferiorly into the anal canal, which extends to the anus. The rectum and anal canal have two AP curves; this fact must be remembered when an enema tube is inserted.

The size, shape, and position of the large intestine vary greatly, depending on body habitus (see Figs. 15.14 and 15.20). In hypersthenic patients, the large intestine is positioned around the periphery of the abdomen and may require more images to show its entire length. The large intestine of asthenic patients, which is bunched together and positioned low in the abdomen, is at the other extreme.

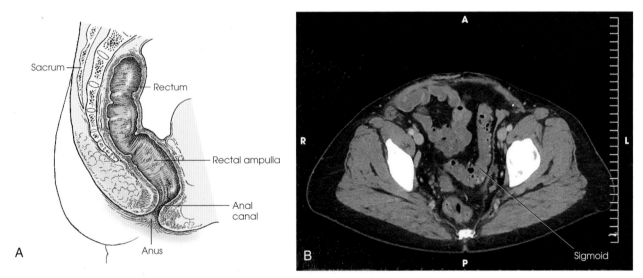

Fig. 15.17 (A) Sagittal section showing direction of anal canal and rectum. (B) Axial CT image of lower pelvis showing rectum and sigmoid colon in relation to surrounding organs.

(B, Courtesy Aimee Rowlett, RT(R)(CT), NEA Baptist Memorial Hospital, Jonesboro, AR.)

Liver and Biliary System

The *liver,* the largest gland in the body, is an irregularly wedge-shaped gland. It is situated with its base on the right and its apex directed anteriorly and to the left (Fig. 15.18). The deepest point of the liver is the inferior aspect just above the right kidney. The diaphragmatic surface of the liver is convex and conforms to the undersurface of the diaphragm. The visceral surface is concave and is molded over the viscera on which it rests. Almost all of the right hypochondrium and a large part of the epigastrium are occupied by the liver. The right portion extends inferiorly into the right lateral region as far as the fourth lumbar vertebra, and the left extremity extends across the left hypochondrium.

At the *falciform ligament,* the liver is divided into a large *right lobe* and a much smaller *left lobe.* Two minor lobes are located on the medial side of the right lobe: the *caudate lobe* on the posterior surface and the *quadrate lobe* on the inferior surface (Fig. 15.19A). The hilum of the liver, called the *porta hepatis,* is situated transversely between the two minor lobes.

The *portal vein* and the *hepatic artery,* both of which convey blood to the liver, enter the porta hepatis and branch out through the liver substance (see Fig. 15.19C). The portal vein ends in the sinusoids, and the hepatic artery ends in capillaries that communicate with sinusoids. In addition to the usual arterial blood supply, the liver receives blood from the portal system.

The portal system, of which the portal vein is the main trunk, consists of the veins arising from the walls of the stomach, from the greater part of the intestinal tract and the gallbladder, and from the pancreas and the spleen. The blood circulating through these organs is rich in nutrients and is carried to the liver for modification before it is returned to the heart. The *hepatic veins* convey the blood from the liver sinusoids to the inferior vena cava.

The liver has numerous physiologic functions. The primary consideration from the radiographic standpoint is the formation of *bile.* The gland secretes bile at the rate of 1 to 3 pints (½ to 1½ L) each day. Bile, the channel of elimination for the waste products of red blood cell destruction, is an excretion and a secretion. As a secretion, it is an important aid in the emulsification and assimilation of fats. The bile is collected from the liver cells by the ducts and is carried to the gallbladder for temporary storage or is poured directly into the duodenum through the common bile duct.

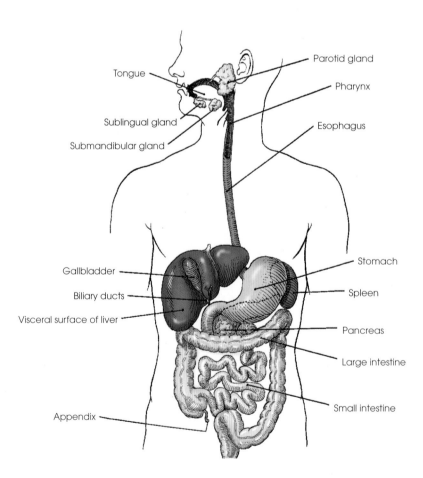

Fig. 15.18 Alimentary tract and accessory organs. To show position of gallbladder in relation to liver, the liver is shown with inferior portion pulled anteriorly and superiorly, placing the liver in an atypical position.

The biliary, or excretory, system of the liver consists of the bile ducts and gallbladder (see Fig. 15.19). Beginning within the lobules as bile capillaries, the ducts unite to form larger and larger passages as they converge, finally forming two main ducts, one leading from each major lobe. The two main *hepatic ducts* emerge at the porta hepatis and join to form the *common hepatic duct,* which unites with the *cystic duct* to form the *common bile duct*. The hepatic and cystic ducts are each about 1½ inches (3.8 cm) long. The common bile duct passes inferiorly for a distance of approximately 3 inches (7.6 cm). The common bile duct joins the pancreatic duct, and they enter together or side by side into an enlarged chamber known as the *hepatopancreatic ampulla,* or *ampulla of Vater*. The ampulla opens into the descending portion of the duodenum. The distal end of the common bile duct is controlled by the *choledochal sphincter* as it enters the duodenum. The hepatopancreatic ampulla is controlled by a circular muscle known as the *sphincter of the hepatopancreatic ampulla,* or *sphincter of Oddi*. During interdigestive periods, the sphincter remains in a contracted state, routing most of the bile into the gallbladder for concentration and temporary storage; during digestion, it relaxes to permit the bile to flow from the liver and gallbladder into the duodenum. The hepatopancreatic ampulla opens on an elevation on the duodenal mucosa known as the *major duodenal papilla*.

A

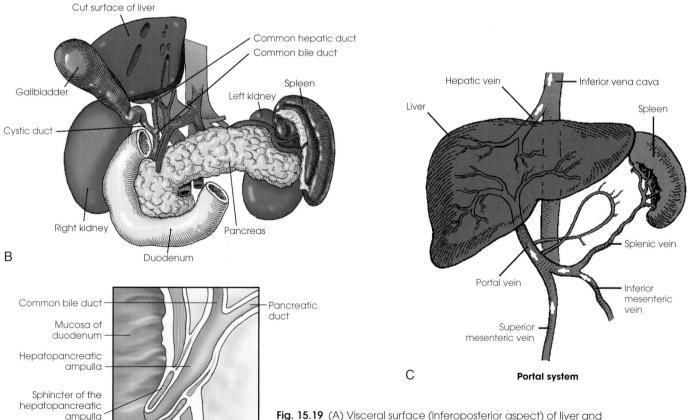

B

C

Portal system

D

Fig. 15.19 (A) Visceral surface (inferoposterior aspect) of liver and gallbladder. (B) Visceral (inferoposterior) surface of gallbladder and bile ducts. (C) Portal system showing hepatic artery and vein and other surrounding vessels. (D) Detail of drainage system into duodenum.

The *gallbladder* is a thin-walled, more or less pear-shaped, musculomembranous sac with a capacity of approximately 2 oz. The gallbladder concentrates bile through absorption of the water content; stores bile during interdigestive periods; and, by contraction of its musculature, evacuates the bile during digestion. The muscular contraction of the gallbladder is activated by a hormone called *cholecystokinin*. This hormone is secreted by the duodenal mucosa and is released into the blood when fatty or acid chyme passes into the intestine. The gallbladder consists of a narrow neck that is continuous with the *cystic duct*; a body or main portion; and a fundus, which is its broad lower portion. The gallbladder is usually lodged in a fossa on the visceral (inferior) surface of the right lobe of the liver, where it lies in an oblique plane inferiorly and anteriorly. Measuring about 1 inch (2.5 cm) in width at its widest part and 3 to 4 inches (7.5 to 10 cm) long, the gallbladder extends from the lower right margin of the porta hepatis to a variable distance below the anterior border of the liver. The position of the gallbladder varies with body habitus; it is high and well away from the midline in hypersthenic persons and low and near the spine in asthenic persons (Fig. 15.20). The gallbladder is sometimes embedded in the liver and frequently hangs free below the inferior margin of the liver.

Pancreas and Spleen

The *pancreas* is an elongated gland situated across the posterior abdominal wall. Extending from the duodenum to the spleen (Fig. 15.21; see Fig. 15.19), the pancreas is about 5½ inches (14 cm) long and consists of a head, neck, body, and tail. The *head,* which is the broadest portion of the organ, extends inferiorly and is enclosed within the curve of the duodenum at the level of the second or third lumbar vertebra. The *body* and *tail* of the pancreas pass transversely behind the stomach and in front of the left kidney, with the narrow tail terminating near the spleen. The pancreas cannot be seen on plain radiographic studies.

The pancreas is an *exocrine* and an *endocrine* gland. The exocrine cells of the pancreas are arranged in lobules with a highly ramified duct system. This exocrine portion of the gland produces *pancreatic juice,* which acts on proteins, fats, and carbohydrates. The endocrine portion of the gland consists of clusters of islet cells, or islets of Langerhans, which are randomly distributed throughout the pancreas. Each islet comprises clusters of cells surrounding small groups of capillaries. These cells produce the hormones *insulin* and *glucagon,* which are responsible for glucose

metabolism. The islet cells do not communicate directly with the ducts but release their secretions directly into the blood through a rich capillary network.

The digestive juice secreted by the exocrine cells of the pancreas is conveyed into the *pancreatic duct* and from there into the duodenum. The pancreatic duct often unites with the common bile duct to form a single passage via the hepatopancreatic ampulla, which opens directly into the descending duodenum.

The *spleen* is included in this section only because of its location; it belongs to the lymphatic system. The spleen is a gland-like but ductless organ that produces lymphocytes and stores and removes dead or dying red blood cells. The spleen is more or less bean-shaped and measures about 5 inches (13 cm) long, 3 inches (7.6 cm) wide, and 1½ inches (3.8 cm) thick. Situated obliquely in the left upper quadrant, the spleen is just below the diaphragm and behind the stomach. It is in contact with the abdominal wall laterally, with the left suprarenal gland and left kidney medially, and with the left colic flexure of the colon inferiorly. The spleen is visualized with and without contrast media.

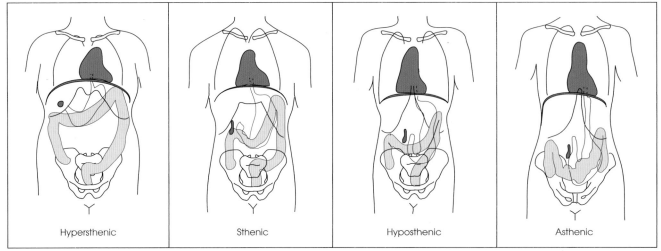

| Hypersthenic | Sthenic | Hyposthenic | Asthenic |

Fig. 15.20 Gallbladder *(green)* position varies with body habitus. Note extreme difference in position of gallbladder between hypersthenic and asthenic habitus. Large intestine is *pink* in these diagrams.

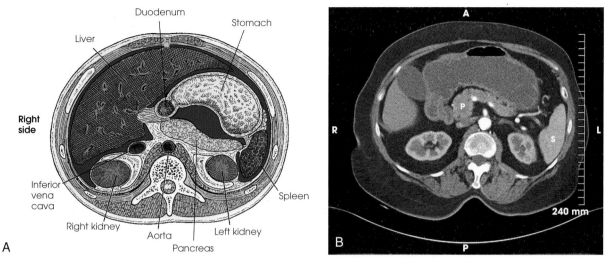

Fig. 15.21 (A) Sectional image of upper abdomen (viewed from the patient's feet upward), showing relationship of digestive system components. (B) Axial CT image of abdomen, demonstrating pancreas *(P)* and the spleen *(S)*.

(Courtesy NEA Baptist Memorial Hospital, Jonesboro, AR.)

ABBREVIATIONS USED IN CHAPTER 15	
BE	Barium enema
CTC	CT colonography
ERCP	Endoscopic retrograde cholangiopancreatography
LES	Lower esophageal sphincter
MBSS	Modified barium swallow study
MPR	Multiplanar reconstruction
TEA	Top of ear attachment
UES	Upper esophageal sphincter
UGI	Upper gastrointestinal
VC	Virtual colonoscopy
VFSS	Videofluoroscopic swallow study

See Addendum B for a summary of all abbreviations used in Volume 2.

SAMPLE EXPOSURE TECHNIQUE CHART ESSENTIAL PROJECTIONS

These techniques were accurate for the equipment used to produce each exposure. However, use caution when applying them in your department because "there is considerable variability in image receptor response owing to varying scatter sensitivity, the use of grids with different grid ratios, collimation, beam filtration, the choice of kilovoltage, source-to-image distance, and image receptor size."[a]

These techniques were accurate for the equipment used to produce each exposure. However, use caution when applying them in your department because generator output characteristics and IR energy sensitivities vary widely.[a]

This chart was created in collaboration with Dennis Bowman, AS, RT(R), Clinical Instructor, Community Hospital of the Monterey Peninsula, Monterey, CA.

http://digitalradiographysolutions.com/

DIGESTIVE SYSTEM, ALIMENTARY CANAL

Part	cm	kVp[b]	SID[c]	Collimation	CR[d] mAs	CR[d] Dose (mGy)[f]	DR[e] mAs	DR[e] Dose (mGy)[f]
Esophagus								
AP and PA[g]	16	120	40″	10″ × 17″ (24 × 43 cm)	8[h]	1.832	4[h]	0.904
Obliques[g]	21	120	40″	10″ × 17″ (24 × 43 cm)	12[h]	3.230	6[h]	1.621
Lateral[g]	30	120	40″	10″ × 17″ (24 × 43 cm)	24[h]	8.230	12[h]	4.085
Stomach and duodenum								
PA and AP[g]	21	120	40″	10″ × 12″ (24 × 30 cm)	10[h]	2.610	5[h]	1.291
PA and AP oblique[g]	24	120	40″	10″ × 12″ (24 × 30 cm)	15[h]	4.495	7.5[h]	2.245
Lateral[g]	27	120	40″	10″ × 12″ (24 × 30 cm)	30[h]	9.770	15[h]	4.860
Small intestine								
PA and AP[g]	21	120	40″	14″ × 17″ (35 × 43 cm)	16[h]	4.320	8[h]	2.160
Large intestine								
PA and AP[g]	21	120	40″	14″ × 17″ (35 × 43 cm)	20[h]	5.420	10[h]	2.700
PA and AP[g] axial	24	120	40″	14″ × 17″ (35 × 43 cm)	32[h]	9.365	16[h]	4.650
PA and AP oblique[g]	24	120	40″	14″ × 17″ (35 × 43 cm)	25[h]	7.310	12.5[h]	3.635
Lower lateral (rectum)[g]	31	120	40″	10″ × 12″ (24 × 30 cm)	60[h]	22.21	30[h]	10.89
AP and PA decubitus (air contrast)[g]	24	120	40″	17″ × 14″ (43 × 35 cm)	25[h]	7.320	12.5[h]	3.640

[a]ACR-AAPM-SIMM Practice Parameters for Digital Radiography, revised 2017.
[b]kVp values are for a high-frequency generator.
[c]40 inches *minimum*; 44 to 48 inches recommended to improve spatial resolution (mAs increase needed, but no increase in patient dose will result).
[d]AGFA CR MD 4.0 General IP, CR 75.0 reader, 400 speed class, with 6:1 (178LPI) grid when needed.
[e]GE Definium 8000, with 13:1 grid when needed.
[f]All doses are skin entrance for average adult (160 to 200 pounds male, 150 to 190 pounds female) at part thickness indicated.
[g]Bucky/Grid.
[h]Large focal spot.

Digestive system
Alimentary canal
Mouth
Pharynx
Esophagus
Stomach
Small intestine
Large intestine (colon)
Anus

Accessory glands
Salivary glands
  Parotid glands
  Parotid ducts
  Submandibular glands
  Submandibular ducts
  Sublingual glands
  Sublingual ducts
Liver
Gallbladder
Pancreas

Mouth
Oral vestibule
Oral cavity
Oropharynx
Hard palate
Soft palate
  Uvula
  Anterior arches
  Posterior arches
  Tonsil
Tongue
  Apex
  Sublingual space
  Frenulum of the
    tongue
  Sublingual fold
  Teeth

Pharynx
Nasopharynx
Soft palate
Hard palate
Uvula
Pharyngeal tonsil
Oropharynx
Hyoid bone
  Laryngeal pharynx

Larynx
Epiglottis
Thyroid cartilage
Piriform recess
Laryngeal cavity
Vestibular folds (false vocal
  cords)
Laryngeal vestibule
Rima glottides
Vocal folds (true vocal
  cords)
  Glottis

Esophagus
Fibrous layer
Muscular layer
Submucosal layer
  Cervical esophagus
  Thoracic esophagus
  Abdominal esophagus
Esophagogastric junction
Cardiac antrum
Cardiac notch

Stomach
Cardia
Fundus
Body
  Rugae
Angular notch

Pyloric portion
  Pyloric antrum
  Pyloric canal
Lesser curvature
Cardiac notch
Greater curvature
Cardiac orifice
Cardiac sphincter
Pyloric orifice
Pyloric sphincter
Chyme

Small intestine
Villi
Duodenum (four regions)
  First (superior)—duodenal
    bulb
  Second (descending)—
    major duodenal papilla
  Third (horizontal)
  Fourth (ascending)—
    duodenojejunal flexure;
    suspensory muscle of
    duodenum
Jejunum
Ileum

Large intestine
Taeniae coli
Haustra
Cecum
Vermiform appendix
Ileocecal valve
Colon
  Ascending colon
  Right colic flexure
  Transverse colon
  Left colic flexure
  Descending colon
  Sigmoid colon

Rectum
  Rectal ampulla
  Anal canal
  Anus

Liver and biliary system
Falciform ligament
Right lobe
Left lobe
Caudate lobe
Quadrate lobe
Porta hepatis
Hepatic artery
Portal vein
Hepatic veins
Hepatic ducts
Common hepatic duct
Cystic duct
Common bile duct
Hepatopancreatic
  ampulla
Sphincter of
  hepatopancreatic
  ampulla
Major duodenal papilla
Gallbladder

Pancreas and spleen
Pancreas
  Head
  Body
  Tail
Exocrine gland
  Pancreatic juice
Endocrine gland
  Islet cells
Pancreatic duct
Spleen

SUMMARY OF PATHOLOGY

Condition	Definition
Achalasia	Failure of smooth muscle of alimentary canal to relax
Appendicitis	Inflammation of the appendix
Barrett esophagus	Peptic ulcer of lower esophagus, often with stricture
Bezoar	Mass in the stomach formed by material that does not pass into the intestine
Biliary stenosis	Narrowing of bile ducts
Calculus	Abnormal concretion of mineral salts, often called a *stone*
Carcinoma	Malignant new growth composed of epithelial cells
Celiac disease or sprue	Malabsorption disease caused by mucosal defect in the jejunum
Cholecystitis	Acute or chronic inflammation of gallbladder
Choledocholithiasis	Calculus in common bile duct
Cholelithiasis	Presence of gallstones
Colitis	Inflammation of the colon
Diverticulitis	Inflammation of diverticula in the alimentary canal
Diverticulosis	Diverticula in the colon without inflammation or symptoms
Diverticulum	Pouch created by herniation of the mucous membrane through the muscular coat
Esophageal varices	Enlarged tortuous veins of lower esophagus, resulting from portal hypertension
Fistula	Abnormal connection between two internal organs or between an organ and the body surface
Foreign body	Foreign material in the airway
Gastritis	Inflammation of lining of stomach
Gastroesophageal reflux	Backward flow of stomach contents into the esophagus
Hiatal hernia	Protrusion of the stomach through the esophageal hiatus of the diaphragm

SUMMARY OF PATHOLOGY—cont'd

Condition	Definition
Hirschsprung disease or congenital aganglionic megacolon	Absence of parasympathetic ganglia, usually in the distal colon, resulting in the absence of peristalsis
Ileus	Failure of bowel peristalsis
Inguinal hernia	Protrusion of the bowel into the groin
Intussusception	Prolapse of a portion of the bowel into the lumen of an adjacent part
Malabsorption syndrome	Disorder in which subnormal absorption of dietary constituents occurs
Meckel diverticulum	Diverticulum of the distal ileum, similar to the appendix
Pancreatic pseudocyst	Collection of debris, fluid, pancreatic enzymes, and blood as a complication of acute pancreatitis
Pancreatitis	Acute or chronic inflammation of the pancreas
Polyp	Growth or mass protruding from a mucous membrane
Pyloric stenosis	Narrowing of pyloric canal causing obstruction
Regional enteritis or Crohn disease	Inflammatory bowel disease, most commonly involving the distal ileum
Salivary duct obstruction	Condition that prevents passage of saliva through the duct
Stenosis	Narrowing or contraction of a passage
Tumor	New tissue growth where cell proliferation is uncontrolled
Ulcer	Depressed lesion on the surface of the alimentary canal
Ulcerative colitis	Recurrent disorder causing inflammatory ulceration in the colon
Volvulus	Twisting of a bowel loop on itself
Zenker diverticulum	Diverticulum located just above the cardiac portion of the stomach

Eponymous (named) pathologies are listed in nonpossessive form to conform to the *AMA manual of style: a guide for authors and editors.* ed 10, Oxford: Oxford University Press; 2009.

Sialography

Sialography is the term applied to radiologic examination of the salivary glands and ducts with the use of a contrast material, usually one of the water-soluble iodinated media. Because of improvements in computed tomography (CT) and magnetic resonance imaging (MRI) techniques, sialography is rarely performed. When the presence of a salivary stone or lesion is suspected, CT or MRI is often the modality of choice. Sialography remains a viable tool, however, when a definitive diagnosis is necessary for a problem related to one of the salivary ducts.[1]

Sialography is used to show such conditions as inflammatory lesions and tumors; to determine the extent of salivary fistulae; and to localize diverticula, strictures, and calculi. Because the glands are paired and the pairs are in such close proximity, only one gland at a time can be examined by the sialographic method (Fig. 15.22).

Sialography is performed as follows:

- Inject the radiopaque medium into the main duct. From there, the contrast material flows into the intraglandular ductules, making it possible to show the surrounding glandular parenchyma and the duct system (Fig. 15.23).
- Obtain preliminary images to detect any condition demonstrable without the use of a contrast medium and to establish the optimal exposure technique.
- About 2 or 3 minutes before the sialographic procedure, give the patient a secretory stimulant to open the duct and its orifice for easier passage of a cannula or catheter. For this purpose, have the patient suck on a wedge of fresh lemon. After the examination, have the patient suck on another lemon wedge to stimulate rapid evacuation of the contrast medium.
- Take an image about 10 minutes after the procedure to verify clearance of the contrast medium, if necessary.

Most physicians inject the contrast medium by manual pressure (i.e., with a syringe attached to the cannula or catheter). Other physicians advocate delivery of the medium by hydrostatic pressure only. The latter method requires the use of a water-soluble iodinated medium, with the contrast solution container (usually a syringe barrel with the plunger removed) attached to a drip stand set at a distance of 28 inches (70 cm) above the level of the patient's mouth. The filling procedure is often performed under fluoroscopic guidance with spot images obtained at various intervals.

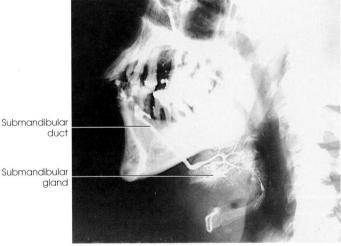

Submandibular duct

Submandibular gland

Fig. 15.22 Sialogram showing opacified submandibular gland.

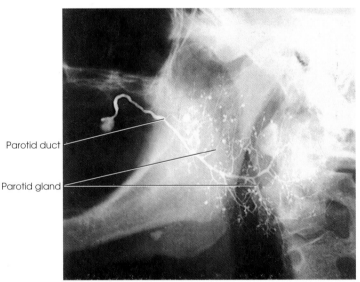

Parotid duct

Parotid gland

Fig. 15.23 Sialogram showing parotid gland in a patient without teeth.

TANGENTIAL PROJECTION

Image receptor: Positioned by manufacturer or department protocol for proper anatomy display orientation; CR plate: 10 × 12 inches (24 × 30 cm) lengthwise.

Position of patient
- Place the patient in a recumbent or a seated position.
- Because the parotid gland lies midway between the anterior and posterior surfaces of the skull, obtain the tangential projection of the glandular region from the posterior or the anterior direction.

Position of part

Supine body position
- With the patient supine, rotate the head slightly toward the side being examined so that the parotid area is perpendicular to the plane of the IR.
- Center the IR to the parotid area.
- With the patient's head resting on the occiput, adjust the head so that the mandibular ramus is parallel with the longitudinal axis of the IR (Fig. 15.24).

Prone body position
- With the patient prone, rotate the head so that the parotid area being examined is perpendicular to the plane of the IR.
- Center the IR to the parotid region.
- With the patient's head resting on the chin, adjust the flexion of the head so that the mandibular ramus is parallel with the longitudinal axis of the IR (Fig. 15.25).
- When the parotid (Stensen) duct does not have to be shown, rest the patient's head on the forehead and nose.
- *Shield gonads.*
- *Respiration:* Improved radiographic quality can be obtained, particularly to show calculi, by having the patient fill the mouth with air and then puff the cheeks out as much as possible. When this cannot be done, ask the patient to suspend respiration for the exposure.

Fig. 15.24 Tangential parotid gland, supine position.

Fig. 15.25 Tangential parotid gland, prone position.

Central ray

- Perpendicular to the plane of the IR, directed along the lateral surface of the mandibular ramus.

Collimation

- Adjust the radiation field to 1 inch (2.5 cm) beyond the skin shadow, superiorly to the top of ear attachment (TEA), and inferiorly below the mandible.

Structures shown

Contrast-filled parotid duct and gland and calcific deposits or swelling (if present) (Figs. 15.26 and 15.27).

The following should be clearly seen:

- Evidence of proper collimation and presence of side marker placed clear of anatomy of interest
- Contrast medium and glandular soft tissue
- Most of the parotid gland lateral to and clear of the mandibular ramus
- Mastoid overlapping only the upper portion of the parotid gland

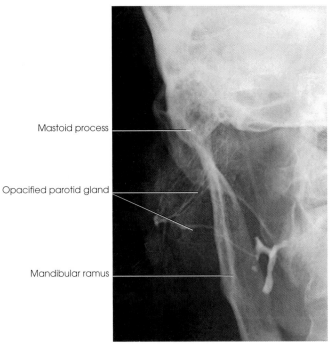

Mastoid process

Opacified parotid gland

Mandibular ramus

Fig. 15.26 Tangential parotid gland showing opacification.

Fig. 15.27 Tangential parotid gland showing opacification.

Digestive System: Salivary Glands, Alimentary Canal, and Biliary System

LATERAL PROJECTION
Right or left position

Image receptor + grid: Positioned by manufacturer or department protocol for proper anatomy display orientation; CR plate: 10 × 12 inches (24 × 30 cm) lengthwise.

Position of patient
- Place the patient in a semiprone or seated and upright position.

Position of part
Parotid gland
- With the affected side closest to the IR, extend the patient's neck so that the space between the cervical area of the spine and the mandibular rami is cleared.
- Center the IR to a point approximately 1 inch (2.5 cm) superior to the mandibular angle.
- Adjust the head so that the MSP plane is rotated approximately 15 degrees toward the IR from a true lateral position.

Submandibular gland
- Center the IR to the inferior margin of the angle of the mandible.
- Adjust the patient's head in a true lateral position (Fig. 15.28).
- An axiolateral or axiolateral oblique projection may also be performed. See Chapter 11 for positioning details.

- Iglauer[2] suggested depressing the floor of the mouth to displace the submandibular gland below the mandible. When the patient's throat is not too sensitive, accomplish this by having the patient place an index finger on the back of the tongue on the affected side.
- *Shield gonads.*
- *Respiration:* suspend.

Central ray
- Perpendicular to the center of the IR and directed (1) at a point 1 inch (2.5 cm) superior to the mandibular angle to show the parotid gland or (2) at the inferior margin of the mandibular angle to show the submandibular gland.

Collimation
- Adjust the radiation field to 1 inch (2.5 cm) beyond the anterior and inferior skin shadows and to MCP posteriorly.

Fig. 15.28 Lateral submandibular gland.

Fig. 15.29 Lateral parotid gland showing opacified gland and parotid duct *(arrow)*.

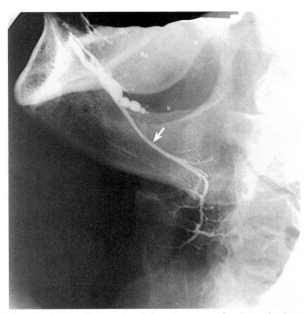

Fig. 15.30 Axiolateral submandibular gland showing opacification of submandibular duct *(arrow)*.

Structures shown

Contrast-filled parotid duct and gland (Fig. 15.29), submandibular duct and gland (Fig. 15.30), surrounding bony and soft tissues, and calcific deposits or swelling (if present).

EVALUATION CRITERIA

The following should be clearly seen:

- Evidence of proper collimation and presence of side marker placed clear of anatomy of interest
- Mandibular rami free of overlap from the cervical vertebrae to show best the parotid gland superimposed over the ramus
- Superimposed mandibular rami and angles, if no tube angulation or head rotation is used for the submandibular gland
- Oblique position for the parotid gland
- Submandibular gland shown without superimposition of contralateral mandibular ramus, on axiolateral projections
- Contrast medium and glandular soft tissue

Modified Barium Swallow Study

One of the most common imaging procedures of the soft palate, pharynx, and larynx is the *x-ray modified barium swallow,* which is listed in the ARRT Radiography Examination Content Specifications[3] as Swallowing Dysfunction Study. This procedure is defined by the American College of Radiology (ACR) as the "videofluoroscopic procedure performed in conjunction with a speech therapist."[4] The technical term used by the American Speech-Language-Hearing Association is *videofluoroscopic swallow study* (VFSS). Fluoroscopy is the modality of choice to demonstrate both the structure and function of the complex anatomy of deglutition and evaluate the presence of any abnormalities, especially those that allow aspiration.

Deglutition

The act of swallowing is performed by the rapid and highly coordinated action of many muscles. The following points are important in radiography of the pharynx and upper esophagus:

- The middle area of the tongue becomes depressed to collect the mass, or bolus, of material to be swallowed.
- The base of the tongue forms a central groove to accommodate the bolus and then moves superiorly and inferiorly along the roof of the mouth to propel the bolus into the pharynx.
- Simultaneously with the posterior thrust of the tongue, the larynx moves anteriorly and superiorly under the root of the tongue, the sphincteric folds nearly closing the laryngeal inlet (orifice).
- The epiglottis divides the passing bolus and drains the two portions laterally into the piriform recesses as it lowers over the laryngeal entrance.

Technical considerations

Imaging and recording of deglutition must occur at 30 frames per second (fps). The fluoroscopic examination may be performed in the department using stationary equipment or in a room equipped with a mobile C-arm. A specialized patient chair is also used to facilitate consistent, safe, and comfortable upright position during imaging (Fig. 15.31). Barium sulfate is the standard contrast agent used for VFSS.

Fig. 15.31 Fluoroscopy room with patient positioning chair set up for modified barium swallow study.

Team Members

The modified barium swallow study (MBSS) requires a coordinated team effort. The speech therapist, radiologic technologist, and radiologist have a role in providing optimum patient care while obtaining a diagnostic study. While the duties of each team member may vary slightly, the general responsibilities for each member are outlined below.

Radiologic technologist

- Prepares the room for the procedure.
- Accompanies patient into the imaging suite.
- Prepares the patient for the procedure by providing a general explanation, removing potential artifacts, provides a gown, if needed.
- Notifies the other team members of the patient's arrival to imaging.
- Assists the patient into the procedure chair or onto the footboard of the upright table.
- Shields patient appropriately.
- Obtains scout image, most commonly a lateral soft tissue neck.

- Moves the fluoroscopy tower into position, while explaining the equipment to the patient.
- In states where allowed, the technologist also operates the fluoroscopy, records the images, and marks each contrast sequence correctly.
- Transfers the recorded images to PACS to allow the speech therapist to review with the patient and the radiologist to dictate the report.
- Prepares the patient for dismissal.
- Assists with cleaning the room.

Speech therapist

- Prepares contrast media, typically a thin and a thick barium, a semi-solid barium (often labeled as "pudding"), barium on a solid, such as a cracker, and barium mixed into a carbonated beverage (Fig. 15.32).
- Administers the contrast medium, in various consistencies, quantities, and using different mechanisms, such as a spoon, cup, and straw.

- Provides the patient specific swallowing instructions.
- Adjusts the patient's head position, such as the "chin tuck" position to evaluate if this position improves the effective seal of the epiglottis over the trachea.
- Consults with radiologist during procedure, particularly when aspiration is present, to adjust the protocol for an accurate assessment and diagnosis.
- Reviews the study with the patient after the procedure is concluded and provides instructions and/or further therapy.
- Assists in cleaning the room after the patient leaves.

Radiologist

- May operate fluoroscopy and perform image recording.
- Observe and comment on findings while viewing the procedure in real time from the control panel monitor.
- Dictates results of the exam for the patient's medical record.

Fig. 15.32 Contrast set up for MBSS. Barium sulfate in various consistencies, a carbonated beverage, and crackers for the solid food swallow test.

Fig. 15.33 Patient positioned for lateral images during MBSS.

⚕ LATERAL PROJECTION
Right or left position

The lateral is often the only projection obtained during an MBSS. The AP may be added based upon information obtained during fluoroscopy of the patient in the lateral position.

Image receptor: Positioned by manufacturer or department protocol for proper anatomy display orientation; CR plate: 10 × 12 inches (24 × 30 cm) lengthwise.

Position of patient
- Seated (or standing) in a true lateral position with MCP perpendicular to the IR.
- Depress the shoulders as much as possible, and adjust them to lie in the same transverse plane.

Position of part
- Assist the speech therapist in adjusting the patient's head into a lateral position.
- Immobilize the head by having the patient look at an object in line with the visual axis. Speech therapist usually dictates the exact alignment of the chin (Fig. 15.33).
- *Shield gonads.*

Central ray
- Perpendicular to the IR.

Collimation
- Adjust the radiation field to the level of the EAM to the jugular notch; include all anterior oropharyngeal structures and the cervical vertebrae posteriorly. Place side marker in the collimated exposure field.

Structures shown

Profile images of the contrast-filled mouth, pharynx, and cervical esophagus in recorded videofluoroscopic images. Proper functioning of the epiglottis during deglutition is best seen in the lateral projection (Fig. 15.34).

EVALUATION CRITERIA

The following should be clearly seen:
- Evidence of proper collimation and presence of side marker placed clear of anatomy of interest
- All soft tissue pharyngolaryngeal structures
- Area from nasopharynx to the uppermost part of the lungs in preliminary studies
- No superimposition of the trachea by the shoulders
- Closely superimposed mandibular shadows

Fig. 15.34 Lateral images from modified barium swallow study. (A) Epiglottis, dotted outline. Thin barium seen on superior surface of epiglottis. (B) Same patient, later in swallowing process. All barium is inferior to epiglottis and in upper esophagus. Normal study. (C) Abnormal study. Epiglottis is curled up, and barium penetrates the upper airway. Chin tuck position performed later in this study and corrected the aspiration.

�֍ AP PROJECTION

MBBS often only utilize the lateral projection. The need for the AP is often determined by specifics in the patient's history or evidence found during lateral imaging.

Position of patient

- Upright position, seated in the procedure chair or standing on the footboard of an upright table.
- If the standing position is used, have the patient distribute the weight of the body equally on the feet.

Position of part

- Center the MSP of the body to the midline of the vertical grid device.
- Adjust the patient's shoulders to lie in the same horizontal plane to prevent rotation of the head and neck and resultant obliquity of the throat structures.
- Center the IR at the level of or just below the laryngeal prominence.
- Assist the speech therapist in the specific head position needed to evaluate deglutition (Fig. 15.35).
- *Shield gonads.*

Central ray

- Perpendicular to the laryngeal prominence.

Collimation

- Adjust the radiation field to the level of the EAM to the jugular notch and 1 inch (2.5 cm) beyond the skin edges on the sides. Place side marker in the collimated exposure field.

Fig. 15.35 Patient positioned for AP images during MBSS.

Structures shown

- Contrast-filled mouth, pharynx, and cervical esophagus in recorded video-fluoroscopic images. Evaluation of unilateral abnormalities are evaluated in the AP projections (Fig. 15.36).

The following should be clearly seen:

- Evidence of proper collimation and presence of side marker placed clear of anatomy of interest
- All soft tissue pharyngolaryngeal structures
- Area from nasopharynx to the uppermost part of the lungs without rotation

Barium retained in esophageal diverticulum (Zenker type)
Barium in upper esophagus

Fig. 15.36 AP images from modified barium swallow study. (A) Early swallow image shows barium retained in Zenker diverticulum and some barium flowing into esophagus. (B) Several swallows later, barium still retained in diverticulum.

Technical Considerations

GASTROINTESTINAL TRANSIT

Peristalsis is the term applied to the contraction waves by which the digestive tube propels its contents toward the rectum. Normally three or four waves per minute occur in the filled stomach. The waves begin in the upper part of the organ and travel toward the pylorus. The average emptying time of a normal stomach is 2 to 3 hours.

Peristaltic action in the intestines is greatest in the upper part of the canal and gradually decreases toward the lower portion. In addition to peristaltic waves, localized contractions occur in the duodenum and the jejunum. These contractions usually occur at intervals of 3 to 4 seconds during digestion. The first part of a "barium meal" normally reaches the ileocecal valve in 2 to 3 hours, and the last portion reaches the ileocecal valve in 4 to 5 hours. The barium usually reaches the rectum within 24 hours.

The specialized procedures commonly used in radiologic examinations of the esophagus, stomach, and intestines are presented in this section. The esophagus connects the pharynx and the stomach and is located in the posterior part of the mediastinum; thus positioning the patient for demonstration of the contrast-filled esophagus is fairly simple, due to its consistent anatomic location. The stomach and intestines vary in size, shape, position, and muscular tonus according to the body habitus (see Fig. 15.14 and 15.20). In addition to normal structural and functional differences, various gastrointestinal abnormalities can cause further changes in location and motility. These variations make the gastrointestinal investigation of every patient an individual study, and meticulous attention must be given to each detail of the examination procedure.

EXAMINATION PROCEDURE

The alimentary canal is typically imaged using only fluoroscopy. The radiographic projections are included in this chapter for student use as these positions are recorded during the fluoroscopic examination. The radiographer is responsible for:

- Preparing the room, equipment, and contrast media prior to the patient's arrival.
- Readying the patient for the procedure, that is, artifact removal, gowning, explanation of procedure.
- Obtaining and recording a thorough history.
- Obtaining a scout image of the anatomy of interest.
- Communicating with and assisting the patient before and after contrast administration.
- Assisting the fluoroscopist during the procedure, as needed.

If radiographic images are requested after the fluoroscopy examination, these images are also the responsibility of the radiographer. Radiographers must be proficient in recognizing the pertinent anatomy shown in each position and projection to provide proper patient assistance in fluoroscopy-only procedures and to obtain accurate radiographic images when requested.

Contrast media

Because the thin-walled alimentary canal does not have sufficient density to be shown through the surrounding structures, demonstration of it on radiographic images requires the use of an artificial contrast medium. *Barium sulfate,* which is a water-insoluble salt of the metallic element barium, is the contrast medium universally used in examinations of the alimentary canal (Fig. 15.37). The barium sulfate used for this purpose is a specially prepared, chemically pure product to which various chemical substances have been added. Barium sulfate is available as a dry powder or as a liquid. The powdered barium has different concentrations and is mixed with plain water. The concentration depends on the part to be examined and the preference of the physician.

Many special barium sulfate products are also available. Products with finely divided barium sulfate particles tend to resist precipitation and remain in suspension longer than regular barium preparations. Some barium preparations contain gums or other suspending or dispersing agents and are referred to as *suspended* or *flocculation-resistant* preparations. The speed with which the barium mixture passes through the alimentary canal depends on the suspending medium, the temperature of the medium, the consistency of the preparation, and the motile function of the alimentary canal.

In addition to barium sulfate, *water-soluble, iodinated contrast media* suitable for opacification of the alimentary canal are available (Fig. 15.38). These preparations are modifications of basic IV urographic media, such as diatrizoate sodium and diatrizoate meglumine.

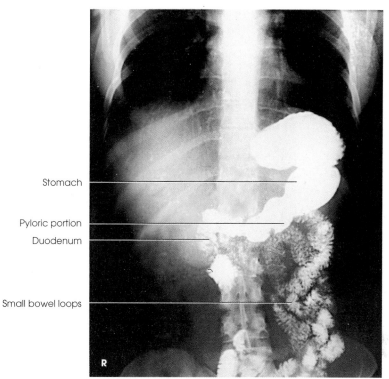

Stomach

Pyloric portion

Duodenum

Small bowel loops

Fig. 15.37 Barium sulfate suspension in stomach, sthenic body habitus.

Fig. 15.38 Water-soluble, iodinated solution in stomach.

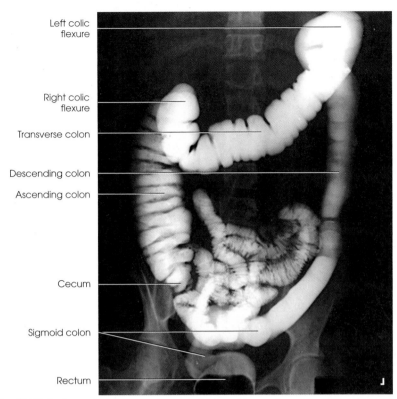

Left colic flexure

Right colic flexure

Transverse colon

Descending colon

Ascending colon

Cecum

Sigmoid colon

Rectum

Fig. 15.39 Barium sulfate suspension administered by rectum, sthenic body habitus.

Fig. 15.40 Water-soluble, iodinated solution administered by mouth.

Iodinated solutions move through the gastrointestinal tract quicker than barium sulfate suspensions (Figs. 15.39 and 15.40). An iodinated solution normally clears the stomach in 1 to 2 hours, and the entire iodinated contrast column reaches and outlines the colon in about 4 hours. An orally administered iodinated medium differs from barium sulfate in the following ways:

1. It outlines the esophagus, but it does not adhere to the mucosa as well as a barium sulfate suspension does.
2. It affords an entirely satisfactory examination of the stomach and duodenum including mucosal delineation.
3. It permits a rapid survey of the entire small intestine but fails to provide clear anatomic detail of this portion of the alimentary canal. This failure results from dilution of the contrast medium and the resultant decrease in opacification.
4. Because of the normal rapid absorption of water through the colonic mucosa, the medium again becomes densely concentrated in the large intestine. As a result of its increased concentration and accelerated transit time, rapid investigation of the large intestine can be performed by the oral route when a patient cannot cooperate for a satisfactory enema study.

A great advantage of water-soluble media is that they are easily removed by aspiration before or during surgery. If a water-soluble, iodinated medium escapes into the peritoneum through a preexisting perforation of the stomach or intestine, no ill effects result. The medium is readily absorbed from the peritoneal cavity and excreted by the kidneys. This provides a definite advantage when perforated ulcers are being investigated.

A disadvantage of iodinated preparations is their strongly bitter taste, which can be masked only to a limited extent. Patients should be forewarned so that they can more easily tolerate ingestion of these agents. In addition, these iodinated contrast media are hyperosmolar, encouraging movement of excess fluid into the gastrointestinal tract lumen.

Radiologic apparatus

Fluoroscopic equipment provides real-time images and recording simultaneously. Remote control fluoroscopic rooms are also available and are used by the fluoroscopist in an adjacent control area (Fig. 15.41). Recorded images and video are available for immediate viewing after the procedure at appropriate workstations.

Compression and palpation of the abdomen are often performed during an examination of the alimentary canal. Many types of compression devices are available. The fluoroscopic unit shown in Fig. 15.42 shows a compression cone in contact with the patient's abdomen. This device is often used during general fluoroscopic examinations.

Other types of commercial compression devices include the pneumatic compression paddle and the F-spoon shown in Fig. 15.43. The compression paddle is often placed under the duodenal bulb or terminal ileum and inflated to place pressure on the abdomen. The balloon region is usually surrounded by a radiopaque ring. The F-spoon is used for the same purpose, but the compression end is completely radiolucent.

Fig. 15.41 Remote control fluoroscopic room, showing patient fluoroscopic table *(background)* and fluoroscopist's control console *(foreground)*. The fluoroscopist views the patient through the large window.

Fig. 15.42 Compression cone in contact with abdomen for fluoroscopy examination.

Fig. 15.43 (A) Compression paddle: inflated *(above)* and noninflated *(below)*; (B) F-spoon; (C) F-spoon with lead glove in position.

Preparation of examining room

The examining room should be completely prepared before the patient enters. In preparing the room, the radiographer should do the following:

- Adjust equipment controls to the appropriate settings.
- Have the footboard and shoulder support available.
- Check for proper operation of the imaging and recording devices.
- Prepare the required type and amount of contrast medium.
- Make appropriate image markers available.

Before beginning the examination, the radiographer must communicate with the patient in the following ways:

- Explain the type and administration route of the contrast media.
  - Use lay terminology, such as "drinking" for orally administered agents.
  - Explain the taste and texture of the contrast agent, such as "chalky and thick" for barium and "bitter" for iodinated agents.
  - For an enema examination, show the tube tip and explain insertion and the potential abdominal sensations that often accompany the flow of contrast into the colon.
- Point out that the lights are dimmed in the room during fluoroscopy, and explain the need for a darkened room during the procedure.

- The fluoroscopist will instruct the patient to move into certain positions and will provide breathing instructions. Assure the patient that you will assist, as needed.
  - If radiographic images are obtained post fluoroscopy, inform the patient of the approximate number of images you will be obtaining when the fluoroscopist leaves the room.
- After you have verified that the patient understands the overall procedure, introduce the patient and the fluoroscopist to each other when the fluoroscopist enters the examining room.

Exposure time

One of the most important considerations in gastrointestinal radiography is the elimination of motion. The highest degree of motor activity is normally found in the stomach and proximal part of the small intestine. Activity gradually decreases along the intestinal tract with the slowest in the distal large bowel. Peristaltic speed also depends on the individual patient's body habitus and is influenced by pathologic changes, use of narcotic pain medication, body position, and respiration. The amount of exposure time for each region must be based on these factors.

In esophageal examinations, the radiographer should observe the following guidelines, if obtaining radiographic images post fluoroscopy:

- Use an exposure time of 0.1 second or less for upright images. The time may be slightly longer for recumbent images because the barium descends more slowly when patients are in a recumbent position.
- Barium passes through the esophagus fairly slowly if it is swallowed at the end of full inspiration. The rate of passage is increased if the barium is swallowed at the end of moderate inspiration. The barium is delayed in the lower part for several seconds, however, if it is swallowed at the end of full expiration.
- Respiration is inhibited for several seconds after the beginning of deglutition, which allows sufficient time for the exposure to be made without the need to instruct the patient to hold his or her breath after swallowing.

In examinations of the stomach and small intestine, the radiographer should observe the following guidelines:

- Use an exposure time no longer than 0.2 second for patients with normal peristaltic activity and never longer than 0.5 second; exposure time should be 0.1 second or less for patients with hypermotility.
- Make exposures of the stomach and intestines at the end of expiration in the routine procedure.

Fig. 15.44 (A) AP spot image of barium-filled fundus of stomach. (B) Spot image of air-contrast colon, showing left colic flexure.

Radiation Protection

The patient receives radiation during fluoroscopy, while the procedure is recorded and images obtained (Fig. 15.44). When radiographic images are a required part of a partial or complete gastrointestinal examination, even more radiation is delivered to the patient. It is taken for granted that properly added filtration is in place at all times in each x-ray tube in the radiology department. It is further assumed that based on the capacity of the machines and the best available accessory equipment, exposure factors are adjusted to deliver the least possible radiation to the patient.

Protection of the patient from unnecessary radiation is a professional responsibility of the radiographer. (See Chapter 1 in Volume 1 of this atlas for specific guidelines.) In this chapter, the *Shield gonads* statement at the end of the *Position of part* section indicates that the patient is to be protected from unnecessary radiation by *restricting the radiation beam using proper collimation to include the primary anatomy of interest*. Placing lead shielding between the gonads and the radiation source when the clinical objectives of the examination are not compromised is also appropriate.

Esophagus
CONTRAST MEDIA STUDIES

The esophagus may be examined by performing a *full-column, single-contrast* study in which only barium or water-soluble, iodinated contrast agent is used to fill the esophageal lumen. A *double-contrast* procedure also may be used. For this study, high-density barium and carbon dioxide crystals (which liberate carbon dioxide when exposed to water) are the two contrast agents. No preliminary preparation of the patient is necessary. These contrast media procedures show intrinsic lesions and extrinsic pathology impressing on the esophagus. Anatomic structures normally indenting the esophagus must be appreciated to identify pathology. Normally indenting structures include the aortic arch, left main stem bronchus, and left atrium (Fig. 15.45).

Barium sulfate mixture

The ACR Practice Parameter (Resolution 29, 2013) recommends using a low-density (60% weight/volume) barium suspension for the single-contrast technique. A high-density barium (210% to 250% weight/volume) is recommended for double-contrast esophageal and gastric examinations.[5] Most barium suspensions are readily available in premixed liquid form, thus providing greater consistency than adding water to a powdered form. Whatever the weight/volume concentration of the barium, the most important criterion is that the barium flows sufficiently to coat the mucosal lining of the upper gastrointestinal (UGI) tract.

Fig. 15.45 Esophagogram images showing luminal indentations from adjacent anatomy. Normally indented structures include aortic arch (*A*), left main stem bronchus (*B*), and left atrium (*C*).

Examination procedures

For a single-contrast examination (Figs. 15.46 through 15.48), the following steps are taken:

- Start the fluoroscopic and spot-image examinations with the patient in the upright position when possible.

- Use the horizontal and Trendelenburg positions as indicated.
- After the fluoroscopic examination of the heart and lungs and when the patient is upright, instruct the patient to take the cup containing the barium suspension into the left hand and to drink it on request.

The radiologist asks the patient to swallow several mouthfuls of the barium so that the act of deglutition can be observed to determine whether any abnormality is present. The radiologist instructs the patient to perform various breathing maneuvers under fluoroscopic observation so that spot images of areas or lesions not otherwise shown can be obtained.

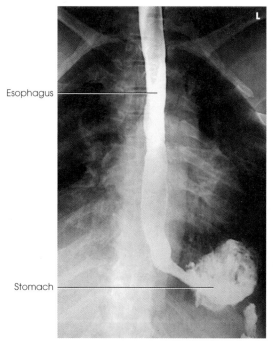

Fig. 15.46 AP esophagus, single-contrast study.

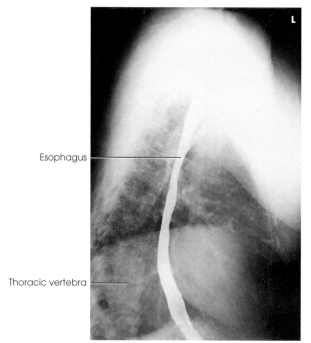

Fig. 15.47 Lateral esophagus, single-contrast study.

Performance of a *double-contrast* esophageal examination (Fig. 15.49) is similar to that of a single-contrast examination. For a double-contrast examination, free-flowing, high-density barium must be used. A gas-producing substance, usually carbon dioxide crystals, can be added to the barium mixture or given by mouth immediately *before* the barium suspension is ingested. Spot images are taken during the examination, and delayed images may be obtained on request.

OPAQUE FOREIGN BODIES

Opaque foreign bodies lodged in the pharynx or in the upper part of the esophagus can usually be shown without the use of a contrast medium. A soft tissue neck or lateral projection of the retrosternal area may be taken for this purpose. A lateral neck image should be obtained at the height of swallowing for the delineation of opaque foreign bodies in the upper end of the intrathoracic esophagus. Swallowing elevates the intrathoracic esophagus a distance of two cervical segments, placing it above the level of the clavicles.

Tufts or pledgets of cotton saturated with a thin barium suspension are sometimes used to show an obstruction or to detect *nonopaque foreign bodies* in the pharynx and upper esophagus (Fig. 15.50).[6]

Fig. 15.48 PA oblique esophagus, RAO position, single-contrast study.

Fig. 15.49 PA oblique distal esophagus, RAO position, double-contrast spot image.

Fig. 15.50 Barium-soaked cotton ball showing nonopaque foreign body in upper esophagus (*arrow*).

AP, PA, OBLIQUE, AND LATERAL PROJECTIONS

Image receptor + grid: Positioned by manufacturer or department protocol for proper anatomy display orientation; CR plate: 14 × 17 inches (35 × 43 cm) lengthwise.

Position of patient

- Position the patient as for chest images (AP, PA, oblique, and lateral; see Chapter 3, Volume 1). Because the RAO position of 35 to 40 degrees (Fig. 15.51) makes it possible to obtain a wider space for an unobstructed image of the esophagus between the vertebrae and the heart, it is usually used in preference to the LAO position. The LPO position has also been recommended.[7]
- Unless the upright position is specified, place the patient in the recumbent position for esophageal studies. The recumbent position is used to obtain more complete contrast filling of the esophagus (especially filling of the proximal part) by having the barium column flow against gravity. The recumbent position is routinely used to show variceal distentions of the esophageal veins because varices are best filled by having the blood flow against gravity. Variceal filling is more complete during increased venous pressure, which may be applied by full expiration or by the Valsalva maneuver.

AP OR PA PROJECTION

The following steps are taken:
- Place the patient in the supine or prone position with the arms above the head in a comfortable position.
- Center the MSP to the grid.
- Turn the head slightly, if necessary, to assist drinking of the barium mixture.
- *Shield gonads.*

AP OR PA OBLIQUE PROJECTION
RAO or LPO position

The steps are as follows:
- Position the patient in the RAO or LPO position with the MSP forming an angle of 35 to 40 degrees from the grid device.
- For the RAO position, adjust the patient's side-down arm at the side and the side-up arm on the pillow by the head. For the LPO position, do the same, with the side-down arm at the side and the side-up arm on the pillow.
- Center the elevated side to the grid through a plane approximately 2 inches (5 cm) lateral to the MSP.
- *Shield gonads.*

LATERAL PROJECTION
Right or left position

The steps are as follows:
- Place the patient's arms forward, with the forearm on the pillow near the head.

- Position the midcoronal plane to the center of the grid.
- *Shield gonads.*

Central ray

- Perpendicular to the midpoint of the IR (the central ray is at the level of T5-T6).

Collimation

- Adjust the radiation field to no larger than 12 × 17 inches (30 × 43 cm). Place side marker in the collimated exposure field.

Structures shown

Contrast-filled esophagus from the lower neck to the esophagogastric junction (Fig. 15.52).

EVALUATION CRITERIA

The following should be clearly seen:

General

- Evidence of proper collimation and presence of side marker placed clear of anatomy of interest
- Esophagus from the lower part of the neck to its entrance into the stomach
- Esophagus filled with barium
- Penetration of the barium

Fig. 15.52 (A) PA oblique esophagus, RAO position. (B) AP oblique esophagus, LPO position.

Fig. 15.51 PA oblique esophagus, RAO position.

AP or PA projection (see Fig. 15.46)
■ Esophagus through the superimposed thoracic vertebrae
■ No rotation of the patient

Oblique projection (see Fig. 15.52)
■ Esophagus between the vertebrae and the heart

Lateral projection (see Fig. 15.47)
■ Proximal esophagus without superimposition of the patient's arm
■ Ribs posterior to the vertebrae superimposed to show that the patient was not rotated

NOTE: The general criteria apply to all projections: AP or PA, oblique, and lateral.

Barium administration and respiration
• Feed the barium sulfate suspension to the patient by spoon, by cup, or through a drinking straw, depending on its consistency.
• Ask the patient to swallow several mouthfuls of barium in rapid succession and then to hold a mouthful until immediately before the exposure.

• To show esophageal varices, instruct the patient (1) to exhale fully and then swallow the barium bolus and avoid inspiration until the exposure has been made, or (2) to take a deep breath and, while holding the breath, swallow the bolus and then perform the Valsalva maneuver (Fig. 15.53A).
• For other conditions, instruct the patient simply to swallow the barium bolus, which is normally done during moderate inspiration (see Fig. 15.53B). Because respiration is inhibited for about 2 seconds after swallowing, the patient does not have to hold his or her breath for the exposure. If the contrast medium is swallowed at the end of full inspiration, make two or three exposures in rapid succession before the contrast medium passes into the stomach. To show the entire esophagus, it is sometimes necessary to make the exposure while the patient is drinking the barium suspension through a straw in rapid and continuous swallows.
• Ask the patient to swallow a barium tablet to evaluate the degree of lumen narrowing with esophageal stricture (Fig. 15.54).

A   B

Fig. 15.53 (A) Spot images showing esophageal varices. (B) Barium bolus clearly shows Schatzki ring *(arrows)*.

(Courtesy Michael J. Kudlas, MEd, RT(R)(QM).)

Fig. 15.54 AP projection showing barium pill in distal esophagus, at the site of luminal stricture.

Gastrointestinal Series

UGI tract images are used to evaluate the distal esophagus, the stomach, and some or all of the small intestine. A UGI examination (Fig. 15.55), usually called a *gastrointestinal* or *UGI series,* may include the following:

1. A preliminary image of the abdomen to delineate the liver, spleen, kidneys, psoas muscles, and bony structures and to detect any abdominal or pelvic calcifications or tumor masses. Detection of calcifications and tumor masses requires that the survey image of the abdomen be taken after preliminary cleansing of the intestinal tract but before administration of the contrast medium.
2. Fluoroscopic recorded images only or a combination of fluoroscopic and radiographic images after contrast administration. Images will include the esophagus, stomach, and duodenum using an ingested opaque mixture, usually barium sulfate.
3. When requested, a small intestine study consisting of images obtained at frequent intervals during passage of the contrast column through the small intestine, at which time the vermiform appendix and the ileocecal region may be examined.

Nonambulatory outpatients or acutely ill patients, such as patients with a bleeding ulcer, are usually examined in the supine position using a fluoroscopic and spot-imaging procedure. Everything possible should be done to expedite the procedure. Any contrast preparation must be ready, and the examination room must be fully prepared before the patient is brought into the radiology department.

PRELIMINARY PREPARATION
Preparation of patient

Because a gastrointestinal series is time-consuming, the patient should be told the approximate time required for the procedure before being assigned an appointment for an examination. The patient also needs to understand the reason for preliminary preparation so that full cooperation can be given.

The stomach must be empty for an examination of the UGI tract (the stomach and small intestine). It is also desirable to have the colon free of gas and fecal material. When the patient is constipated, a non–gas-forming laxative may be administered 1 day before the examination.

An empty stomach is ensured by withholding food and water after midnight for 8 to 9 hours before the examination. When a small intestine study is to be made, food and fluid are withheld after the evening meal.

Because some research suggests that nicotine and chewing gum stimulate gastric secretion and salivation, some physicians tell patients not to smoke or chew gum after midnight on the night before the examination. This restriction is intended to prevent excessive fluid from accumulating in the stomach and diluting the barium suspension enough to interfere with its coating property. Radiographers should verify patient compliance with the preliminary preparation before obtaining the scout abdominal image, and should inform the fluoroscopist of the patient's answer when the scout image is provided for preliminary inspection.

Barium sulfate suspension

The contrast medium generally used in routine gastrointestinal examinations is barium sulfate mixed with water. The preparation must be thoroughly mixed according to the manufacturer's instructions. Specially formulated high-density barium is also available. Advances in the production of barium have all but eliminated the use of a single barium formula for most gastrointestinal examinations performed in the radiology department.

Most physicians use one of the many commercially prepared barium suspensions. These products are available in several flavors, and some are conveniently packaged in individual cups containing the dry ingredients. To these products, the radiographer merely has to add water, recap the cup, and shake it to obtain a smooth suspension. Other barium suspensions are completely mixed and ready to use.

Fig. 15.55 Barium-filled AP stomach and small bowel.

Contrast Studies

Two general procedures are routinely used to examine the stomach: the *single-contrast* method and the *double-contrast* method. A *biphasic* examination is a combination of the single-contrast and double-contrast methods during the same procedure.

SINGLE-CONTRAST EXAMINATION

In the single-contrast method (Fig. 15.56), a barium sulfate suspension is administered during the initial fluoroscopic examination. The ACR recommends a 60% weight/volume barium suspension used for this study.[8] The procedure is as follows:

- Whenever possible, begin the examination with the patient in the upright position.
- The radiologist may first examine the heart and lungs fluoroscopically and observe the abdomen to determine whether food or fluid is in the stomach.
- Give the patient a glass of barium and instruct the patient to drink it as requested by the radiologist. If the patient is in the recumbent position, administer the suspension through a drinking straw.
- The radiologist asks the patient to swallow two or three mouthfuls of barium. During this time, the radiologist examines and exposes any indicated spot images of the esophagus. By manual manipulation of the stomach through the abdominal wall, the radiologist then coats the gastric mucosa.
- Images are obtained with the spot-imaging device or another compression device to show a mucosal lesion of the stomach or duodenum.
- After studying the rugae and as the patient drinks the remainder of the barium suspension, the radiologist observes filling of the stomach and examines the duodenum further. Based on this examination, the following can be accomplished:
  1. Determine the size, shape, and position of the stomach.
  2. Examine the changing contour of the stomach during peristalsis.
  3. Observe the filling and emptying of the duodenal bulb.
  4. Detect any abnormal alteration in the function or contour of the esophagus, stomach, and duodenum.
  5. Record spot images as indicated.

The contrast medium normally begins to pass into the duodenum almost immediately. Nervous tension of the patient may delay transit of the contrast material, however.

Fluoroscopy is performed with the patient in the upright and recumbent positions while the body is rotated and the table is angled, so that all aspects of the esophagus, stomach, and duodenum are shown. Spot images are recorded as indicated. If esophageal involvement is suspected, a study is usually made with a thick barium suspension. In facilities in which subsequent radiographic images of the stomach and duodenum are required, the required projections should be obtained immediately after fluoroscopy before any considerable amount of the barium suspension passes into the jejunum.

Position of patient

The stomach and the duodenum may be examined using PA, AP, oblique, and lateral projections with the patient in the upright and recumbent positions, as indicated by the fluoroscopic findings.

One variation of the supine position is the LPO position. In another variation, the head end of the table is lowered 25 to 30 degrees to show a hiatal hernia. Finally, to show esophageal regurgitation and hiatal hernias, the head end of the table is lowered 10 to 15 degrees and the patient is rotated slightly toward the right side to place the esophagogastric (gastroesophageal) junction in profile to the right of the spine. The medical significance of diagnosing hiatal hernia is a topic that has received much attention in recent years. Some authors report little correlation between the presence of a hiatal hernia and gastrointestinal symptoms. If little correlation exists, radiographic evaluation is of little value in most hiatal hernias.

Fig. 15.56 Barium-filled PA stomach, single-contrast study.

DOUBLE-CONTRAST EXAMINATION

A second approach to examination of the gastrointestinal tract is the *double-contrast* technique (Fig. 15.57). The principal advantages of this method over the single-contrast method are that small lesions are less easily obscured and the mucosal lining of the stomach can be more clearly visualized. For successful results, the patient must be able to move with relative ease throughout the examination.

For double-contrast studies, the procedure is as follows:

- To begin the examination, place the patient on the fluoroscopic table in the upright position.
- Give the patient a gas-producing substance in the form of a powder, crystals, pills, or a carbonated beverage.
- Give the patient a small amount of commercially available, high-density barium suspension. For even coating of the stomach walls, the barium must flow freely and have low viscosity. Many high-density barium products are available; these suspensions have weight/volume ratios of up to 250%.
- Place the patient in the recumbent position, and instruct him or her to turn from side to side or to roll over a few times. This movement serves to coat the mucosal lining of the stomach as the carbon dioxide continues to expand. The patient may feel the need to belch but should refrain from doing so until the examination is finished to ensure that an optimal amount of contrast material (gas) remains for the duration of the examination.
- Just before the examination, the patient may be given glucagon or other anticholinergic medications intravenously or intramuscularly to relax the gastrointestinal tract.[9] These medications improve visualization by inducing greater distention of the stomach and intestines. Before administering these agents, the radiologist must consider numerous factors, including side effects, contraindications, availability, and cost.

Radiographic imaging procedure

The conventional images obtained after the fluoroscopic examination may be the same as images obtained for the single-contrast examination. Often the images with the greatest amount of diagnostic information are the spot images taken during fluoroscopy. In most cases, the radiologist will have already obtained most of the necessary diagnostic images. Nonfluoroscopic images may be unnecessary.

BIPHASIC EXAMINATION

The *biphasic* gastrointestinal examination incorporates the advantages of single-contrast and double-contrast UGI examinations, with both examinations performed during the same procedure. The patient first undergoes a double-contrast examination of the UGI tract. When this study is completed, the patient is given an approximately 15% weight/volume barium suspension, and a single-contrast examination is performed. This biphasic approach increases the accuracy of diagnosis without significantly increasing the cost of the examination.

Barium in fundus

Air-filled, barium-coated stomach

Fig. 15.57 Double-contrast stomach spot images.

★ PA PROJECTION

Image receptor + grid: Positioned by manufacturer or department protocol for proper anatomy display orientation; CR plate: 10 × 12 inches (24 × 30 cm) or 14 × 17 inches (35 × 43 cm) lengthwise.

Position of patient

- For radiographic studies of the stomach and duodenum, place the patient in the recumbent position. The upright position is sometimes used to show the relative position of the stomach.
- When adjusting thin patients in the prone position, support the weight of the body on pillows or other suitable pads positioned under the thorax and pelvis. This adjustment keeps the stomach or duodenum from pressing against the vertebrae, with resultant pressure-filling defects.

Position of part

- Adjust the patient's position recumbent or upright so that the midline of the grid coincides with a sagittal plane passing halfway between the vertebral column and the left lateral border of the abdomen (Fig. 15.58).
- Center the IR about 1 to 2 inches (2.5 to 5 cm) above the lower rib margin at the level of L1-L2 when the patient is prone (Figs. 15.59 and 15.60).
- For upright images, center the IR 3 to 6 inches (7.6 to 15 cm) lower than L1-L2. The greatest visceral movement between prone and upright positions occurs in asthenic patients.
- *Shield gonads.*
- *Respiration:* Suspend at the end of expiration unless otherwise requested.

Central ray

- Perpendicular to the center of the IR.

Collimation

- Adjust the radiation field to no larger than 10 × 12 inches (24 × 30 cm) for smaller patients or 11 × 14 inches (28 × 35 cm) for larger patients. Place side marker in the collimated exposure field.

Structures shown

A PA projection of the contour of the barium-filled stomach and duodenal bulb is shown. The upright position shows the size, shape, and relative position of the filled stomach, but it does not adequately show the unfilled fundic portion of the organ. In the prone position, the stomach moves superiorly 1 1/2 to 4 inches (3.8 to 10 cm) according to the patient's body habitus (Figs. 15.61–15.64). At the same time, the stomach spreads horizontally, with a comparable decrease in its length. (Note that the fundus usually fills in asthenic patients.)

Fig. 15.58 PA stomach and duodenum.

Fig. 15.59 Single-contrast PA stomach and duodenum.

Fig. 15.60 Double-contrast PA stomach and duodenum.

The pyloric canal and the duodenal bulb are well shown in patients with an asthenic or hyposthenic habitus. These structures are often partially obscured in patients with a sthenic habitus and, except in the PA axial projection, are completely obscured by the prepyloric portion of the stomach in patients with a hypersthenic habitus.

The following should be clearly seen:
- Evidence of proper collimation and presence of side marker placed clear of anatomy of interest
- Entire stomach and duodenal loop
- Stomach centered at the level of the pylorus
- No rotation of the patient
- Penetration of the contrast medium
- Surrounding anatomy

NOTE: A 14- × 17-inch (35- × 43-cm) exposure field is often used when the distal esophagus or the small bowel is to be visualized along with the stomach.

Fig. 15.61 Hypersthenic patient.

Fig. 15.62 Sthenic patient.

Fig. 15.63 Hyposthenic patient.

Fig. 15.64 Asthenic patient.

PA AXIAL PROJECTION

Image receptor + grid: Positioned by manufacturer or department protocol for proper anatomy display orientation; CR plate: 10 × 12 inches (24 × 30 cm) or 14 × 17 inches (35 × 43 cm) lengthwise.

Position of patient

- Place the patient in the prone position.

Position of part

- Adjust the patient's body so that the MSP is centered to the grid.
- For a sthenic patient, center the IR at the level of L2 (Fig. 15.65), at about 1 to 2 inches (2.5 to 5 cm) above the lower rib margin; center it higher for a hypersthenic patient and lower for an asthenic patient.
- *Shield gonads.*
- *Respiration:* Suspend respiration at the end of expiration unless otherwise requested.

Central ray

- Directed to the midpoint of the IR at an angle of 35 to 45 degrees cephalad. Gugliantini[10] recommended cephalic angulation of 20 to 25 degrees to show the stomach in infants.

Collimation

- Adjust the radiation field to be no larger than 14 × 17 inches (35 × 43 cm). Place side marker in the collimated exposure field.

Structures shown

Gordon[11] developed the PA axial projection to "open up" the high, horizontal (hypersthenic-type) stomach to show the greater and lesser curvatures, the antral portion of the stomach, the pyloric canal, and the duodenal bulb. The resultant image gives a hypersthenic stomach much the same configuration as the average sthenic type of stomach (Fig. 15.66).

The following should clearly be seen:

- Evidence of proper collimation and presence of side marker placed clear of anatomy of interest
- Entire stomach and proximal duodenum
- Stomach centered at the level of the pylorus
- Penetration of the contrast medium
- Surrounding anatomy

Fig. 15.65 PA axial stomach.

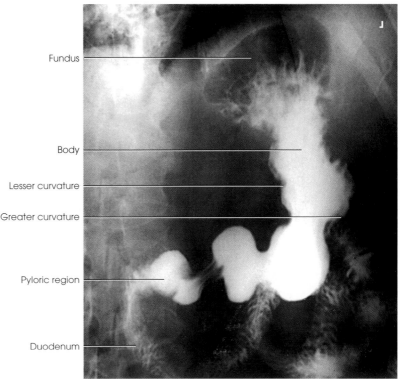

Fig. 15.66 PA axial stomach, sthenic habitus.

Stomach and Duodenum

225

🕊 PA OBLIQUE PROJECTION
RAO position

Image receptor + grid: Positioned by manufacturer or department protocol for proper anatomy display orientation; CR plate: 10 × 12 inches (24 × 30 cm) or 14 × 17 inches (35 × 43 cm) lengthwise.

Position of patient
- Place the patient in the recumbent position.

Position of part
- After the PA projection, instruct the patient to rest the head on the right cheek and to place the right arm along the side of the body.
- Have the patient raise his or her left side and support the body on the left forearm and flexed left knee.
- Adjust the patient's position so that a sagittal plane passing midway between the vertebrae and the lateral border of the elevated side coincides with the midline of the grid (Fig. 15.67).
- Center the IR about 1 to 2 inches (2.5 to 5 cm) above the lower rib margin, at the level of L1-L2, when the patient is prone.

- Make the final adjustment in body rotation. The approximately 40 to 70 degrees of rotation required to give the best image of the pyloric canal and duodenum depends on the size, shape, and position of the stomach. Generally, hypersthenic patients require a greater degree of rotation than sthenic and asthenic patients.
- The RAO position is used for serial studies of the pyloric canal and the duodenal bulb because gastric peristalsis is usually more active when the patient is in this position.
- *Shield gonads.*
- *Respiration:* Suspend at the end of expiration unless otherwise requested.

Central ray
- Perpendicular to the center of the IR.

Collimation
- Adjust the radiation field to no larger than 10 × 12 inches (24 × 30 cm) for smaller patients and no larger than 11 × 14 inches (28 × 35 cm) for larger patients. Place side marker in the collimated exposure field.

Fig. 15.67 PA oblique stomach and duodenum, RAO position.

Structures shown

Entire stomach and duodenal loop demonstrated. Provides the best image of the pyloric canal and duodenal bulb in sthenic patients (Figs. 15.68 and 15.69).

Because gastric peristalsis is generally more active with the patient in the RAO position, a serial study of several exposures is sometimes obtained at intervals of 30 to 40 seconds to delineate the pyloric canal and duodenal bulb.

The following should be clearly seen:

- Evidence of proper collimation and presence of side marker placed clear of anatomy of interest
- Entire stomach and duodenal loop
- No superimposition of the pylorus and duodenal bulb
- Duodenal bulb and loop in profile
- Stomach centered at the level of the pylorus
- Penetration of the contrast medium
- Surrounding anatomy

Fundus

Greater curvature

Duodenal bulb

Pylorus

Fig. 15.68 Single-contrast PA oblique stomach and duodenum, RAO position.

Fig. 15.69 Double-contrast PA oblique stomach and duodenum. Note esophagus entering stomach *(arrow)*.

⚸ AP OBLIQUE PROJECTION
LPO position

Image receptor + grid: Positioned by manufacturer or department protocol for proper anatomy display orientation; CR plate: 10 × 12 inches (24 × 30 cm) or 14 × 17 inches (35 × 43 cm) lengthwise.

Position of patient
- Place the patient in the supine position.

Position of part
- Have the patient abduct the left arm and place the hand near the head, or place the extended arm alongside the body.
- Place the right arm alongside the body or across the upper chest, as preferred.
- Have the patient turn toward the left, resting on the left posterior body surface.
- Flex the patient's right knee, and rotate the knee toward the left for support.
- Place a positioning sponge against the patient's elevated back for immobilization.
- Adjust the patient's position so that a sagittal plane passing approximately midway between the vertebrae and the left lateral margin of the abdomen is centered to the IR.

- Adjust the center of the IR at the level of the body of the stomach. Centering should be adjusted at a point midway between the xiphoid process and the lower margin of the ribs (Fig. 15.70).
- The degree of rotation required to show the stomach best depends on the patient's body habitus. An average angle of 45 degrees should be sufficient for a sthenic patient, but the degree of angulation can vary from 30 to 60 degrees.
- *Shield gonads.*
- *Respiration:* Suspend at the end of expiration unless otherwise instructed.

Fig. 15.70 AP oblique stomach and duodenum, LPO position.

Central ray

- Perpendicular to the center of the IR.

Collimation

- Adjust the radiation field to no larger than 10 × 12 inches (24 × 30 cm) for smaller patients and 11 × 14 inches (28 × 35 cm) for larger patients. Place side marker in the collimated exposure field.

Structures shown

The fundic portion of the stomach (Fig. 15.71). Because of the effect of gravity, the pyloric canal and the duodenal bulb are not as filled with barium as they are in the opposite and complementary position (the RAO position; see Figs. 15.67 to 15.69).

EVALUATION CRITERIA

The following should be clearly seen:
- Evidence of proper collimation and presence of side marker placed clear of anatomy of interest
- Entire stomach and duodenal loop
- Fundic portion of stomach
- No superimposition of pylorus and duodenal bulb
- Body of the stomach centered to the image
- Penetration of the contrast medium
- Surrounding anatomy
- Body and pyloric antrum with double-contrast visualization

Fig. 15.71 Double-contrast AP oblique stomach and duodenum, LPO position.

⚭ LATERAL PROJECTION
Right position

Image receptor + grid: Positioned by manufacturer or department protocol for proper anatomy display orientation; CR plate: 10 × 12 inches (24 × 30 cm) or 14 × 17 inches (35 × 43 cm) lengthwise.

Position of patient

- Place the patient in the *upright left lateral position* to show the left retrogastric space and in the *recumbent right lateral position* to show the right retrogastric space, duodenal loop, and duodenojejunal junction.

Position of part

- With the patient in the upright or recumbent position, adjust the body so that a plane passing midway between the midcoronal plane and the anterior surface of the abdomen coincides with the midline of the grid.
- Center the IR at the level of L1-L2 for the recumbent position (about 1 to 2 inches [2.5 to 5 cm] above the lower rib margin) and at L3 for the upright position.
- Adjust the body in a true lateral position (Fig. 15.72).
- *Shield gonads.*
- *Respiration:* Suspend at the end of expiration unless otherwise requested.

Fig. 15.72 Right lateral stomach and duodenum.

Central ray
- Perpendicular to the center of the IR

Collimation
- Adjust the radiation field to no larger than 10 × 12 inches (24 × 30 cm) for smaller patients and no larger than 11 × 14 inches (28 × 35 cm) for larger patients. Place side marker in the collimated exposure field.

Structures shown
The anterior and posterior aspects of the stomach, the pyloric canal, and the duodenal bulb (Figs. 15.73 and 15.74). The right lateral projection commonly affords the best image of the pyloric canal and the duodenal bulb in patients with a hypersthenic habitus.

The following should be clearly seen:
- Evidence of proper collimation and presence of side marker placed clear of anatomy of interest
- Entire stomach and duodenal loop
- No rotation of the patient, as shown by the vertebrae
- Stomach centered at the level of the pylorus
- Penetration of the contrast medium
- Surrounding anatomy

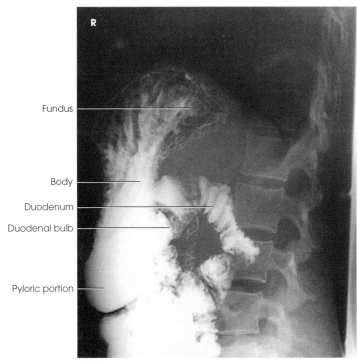

Fundus

Body

Duodenum

Duodenal bulb

Pyloric portion

Fig. 15.73 Single-contrast right lateral stomach and duodenum.

Fig. 15.74 Double-contrast right lateral stomach and duodenum.

🐦 AP PROJECTION

Image receptor + grid: Positioned by manufacturer or department protocol for proper anatomy display orientation; CR plate: 10 × 12 inches (24 × 30 cm) for small hiatal hernias; 14 × 17 inches (35 × 43 cm) lengthwise for large diaphragmatic herniations or for the stomach and small bowel.

Position of patient

- Place the patient in the supine position. The stomach moves superiorly and to the left in this position, and, except in thin patients, its pyloric end is elevated so that the barium flows into and fills its cardiac or fundic portions or both. Filling of the fundus displaces the gas bubble into the pyloric end of the stomach, where it allows double-contrast delineation of posterior wall lesions when a single-contrast examination is performed. If the patient is thin, the intestinal loops do not move superior enough to tilt the stomach for fundic filling. Rotating the patient's body toward the left or angling the head end of the table downward is necessary.
- Tilt the table to full or partial Trendelenburg angulation to show diaphragmatic herniations (Fig. 15.75). In the Trendelenburg position, the involved organ or organs, which may appear to be normally located in all other body positions, shift upward and protrude through the hernial orifice (most commonly through the esophageal hiatus).

NOTE: Valsalva maneuver may be used in conjunction with or as an alternative to the Trendelenburg position.

Position of part

- Adjust the position of the patient so that the midline of the grid coincides (1) with the midline of the body when a 14- × 17-inches (35 × 43-cm) exposure field (or CR plate) is used (see Fig. 15.75) or (2) with a sagittal plane passing midway between the midline and the left lateral margin of the abdomen when a 10- × 12-inch (24 × 30-cm) exposure field (or CR plate) is used (Fig. 15.76). Longitudinal centering of the larger exposure field depends on the extent of hernial protrusion into the thorax and is determined during fluoroscopy.
- For the stomach and duodenum, center the 10- × 12-inch (24- × 30-cm) exposure field/IR at a level midway between the xiphoid process and the lower rib margin (approximately L1-L2). For the 14- × 17-inch (35- × 43-cm) exposure field/IR, center it at the same level and adjust up or down slightly, depending on whether the diaphragm or the small bowel needs to be seen.
- *Shield gonads.*
- *Respiration:* Suspend at the end of expiration unless otherwise requested.

Central ray

- Perpendicular to the center of the IR.

Collimation

- Adjust the radiation field to no larger than 10 × 12 inches (24 × 30 cm) when the stomach alone is of interest; no larger than 14 × 17 inches (35 × 43 cm) when the small bowel is to be included. Place side marker in the collimated exposure field.

Structures shown

Stomach. A well-filled fundic portion and usually a double-contrast delineation of the body, pyloric portion, and duodenum (Fig. 15.77). Because of the elevation and superior displacement of the stomach, this projection affords the best AP projection of the retrogastric portion of the duodenum and jejunum.

Diaphragm. An AP projection of the abdominothoracic region shows the organ or organs involved in, and the location and extent of, any gross hernial protrusion through the diaphragm (Figs. 15.78 and 15.79).

The following should be clearly seen:

- Evidence of proper collimation and presence of side marker placed clear of anatomy of interest
- Entire stomach and duodenal loop
- Double-contrast visualization of the gastric body, pylorus, and duodenal bulb
- Retrogastric portion of the duodenum and jejunum
- Lower lung fields on 14- × 17-inch (35- × 43-cm) images to show diaphragmatic hernias
- Stomach centered at the level of the pylorus on 10- × 12-inch (24- × 30-cm) images
- No rotation of the patient
- Penetration the contrast medium
- Surrounding soft tissues

Fig. 15.75 AP stomach and duodenum with table in partial Trendelenburg position.

Fig. 15.76 AP stomach and duodenum.

Fundus

Body

Pyloric portion
Duodenal loop

Fig. 15.77 AP stomach and duodenum, sthenic habitus.

Fig. 15.78 AP stomach and duodenum, showing hiatal hernia above level of diaphragm *(arrow)*.

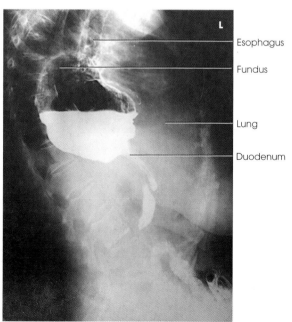

Esophagus

Fundus

Lung

Duodenum

Fig. 15.79 Upright left lateral stomach showing hiatal hernia.

(Comparison lateral images are shown in Figs. 15.73 and 15.74.)

PA OBLIQUE PROJECTION
WOLF METHOD (FOR HIATAL HERNIA)
RAO position

Image receptor + grid: Positioned by manufacturer or department protocol for proper anatomy display orientation; CR plate: 14 × 17 inches (35 × 43 cm) lengthwise.

The Wolf method[12] is a modification of the Trendelenburg position. The technique was developed for the purpose of applying greater intra-abdominal pressure than is provided by body angulation alone and ensuring more consistent results in the radiographic demonstration of small, sliding gastroesophageal herniations through the esophageal hiatus.

The Wolf method requires the use of a semicylindric radiolucent compression device measuring 22 inches (55 cm) in length, 10 inches (24 cm) in width, and 8 inches (20 cm) in height. (The compression sponge depicted in Fig. 15.80 is slightly smaller than the one described by Wolf.)

Wolf and Guglielmo[13] stated that this compression device not only provides Trendelenburg angulation of the patient's trunk, but it also increases intra-abdominal pressure enough to permit adequate contrast filling and maximal distention of the entire esophagus. A further advantage of the device is that it does not require angulation of the table; the patient can hold the barium container and ingest the barium suspension through a straw with comparative ease.

NOTE: Valsalva maneuver also increases intra-abdominal pressure and may be used instead of the Wolf method.

Position of patient
- Place the patient in the prone position on the radiographic table.

Position of part
- Instruct the patient to assume a modified knee-chest position during placement of the compression device.
- Place the compression device horizontally under the abdomen and just below the costal margin.
- Adjust the patient in a 40- to 45-degree RAO position, with the thorax centered to the midline of the grid.
- Instruct the patient to ingest the barium suspension in rapid, continuous swallows.
- To allow for complete filling of the esophagus, make the exposure during the third or fourth swallow.
- *Shield gonads.*
- *Respiration:* Suspend at the end of expiration.

Fig. 15.80 PA oblique stomach with compression sponge, RAO position.

Central ray

- Perpendicular to the long axis of the patient's back and centered at the level of T6 or T7. This position usually results in 10- to 20-degree caudad angulation of the central ray.

Collimation

- Adjust the radiation field to no larger than 14 × 17 inches (35 × 43 cm). Place side marker in the collimated exposure field.

Structures shown

The relationship of the stomach to the diaphragm and is useful in diagnosing a hiatal hernia (Fig. 15.81).

The following should be clearly seen:

- Evidence of proper collimation and presence of side marker placed clear of anatomy of interest
- Middle or distal aspects of the esophagus and the upper aspect of the stomach
- Esophagus visible between the vertebral column and the heart
- Penetration of the contrast medium
- Surrounding anatomy

Fig. 15.81 Comparison PA axial oblique images in one patient. (A) Without abdominal compression: no evidence of hernia. (B) With abdominal compression: obvious large sliding hernia *(arrow)*.

Radiologic examinations of the small intestine are performed by administering a barium sulfate preparation (1) by *mouth*; (2) by complete *reflux filling* with a large-volume barium enema (BE); or (3) by direct injection into the bowel through an intestinal tube—a technique that is called *enteroclysis,* or small intestine enema. The latter two methods are used when the oral method fails to provide conclusive information.[14] Enteroclysis is technically difficult, so its use is usually limited to larger medical facilities.

PREPARATION FOR EXAMINATION

Preferably, the patient has a soft or low-residue diet for 2 days before the small intestine study. Because of economics, however, it often is impossible to delay the examination for 2 days. Food and fluid are usually withheld after the evening meal of the day before the examination, and breakfast is withheld on the day of the study. A cleansing enema may be administered to clear the colon; however, an enema is not always recommended for enteroclysis because enema fluid may be retained in the small intestine. The barium formula varies depending on the method of examination. The patient's bladder should be empty before and during the procedure to avoid displacing or compressing the ileum.

ORAL METHOD OF EXAMINATION

The radiographic examination of the small intestine is usually termed a *small bowel series* because several identical images are done at timed intervals. The oral examination, or ingestion of barium through the mouth, is usually preceded by a preliminary image of the abdomen. Each image of the small intestine is identified with a time marker indicating the interval between its exposure and ingestion of barium. Studies are made with the patient in the supine or the prone position. The supine position is used (1) to take advantage of the superior and lateral shift of the barium-filled stomach for visualization of retrogastric portions of the duodenum and jejunum and (2) to prevent possible compression overlapping of loops of the intestine. The prone position is used to compress the abdominal contents; this enhances radiographic image quality. For the final images in thin patients, it may be necessary to angle the table into the Trendelenburg position to "unfold" low-lying and superimposed loops of the ileum.

The first exposure of the small intestine is usually taken 15 minutes after the patient drinks the barium. The interval to the next exposure varies from 15 to 30 minutes depending on the average transit time of the barium sulfate preparation used. Regardless of the barium preparation used, the radiologist inspects the images as they are processed and varies the procedure according to requirements for the individual patient. Fluoroscopic and radiographic studies (spot or conventional) may be made of any segment of the bowel as the loops become opacified.

Some radiologists request that a glass of ice water (or another routinely used food stimulant) be given to a patient with hypomotility after 3 or 4 hours of administrating barium sulfate to accelerate peristalsis. Others give patients a water-soluble gastrointestinal contrast medium, tea, or coffee to stimulate peristalsis. Other radiologists administer peristaltic stimulants every 15 minutes through the transit time. With these methods, transit of the medium is shown fluoroscopically, spot and conventional radiographic images are exposed as indicated, and the examination is usually completed in 30 to 60 minutes.

⚜ PA OR AP PROJECTION

Image receptor + grid: Positioned by manufacturer or department protocol for proper anatomy display orientation; CR plate: 14 × 17 inches (35 × 43 cm) lengthwise.

Position of patient
- Place the patient in the prone or supine position.

Position of part
- Adjust the patient so that the MSP is centered to the grid.
- For a sthenic patient, center the IR at the level of L2 for images taken within 30 minutes after the contrast medium is administered (Fig. 15.82).
- For delayed images, center the IR at the level of the iliac crests.
- *Shield gonads.*
- *Respiration:* Suspend at the end of expiration unless otherwise requested.

Central ray
- Perpendicular to the midpoint of the IR (L2) for early images or at the level of the iliac crests for delayed sequence exposures.

Collimation
- Adjust the radiation field to no larger than 14 × 17 inches (35 × 43 cm). For smaller patients, collimate to within 1 inch (2.5 cm) of shadow of the abdomen flanks. Place side marker in the collimated exposure field.

Structures shown
The small intestine progressively filling until barium reaches the ileocecal valve (Figs. 15.83–15.86). When barium has reached the ileocecal region, fluoroscopy may be performed, and compression radiographic images may be obtained (Fig. 15.87). The examination is usually completed when the barium is visualized in the cecum, typically within about 2 hours for a patient with normal intestinal motility.

EVALUATION CRITERIA

The following should be clearly seen:
- Evidence of proper collimation and presence of side marker placed clear of anatomy of interest
- Entire small intestine on each image
- Stomach on initial images
- Time marker
- Vertebral column centered on the image
- No rotation of the patient
- Penetration of the contrast medium
- Complete examination when barium reaches the cecum

Fig. 15.82 AP small intestine.

Fig. 15.83 Immediate AP small intestine.

Fig. 15.84 AP small intestine at 15 minutes.

Fig. 15.85 AP small intestine at 30 minutes, showing stomach *(st)* and small intestine *(si)*.

Fig. 15.86 AP small intestine at 1 hour, showing barium-filled cecum.

Fig. 15.87 Ileocecal studies.

Ileocecal valve
Cecum
Appendix
Ileum

COMPLETE REFLUX EXAMINATION

For a complete reflux examination of the small intestine,[15,16] the patient's colon and small intestine are filled by a BE administered to show the colon and small bowel. Before the examination, glucagon may be administered to relax the intestine. Diazepam (Valium) may also be given to diminish patient discomfort during initial filling of the bowel. A 15% ± 5% weight/volume barium suspension is often used, and a large amount of the suspension (about 4500 mL) is required to fill the colon and small intestine.

A retention enema tip is used, and the patient is placed in the supine position for the examination. The barium suspension is allowed to flow until it is observed in the duodenal bulb. The enema bag is lowered to the floor to drain the colon before images of the small intestine are obtained (Fig. 15.88).

ENTEROCLYSIS PROCEDURE

Enteroclysis (the injection of nutrient or medicinal liquid into the bowel) is a radiographic procedure in which contrast medium is injected into the duodenum under fluoroscopic control for examination of the small intestine. Contrast medium is injected through a specially designed enteroclysis catheter, historically a Bilbao or Sellink tube.

Before the procedure is begun, the patient's colon must be thoroughly cleansed. Enemas are not recommended as preparation for enteroclysis because some enema fluid may be retained in the small intestine. Under fluoroscopic control, the enteroclysis catheter with a stiff guidewire is advanced to the end of the duodenum at the duodenojejunal flexure, near the ligament of Treitz. The retention balloon, if present, is filled with sterile water or saline. Barium is instilled through the tube at a rate of approximately 100 mL/min (Fig. 15.89). Spot images, with and without compression, are taken as required. In some patients, air is injected after contrast fluid has reached the distal small intestine (Fig. 15.90). When CT is to be performed, an iodinated contrast medium (Figs. 15.91 and 15.92) or tap water (Figs. 15.93 and 15.94) may be used.

After fluoroscopic examination of the patient's small intestine, images of the small intestine may be requested. The projections most often requested include AP, PA, oblique, and lateral. Recumbent and upright images may be requested. (Positioning descriptions involving the abdomen are presented in Chapter 4.)

Fig. 15.88 Normal retrograde reflux examination of small intestine.

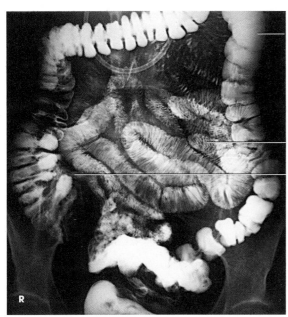

Fig. 15.89 Enteroclysis procedure with barium visualized in colon.

Barium in colon

Small intestine

Terminal ileum

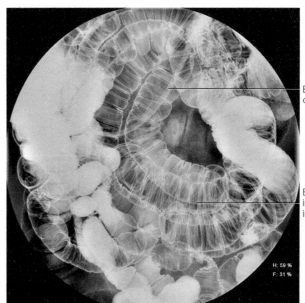

Fig. 15.90 Air-contrast enteroclysis.

Enteroclysis catheter

Barium air in small intestine

Fig. 15.91 Enteroclysis with iodinated contrast medium. Filled retention balloon is seen in duodenum *(arrow)*.

(Courtesy Michelle Alting, AS, RT(R).)

Fig. 15.92 Axial CT enteroclysis of the patient in Fig. 15.91.

Colon　　　　　　　　　　　Small intestine

Fig. 15.93 Axial CT enteroclysis with tap water and intravenous iodinated contrast medium. Intraluminal water *(dark gray)* is clearly delineated from bowel wall *(light gray)*.

Spleen

Kidney

Colon

Small intestine

Fig. 15.94 Sagittal reconstruction of CT enteroclysis from Fig. 15.93.

INTUBATION EXAMINATION PROCEDURES

Gastrointestinal intubation is a procedure in which a long, specially designed tube is inserted through the nose and passed into the stomach. From there, the tube is carried inferiorly by peristaltic action. Gastrointestinal intubation is used for therapeutic and diagnostic purposes.

When gastrointestinal intubation is used therapeutically, the tube is connected to a suction system for continuous siphoning of gas and fluid contents of the gastrointestinal tract. The purpose of the maneuver is to prevent or relieve postoperative distention or to deflate or decompress an obstructed small intestine.

Although used much less frequently than in the past, a *Miller-Abbott* double-lumen, single-balloon tube (or other similar tubing) can be used to intubate the small intestine. Just above the tip of the Miller-Abbott tube is a small, thin rubber balloon. Marks on the tube, beginning at the distal end, indicate the extent of the tube's passage and are read from the edge of the nostril. The marks are graduated in centimeters up to 85 cm and are given in feet thereafter. The lumen of the tube is asymmetrically divided into (1) a small balloon lumen that communicates with the balloon only and is used for inflation and deflation of the balloon and for injection of mercury to weight the balloon and (2) a large aspiration lumen that communicates with the gastrointestinal tract through perforations near and at the distal end of the tube. Gas and fluids are withdrawn through the aspiration lumen, and liquids are injected through it.

The introduction of an intestinal tube is an unpleasant experience for a patient, especially one who is acutely ill. Depending on the condition of the patient, the tube is more readily passed if the patient can sit erect and lean slightly forward, or if the patient can be elevated almost to a sitting position.

With the intestinal tube in place, the patient is turned to an RAO position, a syringe is connected to the balloon lumen, and mercury is poured into the syringe and allowed to flow into the balloon. Air is slowly withdrawn from the balloon. The tube is secured with an adhesive strip beside the nostril to prevent regurgitation or advancement of the tube. The stomach is aspirated by using a syringe or by attaching the large port of the lumen to the suction apparatus.

With the tip of the tube situated close to the pyloric sphincter and the patient in the RAO position (a position in which gastric peristalsis is usually more active), the tube should pass into the duodenum in a reasonably short time. Without intervention, this process sometimes takes many hours. Having the patient drink ice water to stimulate peristalsis is often successful. When this measure fails, the examiner guides the tube into the duodenum by manual manipulation under fluoroscopic observation. After the tube enters the duodenum, it is inflated again to provide a bolus that peristaltic waves can more readily move along the intestine.

When the tube is inserted for decompression of an intestinal obstruction and possible later radiologic investigation, the adhesive strip is removed and replaced with an adhesive loop attached to the forehead. The tube can slide through the loop without tension as it advances toward the obstructed site. The patient is then returned to the hospital room. Radiographic images of the abdomen may be taken to check the progress of the tube and the effectiveness of decompression. Simple obstructions are sometimes relieved by suction; others require surgical intervention.

If passage of the intestinal tube is arrested, suction is discontinued, and the patient is returned to the radiology department for a Miller-Abbott tube study. The contrast medium used for studies of a localized segment of the small intestine may be a water-soluble, iodinated solution (Fig. 15.95A), or a thin barium sulfate suspension. Under fluoroscopic observation, the contrast agent is injected through the large lumen of the tube with a syringe. Spot and conventional images are obtained as indicated.

When the intestinal tube is introduced for the purpose of performing a small intestine enema, the tube is advanced into the proximal loop of the jejunum and is secured at this level with an adhesive strip taped beside the nose. Medical opinion varies regarding the quantity of barium suspension required for this examination (see Fig. 15.95B). The medium is injected through the aspiration lumen of the tube in a continuous, low-pressure flow. Spot and conventional images are exposed as indicated. Except for the presence of the tube in the upper jejunum, resultant images resemble those obtained by the oral method.

Fig. 15.95 (A) Miller-Abbott tube study with water-soluble medium. (B) Small bowel examination by Miller-Abbott tube with injection of barium sulfate.

CONTRAST MEDIA STUDIES

The two basic radiologic methods of examining the large intestine by means of contrast media enemas are (1) the *single-contrast* method (Fig. 15.96), in which the colon is examined with a barium sulfate suspension or water-soluble iodide only; and (2) the *double-contrast* method (Fig. 15.97), which may be performed as a two-stage or single-stage procedure. In the *two-stage, double-contrast procedure,* the colon is examined with a barium sulfate suspension and then, immediately after evacuation of the barium suspension, with an air enema or another gaseous enema. In the *single-stage, double-contrast procedure,* the fluoroscopist selectively injects the barium suspension and the gas.

Positive contrast medium shows the anatomy and tonus of the colon and most of the abnormalities to which it is subject. The addition of the air (negative) contrast distends the lumen of the bowel for optimum visualization of the barium-coated mucosal lining of the colon. Double-contrast, or air-contrast studies, allow for demonstration of small intraluminal lesions, such as polypoid tumors.

A more recent development in radiographic examination of the large intestine is *computed tomography colonography* (CTC), also called *virtual colonoscopy* (VC)—a procedure used as a primary screening tool for colorectal cancer or after a failed conventional colonoscopy. This software-driven technique combines helical CT and virtual reality software to create three-dimensional and multiplanar images of the colonic mucosa. Examples of currently available CTC techniques include the perspective-filet or virtual dissection view, the three-dimensional topographic view, the multiplanar reformatted (MPR) view, and the colonoscopic-like endoluminal view (Figs. 15.98 through 15.100).

Contrast media

Commercially prepared barium sulfate products are generally used for routine retrograde examinations of the large intestine. Some of these products are referred to as *colloidal preparations* because they have finely divided barium particles that resist precipitation, whereas others are referred to as suspended or *flocculation-resistant preparations* because they contain some form of suspending or dispersing agent.

The newest barium products available are referred to as *high-density barium sulfate*. These products absorb a greater percentage of radiation, similar to older "thick" barium products. High-density barium is particularly useful for double-contrast studies of the alimentary canal in which uniform coating of the lumen is required.

Air is the gaseous medium usually used in the double-contrast enema study. The procedure is generally called an *air-contrast study.* Carbon dioxide may also be used because it is more rapidly absorbed than the nitrogen in air when evacuation of the gaseous medium is incomplete. Use of air as a contrast medium for radiographic evaluation of the colon is not limited to the double-contrast enema procedure. Air or carbon dioxide insufflation of the colon is used to perform CTC or VC.

Fig. 15.96 Large intestine, single-contrast study.

Fig. 15.97 Large intestine, double-contrast study.

Water-soluble, iodinated contrast media enemas are performed when colon perforation or leak is suspected. These iodinated contrast agents are administered orally to selected patients when retrograde filling of the colon with barium is impossible or is contraindicated. A disadvantage of iodinated solutions is that evacuation often is insufficient for satisfactory double-contrast visualization of the mucosal pattern. When a patient is unable to cooperate for a successful enema study, orally administered iodinated medium allows satisfactory examination of the colon. With these oral agents, transit time from ingestion to colonic filling is fast, averaging 3 to 4 hours. Iodinated solutions are practically nonabsorbable from the gastrointestinal mucosa. As a result, the oral dose reaches and outlines the entire large bowel. In contrast to an ingested barium sulfate suspension, this medium is not subject to drying, flaking, and unequal distribution in the colon. It frequently delineates the intestine almost as well as the BE does.

Fig. 15.98 Examples of CTC or VC. (A) Perspective-filet or virtual dissection view, showing diverticulum *(arrow)*. (B) Three-dimensional topographic view: *Purple line* in the sigmoid shows length of filet in (A). (C) Axial MPR, showing same diverticulum as in A *(arrow)*. (D) Endoluminal view showing opening *(arrow)* of diverticulum from A.

(D, Courtesy J. Louis Rankin, BS, RT(R)(MR).)

Fig. 15.99 Endoluminal CTC image, showing two tubular adenomas *(arrows)*.

Fig. 15.100 Axial MPR image of upper tubular adenoma *(arrow)* from Fig. 15.99.

Preparation of intestinal tract

Medical opinion about preparation measures varies. Members of the medical profession usually agree, however, that the large intestine must be completely emptied of its contents to render all portions of its inner wall visible for inspection. When coated with a barium sulfate suspension, retained fecal masses are likely to simulate the appearance of polypoid or other small tumor masses (Fig. 15.101); this makes thorough cleansing of the entire colon a matter of prime importance. Preliminary preparation of the intestinal tract of patients who have a condition such as severe diarrhea, gross bleeding, or symptoms of obstruction is limited. Other patients are prepared, with modification as indicated, according to specifications established by the examining physician. The preliminary preparation usually includes dietary restrictions ("clear" liquids only) and a bowel cleansing regimen. Methods of bowel cleansing include the following:

- Complete intestinal tract cleansing kits
- Gastrointestinal lavage preparations
- Cleansing enema

Standard barium enema apparatus

Disposable soft plastic enema tips and enema bags are commercially available in different sizes. A soft rubber rectal catheter of small caliber should be used in patients who have inflamed hemorrhoids, fissures, a stricture, or other abnormalities of the anus.

Disposable rectal *retention tips* (Fig. 15.102, *inset*) have a double-lumen tube with a thin balloon at its distal end. Because of the danger of intestinal wall damage, the retention tip must be inserted with extreme care. The enema retention tip is used in a patient who has a relaxed anal sphincter or another condition that makes it difficult or impossible to retain an enema. Some radiologists routinely use retention enema tips and inflate them if necessary.

The disposable rectal retention tip has a balloon cuff that fits snugly against the enema nozzle before inflation and after deflation so that it can be inserted and removed with little discomfort to the patient. A reusable squeeze inflator is recommended to limit air capacity to approximately 90 mL. One complete squeeze of the inflator provides adequate distention of the retention balloon without danger of overinflation. Disposable retention tips are available for double-contrast and single-contrast enemas. For the safety of the patient, any retention balloon must be inflated with caution, using fluoroscopy, just before the examination.

Fig. 15.101 Single-contrast, barium-filled colon, showing fecal material that simulates or masks pathologic condition *(arrows)*.

Fig. 15.102 Disposable retention enema tip. Uninflated balloon fits snugly. The bulb used to instill air into the colon is labeled *A.* The cuff used to inflate the retention balloon is labeled *B. (Inset)* Balloon cuff inflated with 90 mL of air (one complete squeeze of inflator).

For performance of a double-contrast BE examination, a special rectal tip is necessary to instill air in the colon (Fig. 15.103). The cuff for the inflation of the retention bulb is labeled as A, and the bulb for administering air into the colon is labeled B. The tubing to administer the air contrast during the procedure lies in the center of the lumen of the enema tip. Barium flows through the holes in the side of the tip, while air is pumped through the tubing.

Fig. 15.103 Air-contrast enema kit filled with barium. *Arrow* indicates bulb used to administer air into the colon. An asterisk *(*)* marks the retention tip inflator cuff.

Preparation of barium suspensions

Commercially prepared, premixed liquid barium preparations that can be poured into the disposable enema kit bag are recommended by the ACR. Most enema bags have a capacity of 3000 mL with graduated markings along the sides. Most BE exams require 1000 to 2000 mL of premixed liquid barium. For single-contrast exams, a low-density (15% to 20% weight/volume) barium suspension is recommended. Optimal imaging in double-contrast exams of the colon requires high-density barium (80% to 100% weight/volume). When water-soluble contrast is required, 60% to 76% density (300 to 370 mg of iodine/mL) provides adequate opacification.[17,18] Powdered barium is also available in single-contrast disposable kit bags. Water is added, and the solution is mixed by shaking the bag. Instructions for mixing a barium preparation vary according to the manufacturer and the type of barium used. The best recommendation is to *precisely* follow the manufacturer's instructions regarding the amount and temperature of added water to attain appropriate consistency.

Preparation and care of patient

In no radiologic examination is the full cooperation of the patient more essential to success than in the retrograde examination of the colon. Few patients who are physically able to retain the enema fail to do so when they understand the procedure and realize that in large measure the success of the examination depends on them. The radiographer should observe the following guidelines in preparing a patient for retrograde examination of the colon:

- Take time to explain the procedural differences between an ordinary cleansing enema and a diagnostic enema: (1) With the diagnostic enema, the fluoroscopist examines all portions of the bowel as it is being filled with contrast medium under fluoroscopic observation; (2) this part of the examination involves palpation of the abdomen, rotation of the body as required to visualize different segments of the colon, and taking of spot images without and, when indicated, with compression; (3) a series of large radiographic images are taken before the colon can be evacuated.
- Assure the patient that retention of the diagnostic enema preparation is comparatively easy because its flow is controlled under fluoroscopic observation.

- Instruct the patient to (1) keep the anal sphincter tightly contracted against the tubing to hold it in position and prevent leakage; (2) relax the abdominal muscles to prevent intra-abdominal pressure; and (3) concentrate on deep oral breathing to reduce the incidence of colonic spasm and resultant cramps.
- Assure the patient that the flow of the enema would be stopped for the duration of any cramping.

A patient who has not had a previous colonic examination is usually fearful of being embarrassed by inadequate draping and failure to retain the enema for the required time. The radiographer can dispel or greatly relieve the patient's anxiety by taking the following steps:

- Assure the patient that he or she will be properly covered.
- Assure the patient that although there is little chance of "mishap," he or she will be well protected, and there is no need to feel embarrassed should one occur.
- Keep a bedpan in the examining room for a patient who cannot or may not be able to make the trip to the toilet.

The preliminary preparation required for a retrograde study of the colon is strenuous for the patient. The examination itself further depletes the patient's strength. Feeble patients, particularly elderly patients, are likely to become weak and faint from the exertion of the preparation, the examination, and the effort made to expel the enema. The strenuous nature of these procedures presents an increased risk for patients with a history of heart disease. An emergency call button should be available in the lavatory so that the patient can summon help if necessary. Although the patient's privacy must be respected, the radiographer or an aide should frequently inquire to ensure that the patient is all right.

Insertion of enema tip

In preparation for insertion of the enema tip, the following steps are taken:

- Instruct the patient to turn onto the left side, roll forward about 35 to 40 degrees, and rest the flexed right knee on the table, above and in front of the slightly flexed left knee (Sims position). This position relaxes the abdominal muscles, which decreases intra-abdominal pressure on the rectum and makes relaxation of the anal sphincter less difficult.

- Adjust the IV pole so that the enema contents are no higher than 24 inches (61 cm) above the level of the anus.
- Adjust the overlapping back of the gown or other draping to expose the anal region only, but keep the patient otherwise well covered. The anal orifice is commonly partially obscured by distended hemorrhoids or a fringe of undistended hemorrhoids. Sometimes there is a contraction or other abnormality of the orifice. It is necessary for the anus to be exposed and sufficiently well lighted for the orifice to be clearly visible, so that the enema tip can be inserted without injury or discomfort.
- Run a little of the barium mixture into a waste basin to free the tubing of air, and then lubricate the rectal tube well with a water-soluble lubricant.
- Advise the patient to relax and take deep breaths so that no discomfort is felt when the tube is inserted.
- Elevate the right buttock laterally to open the gluteal fold.
- As the abdominal muscles and anal sphincter are relaxed during the expiration phase of a deep breath, insert the rectal tube gently and slowly into the anal orifice. Following the angle of the anal canal, direct the tube anteriorly 1 to 1 1/2 inches (2.5 to 3.8 cm). Then, while following the curve of the rectum, direct the tube slightly superiorly.
- Insert the tube for a total distance of no more than 4 inches (10 cm). Insertion for a greater distance not only is unnecessary but also may injure the rectum.
- If the tube cannot be entered easily, ask the patient to assist if he or she is capable.
- *Never* forcibly insert a rectal tube because the patient may have distended internal hemorrhoids or another condition that makes forced insertion of the tube dangerous.
- After the enema tip is inserted, hold it in position to prevent slipping while the patient turns to the supine or prone position for fluoroscopy, according to the preference of the fluoroscopist. The retention cuff may be inflated at this time.
- Adjust the protective underpadding and relieve any pressure on the tubing, so that the enema mixture flows freely.

SINGLE-CONTRAST BARIUM ENEMA

Administration of contrast medium

After preparing the patient for the examination, the radiographer observes the following steps:

- Notify the radiologist as soon as everything is ready for the examination.
- If the patient has not been introduced to the radiologist, make the introduction at this time.
- At the radiologist's request, release the control clip and ensure the enema flow.
- When occlusion of the enema tip occurs, displace soft fecal material by withdrawing the rectal tube about 1 inch (2.5 cm). Before reinserting the tip, temporarily elevate the enema bag to increase fluid pressure.

The rectal ampulla fills slowly. Unless the barium flow is stopped for a few seconds after the rectal ampulla is full, the suspension flows through the sigmoid and descending portions of the colon at a fairly rapid rate, frequently causing a severe cramp and acute stimulation of the defecation impulse. The flow of the barium suspension is usually stopped for several seconds at frequent intervals during fluoroscopically controlled filling of the colon.

During the fluoroscopic procedure, the radiologist rotates the patient to inspect all segments of the bowel. The radiologist takes spot images as indicated and determines the positions to be used for subsequent radiographic studies. On completion of the fluoroscopic examination, the enema tip is usually removed so the patient can be maneuvered more easily, and so the tip is not accidentally displaced during the imaging procedure. A retention tube is not removed until the patient is placed on a bedpan or the toilet.

After the needed images have been obtained (Fig. 15.104), the patient is escorted to a toilet or placed on a bedpan and is instructed to expel as much of the barium suspension as possible. A postevacuation image is then taken (Fig. 15.105). If this image shows evacuation to be inadequate for satisfactory delineation of the mucosa, the patient may be given a hot beverage (tea or coffee) to stimulate further evacuation.

Positioning of opacified colon

The most commonly obtained projections for single-contrast BE are PA or AP and PA obliques, axial for the sigmoid, and lateral to show the rectum.

Left colic flexure
Right colic flexure
Transverse colon
Descending colon
Ascending colon
Terminal ileum
Cecum
Sigmoid
Rectum
Air-filled retention tip

Fig. 15.104 Single-contrast BE image, sthenic habitus.

Fig. 15.105 Postevacuation image showing mucosal pattern *(arrows).* Hyposthenic habitus.

DOUBLE-CONTRAST BARIUM ENEMA

Two approaches to administering double-contrast BEs are currently in use. The first technique is a *two-stage procedure*, described by Welin,[19] which is detailed in the 13th and previous editions of *Merrill's Atlas*. The second approach is the *single-stage, double-contrast examination*. The popularity of this approach can be attributed primarily to more recent advancements in the manufacture of high-density barium sulfate.

Single-stage procedure

In performing the single-stage, double-contrast enema, certain requirements must be met to ensure an adequate examination. The most important requirement is that the patient's colon must be exceptionally clean. Residual fecal material can obscure small polyps or tumor masses. A second requirement is that a suitable barium suspension must be used. A barium mixture that clumps or flakes neither clearly shows the lumen nor properly drains from the colon.

Fig. 15.106 Spot images, double-contrast BE. (A) Lateral rectum. (B) Axial sigmoid. (C) Hepatic flexure. (D) Splenic flexure. (E) Cecum.

(Courtesy NEA Baptist Memorial Hospital, Jonesboro, AR.)

Currently available, premixed liquid barium products are generally more uniform for radiographic use than most barium suspensions mixed in the health care institution. A barium product with a density of 80% to 100% weight/volume may be used for a single-stage, double-contrast examination of the colon. The most important criterion is that the barium flows sufficiently to coat the walls of the colon.

With advances in the manufacture of high-density barium, high-quality double-contrast colon images can be consistently obtained during one filling of the colon. In the single-stage procedure, barium and air are instilled in a single procedure. Miller[20] described a *7-pump* method for performing single-stage, double-contrast examinations. This method reduces cost, saves time, and reduces radiation exposure to the patient. (A more complete description of the 7-pump method is provided in the seventh edition or earlier editions of this atlas.)

Barium is instilled and the patient assisted in rotating to coat the mucosal lining. Air is pumped in slowly to expand the lumen. Fluoroscopy is performed to check the location of the barium, and additional air is instilled under fluoroscopic control. The entire colon is coated and expanded with air by slowly rotating the patient into various positions while imaging every portion of the colon. The ACR recommends images be obtained to attempt to demonstrate all segments of the colon in double contrast. Suggested views include the following:
- Spot images of the rectum, sigmoid colon, both flexures, and cecum in double contrast (Fig. 15.106).
- Large format images obtained with the patient supine and prone to include the entire colon.
- An axial of the sigmoid colon.
- Lateral of the rectum, either cross-table lateral or vertical beam, preferably with the enema tip removed.
- Both lateral decubitus positions of the entire colon (Fig. 15.107).
- Both flexures imaged with the patient upright or semi-upright.
- Postevacuation image.

The ACR uses the following criteria to ensure consistent quality in double-contrast BE examinations:
- Entire colon sufficiently coated with barium.
- The colon well distended with air.
- Each portion of the colon demonstrated in double-contrast on a minimum of two images taken in different positions, whenever possible.
- Demonstration of the entire colon, proven when the ileocecal valve, terminal ileum, or appendix is seen.[21]

Fig. 15.107 (A) Right lateral decubitus position. (B) Left lateral decubitus position.

(Courtesy NEA Baptist Memorial Hospital, Jonesboro, AR.)

OPACIFIED COLON

Radiographic studies of the adult colon are made using a 14- × 17-inch (35- × 43-cm) exposure field or CR plate. Except for axial projections, these IRs may be centered at the level of the iliac crests on patients of sthenic build—higher for hypersthenic patients and lower for asthenic patients. AP and PA projections of the colon and abdomen may require two exposures, with the exposure field or CR plate crosswise: The first is centered high enough to include the diaphragm, and the second is centered low enough to include the rectum. Localized studies of the rectum and rectosigmoid junction are often exposed using a 10- × 12-inch (24-× 30-cm) exposure field or CR plate centered at or slightly above the level of the pubic symphysis. Preevacuation images of the colon include one or more images to show otherwise obscured flexed and curved areas of the large intestine.

Depending on the preference of the radiologist, the radiographic projections taken after fluoroscopy vary considerably. Any combination of the following images may be taken to complete the examination.

★ PA PROJECTION

Image receptor + grid: Positioned by manufacturer or department protocol for proper anatomy display orientation; CR plate: 14 × 17 inches (35 × 43 cm) lengthwise.

Position of patient
- Place the patient in the prone position.

Position of part
- Center the MSP to the grid.
- Adjust the center of the IR at the level of the iliac crests (Fig. 15.108).
- In addition to positioning for the PA projection, place the fluoroscopic table in a slight Trendelenburg position if necessary. This table position helps separate redundant and overlapping loops of the bowel by "spilling" them out of the pelvis.
- *Shield gonads.*
- *Respiration:* Suspend.

Central ray
- Perpendicular to the IR to enter the midline of the body at the level of the iliac crests.

Collimation
- Adjust the radiation field to no larger than 14 × 17 inches (35 × 43 cm). For smaller patients, collimate to within 1 inch (2.5 cm) of shadow of the abdomen flanks. Place side marker in the collimated exposure field.

Structures shown
The entire colon with the patient prone (Figs. 15.109–15.111).

EVALUATION CRITERIA
The following should be clearly seen:
- Evidence of proper collimation and presence of side marker placed clear of anatomy of interest
- Entire colon including the flexures and the rectum (two images may be necessary for hypersthenic patients)
- Vertebral column centered so that ascending and descending portions of the colon are included
- Penetration of the contrast medium

Fig. 15.108 PA large intestine.

Fig. 15.109 Single-contrast PA large intestine.

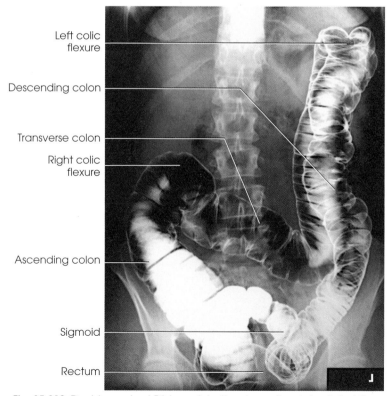

Left colic
flexure

Descending colon

Transverse colon

Right colic
flexure

Ascending colon

Sigmoid

Rectum

Fig. 15.110 Double-contrast PA large intestine, hyposthenic body habitus.

Fig. 15.111 Postevacuation PA large intestine. *Arrows* mark mucosal patterns evident in postevacuation images.

🐦 PA AXIAL PROJECTION

Image receptor + grid: Positioned by manufacturer or department protocol for proper anatomy display orientation; CR plate: 10 × 12 inches (24 × 30 cm) or 14 × 17 inches (35 × 43 cm) lengthwise.

Position of patient

- Place the patient in the prone position.

Position of part

- Center the MSP to the grid.
- Adjust the center of the IR at the level of the iliac crests (Fig. 15.112).
- *Shield gonads.*
- *Respiration:* Suspend.

Central ray

- Directed 30 to 40 degrees caudad to enter the midline of the body at the level of the anterior superior iliac spine (ASIS).

Collimation

- Adjust the radiation field to no larger than 14 × 17 inches (35 × 43 cm) or 10 × 12 inches (24 × 30). Place side marker in the collimated exposure field.

Structures shown

The rectosigmoid area of the colon (Figs. 15.113 and 15.114).

NOTE: This axial projection is sometimes performed with the patient in the RAO position, to further reduce superimposition in the rectosigmoid area.

The following should be clearly seen:

- Evidence of proper collimation and presence of side marker placed clear of anatomy of interest
- Rectosigmoid area centered to image when a 10- × 12-inch (24- × 30-cm) exposure field/IR is used
- Rectosigmoid area with less superimposition than in PA projection because of angulation of the central ray
- Transverse colon and both flexures not always included
- Penetration of the contrast medium

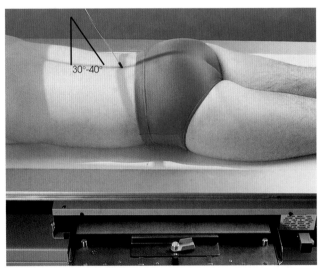

Fig. 15.112 PA axial large intestine.

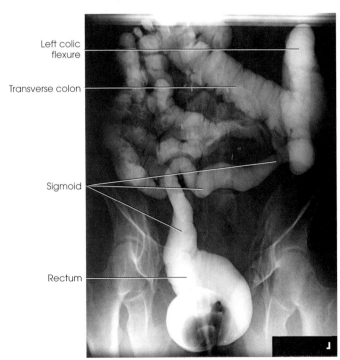

Left colic flexure

Transverse colon

Sigmoid

Rectum

Fig. 15.113 Single-contrast PA axial (30-degree angulation) large intestine.

Fig. 15.114 Double-contrast PA axial (40-degree angulation) large intestine.

⚜ PA OBLIQUE PROJECTION
RAO position

Image receptor + grid: Positioned by manufacturer or department protocol for proper anatomy display orientation; CR plate: 14 × 17 inches (35 × 43 cm) lengthwise.

Position of patient
• Place the patient in the prone position.

Position of part
• With the patient's right arm by the side of the body and the left hand by the head, have the patient roll onto the right hip to obtain a 35- to 45-degree rotation from the radiographic table.
• Flex the patient's left knee to provide stability.
• Center the patient's body to the midline of the grid.
• Adjust the center of the IR at the level of the iliac crests (Fig. 15.115).
• *Shield gonads.*
• *Respiration:* suspend.

Central ray
• Perpendicular to the IR and entering approximately 1 to 2 inches (2.5 to 5 cm) lateral to the midline of the body on the elevated side at the level of the iliac crest.

Collimation
• Adjust the radiation field to no larger than 14 × 17 inches (35 × 43 cm). For smaller patients, collimate to within 1 inch (2.5 cm) of shadow of the abdomen flanks. Place side marker in the collimated exposure field.

Structures shown
The right colic flexure, the ascending portion of the colon, and the sigmoid portion of the colon (Figs. 15.116 and 15.117).

The following should be clearly seen:
■ Evidence of proper collimation and presence of side marker placed clear of anatomy of interest
■ Entire colon
■ Right colic flexure less superimposed or open compared with the PA projection
■ Ascending colon, cecum, and sigmoid colon
■ Penetration of the contrast media

Fig. 15.115 PA oblique large intestine, RAO position.

Fig. 15.116 Single-contrast PA oblique large intestine, RAO position.

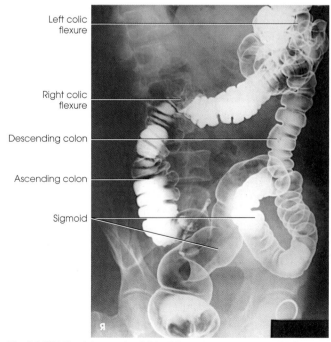

Left colic flexure

Right colic flexure

Descending colon

Ascending colon

Sigmoid

Fig. 15.117 Double-contrast PA oblique large intestine, RAO position.

⚜ PA OBLIQUE PROJECTION
LAO position

Image receptor + grid: Positioned by manufacturer or department protocol for proper anatomy display orientation; CR plate: 14 × 17 inches (35 × 43 cm) lengthwise.

Position of patient
• Place the patient in the prone position.

Position of part
• With the patient's left arm by the side of the body and the right hand by the head, have the patient roll onto the left hip to obtain a 35- to 45-degree rotation from the radiographic table.
• Flex the patient's right knee to provide stability.
• Center the patient's body to the midline of the grid.
• Adjust the center of the IR at the level of the iliac crest (Fig. 15.118).
• *Shield gonads.*
• *Respiration*: Suspend.

Central ray
• Perpendicular to the IR and entering approximately 1 to 2 inches (2.5 to 5 cm) lateral to the midline of the body on the elevated side at the level of the iliac crest.

Collimation
• Adjust the radiation field to no larger than 14 × 17 inches (35 × 43 cm). For smaller patients, collimate to within 1 inch (2.5 cm) of shadow of the abdomen flanks. Place side marker in the collimated exposure field.

Structures shown
The left colic flexure and the descending portion of the colon (Figs. 15.119 and 15.120).

The following should be clearly seen:
■ Evidence of proper collimation and presence of side marker placed clear of anatomy of interest
■ Entire colon
■ Left colic flexure less superimposed or open compared with the PA projection
■ Descending colon
■ Penetration of the contrast medium

Fig. 15.118 PA oblique large intestine, LAO position.

Fig. 15.119 Single-contrast PA oblique large intestine, LAO position.

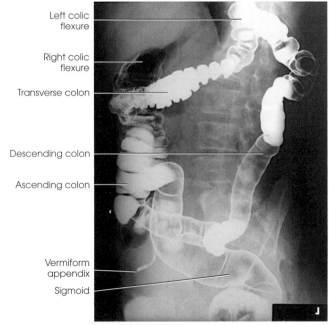

Left colic flexure

Right colic flexure

Transverse colon

Descending colon

Ascending colon

Vermiform appendix

Sigmoid

Fig. 15.120 Double-contrast PA oblique large intestine, LAO position.

⋏ LATERAL PROJECTION
Right or left position

Image receptor + grid: Positioned by manufacturer or department protocol for proper anatomy display orientation; CR plate: 10 × 12 inches (24 × 30 cm) lengthwise.

Position of patient
- Place the patient in the lateral recumbent position on the left or the right side.

Position of part
- Center the midcoronal plane to the center of the grid.
- Flex the patient's knees slightly for stability, and place a support between the knees to keep the pelvis lateral.
- Adjust the patient's shoulders and hips to be perpendicular (Fig. 15.121).
- Adjust the center of the IR to the ASIS.
- *Shield gonads.*
- *Respiration*: Suspend.

Central ray
- Perpendicular to the IR to enter the midcoronal plane at the level of the ASIS.

Collimation
- Adjust the radiation field to no larger than 10 × 12 inches (24 × 30 cm). Place side marker in the collimated exposure field.

Structures shown
The rectum and the distal sigmoid portion of the colon (Figs. 15.122 and 15.123).

EVALUATION CRITERIA
The following should be clearly seen:
- Evidence of proper collimation and presence of side marker placed clear of anatomy of interest
- Rectosigmoid area in the center of the image
- No rotation of the patient
- Superimposed hips and femora
- Superior portion of colon not included when the rectosigmoid region is the area of interest
- Penetration of the contrast medium

Fig. 15.121 Left lateral rectum.

Sigmoid
Sacrum
Rectum
Pubic symphysis

Fig. 15.122 Single-contrast left lateral rectum.

Fig. 15.123 Double-contrast left lateral rectum.

✿ AP PROJECTION

Image receptor + grid: Positioned by manufacturer or department protocol or proper anatomy display orientation; CR plate: 14 × 17 inches (35 × 43 cm) lengthwise.

Position of patient
• Place the patient in the supine position.

Position of part
• Center the MSP to the grid.
• Adjust the center of the IR at the level of the iliac crests (Fig. 15.124).
• *Shield gonads.*
• *Respiration*: suspend.

Central ray
• Perpendicular to the IR to enter the midline of the body at the level of the iliac crests.

Collimation
• Adjust the radiation field to no larger than 14 × 17 inches (35 × 43 cm). For smaller patients, collimate to within 1 inch (2.5 cm) of shadow of the abdomen flanks. Place side marker in the collimated exposure field.

Structures shown
The entire colon with the patient supine (Figs. 15.125 and 15.126).

EVALUATION CRITERIA

The following should be clearly seen:
■ Evidence of proper collimation and presence of side marker placed clear of anatomy of interest
■ Entire colon including the splenic flexure and the rectum (two images may be necessary for hypersthenic patients)
■ Vertebral column centered so that the ascending colon and the descending colon are completely included
■ Penetration of the contrast medium

Fig. 15.124 AP large intestine.

Fig. 15.125 Single-contrast AP large intestine, sthenic habitus.

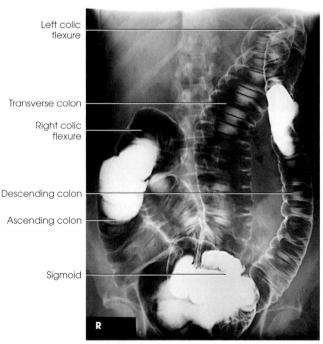

Left colic flexure

Transverse colon

Right colic flexure

Descending colon

Ascending colon

Sigmoid

Fig. 15.126 Double-contrast AP large intestine, asthenic habitus.

Digestive System: Salivary Glands, Alimentary Canal, and Biliary System

✤ AP AXIAL PROJECTION

Image receptor + grid: Positioned by manufacturer or department protocol for proper anatomy display orientation; CR plate: 10 × 12 inches (24 × 30 cm) or 14 × 17 inches (35 × 43 cm) lengthwise.

Position of patient
• Place the patient in the supine position.

Position of part
• Center the MSP to the grid.
• Adjust the center of the IR at a level approximately 2 inches (5 cm) above the level of the iliac crests (Fig. 15.127).
• *Shield gonads.*
• *Respiration*: Suspend.

Central ray
• Directed 30 to 40 degrees cephalad to enter the midline of the body approximately 2 inches (5 cm) below the level of the ASIS.
• Directed to enter the inferior margin of the pubic symphysis when a collimated image is desired to show the rectosigmoid region.

Collimation
• Adjust the radiation field to no larger than 14 × 17 inches (35 × 43 cm) or 10 × 12 inches (24 × 30 cm). Place side marker in the collimated exposure field.

Structures shown
The rectosigmoid area of the colon (Figs. 15.128 and 15.129). A similar image is obtained when the patient is prone (see Figs. 15.113 and 15.114).

NOTE: This axial projection is sometimes performed with the patient in the LPO position, to further reduce superimposition in the rectosigmoid area.

The following should be clearly seen:
■ Evidence of proper collimation and presence of side marker placed clear of anatomy of interest
■ Rectosigmoid area centered when a 10- × 12-inch (24- × 30-cm) IR is used
■ Rectosigmoid area with less superimposition than in the AP projection because of the angulation of the central ray
■ Transverse colon and flexures not included
■ Penetration of the contrast medium

Fig. 15.127 AP axial large intestine.

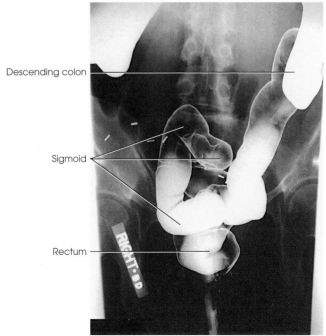

Fig. 15.128 Single-contrast AP axial large intestine.

Fig. 15.129 Double-contrast AP axial large intestine.

Descending colon

Sigmoid

Rectum

🌟 AP OBLIQUE PROJECTION
LPO position

Image receptor + grid: Positioned by manufacturer or department protocol for proper anatomy display orientation; CR plate: 14 × 17 inches (35 × 43 cm) lengthwise.

Position of patient
• Place the patient in the supine position.

Position of part
• With the patient's left arm by the side of the body and the right arm across the superior chest, have the patient roll onto the left hip to obtain a 35- to 45-degree rotation from the table.
• Use a positioning sponge and flex the patient's right knee for stability, if necessary.
• Center the patient's body to the midline of the grid.
• Adjust the center of the IR at the level of the iliac crests (Fig. 15.130).
• *Shield gonads.*
• *Respiration*: Suspend.

Central ray
• Perpendicular to the IR to enter approximately 1 to 2 inches (2.5 to 5 cm) lateral to the midline of the body on the elevated side at the level of the iliac crest.

Collimation
• Adjust the radiation field to no larger than 14 × 17 inches (35 × 43 cm). For smaller patients, collimate to within 1 inch (2.5 cm) of shadow of the abdomen flanks. Place side marker in the collimated exposure field.

Structures shown
The right colic flexure and the ascending and sigmoid portions of the colon (Figs. 15.131 and 15.132).

The following should be clearly seen:
■ Evidence of proper collimation and presence of side marker placed clear of anatomy of interest
■ Entire colon
■ Right colic flexure less superimposed or open compared with the AP projection
■ Ascending colon, cecum, and sigmoid colon
■ Penetration of the contrast medium

Fig. 15.130 AP oblique large intestine, LPO position.

Fig. 15.131 Single-contrast AP oblique large intestine, LPO position.

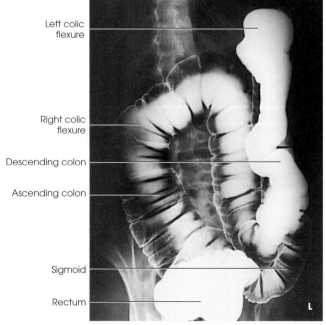

Left colic flexure

Right colic flexure

Descending colon

Ascending colon

Sigmoid

Rectum

Fig. 15.132 Double-contrast AP oblique large intestine, LPO position.

⚚ AP OBLIQUE PROJECTION
RPO position

Image receptor + grid: Positioned by manufacturer or department protocol for proper anatomy display orientation; CR plate: 14 × 17 inches (35 × 43 cm) lengthwise.

Position of patient
- Place the patient in the supine position.

Position of part
- With the patient's right arm by the side of the body and the left arm across the superior chest, have the patient roll onto the right hip to obtain a 35- to 45-degree rotation from the radiographic table.
- Use a positioning sponge and flex the patient's right knee for stability, if needed.
- Center the patient's body to the midline of the grid.
- Adjust the center of the IR at the level of the iliac crests (Fig. 15.133).
- *Shield gonads.*
- *Respiration:* suspend.

Central ray
- Perpendicular to the IR to enter approximately 1 to 2 inches (2.5 to 5 cm) lateral to the midline of the body on the elevated side at the level of the iliac crest.

Collimation
- Adjust the radiation field to no larger than 14 × 17 inches (35 × 43 cm). For smaller patients, collimate to within 1 inch (2.5 cm) of shadow of the abdomen flanks. Place side marker in the collimated exposure field.

Structures shown
The left colic flexure and the descending colon (Figs. 15.134 and 15.135).

The following should be clearly seen:
- Evidence of proper collimation and presence of side marker placed clear of anatomy of interest
- Entire colon
- Left colic flexure and descending colon
- Penetration of the contrast medium

Fig. 15.133 AP oblique large intestine, RPO position.

Fig. 15.134 Single-contrast AP oblique large intestine, RPO position.

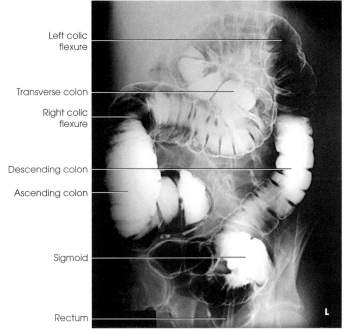

Left colic flexure

Transverse colon

Right colic flexure

Descending colon

Ascending colon

Sigmoid

Rectum

Fig. 15.135 Double-contrast AP oblique large intestine, RPO position.

Decubitus Positions

When a patient is being prepared for an examination in a decubitus position, the following general guidelines are observed:

- Take all decubitus images (1) with the patient lying on the fluoroscopic table and a grid IR firmly supported behind the patient's body; (2) with the patient lying on a patient cart with the body against an upright table or chest device; or (3) with the patient lying on a table or cart and a specially designed vertical grid device behind the patient.

- To ensure that the side on which the patient is lying is shown, elevate the patient on a suitable radiolucent support. If this is not done, the image records artifacts from the mattress or from the table edge and superimposes these images over the portion of the patient's colon on the "down" side.

- For all decubitus procedures, *exercise extreme caution* to ensure that the *wheels of the cart are securely locked* so that the patient will not fall.

- For lateral decubitus images, have the patient put the back or abdomen against the vertical grid device. Most patients find it more comfortable to have their back against the vertical grid device than to have their abdomen against the same device.

- If both lateral decubitus images are requested (which is often the case with air-contrast examinations), take one image with the patient's anterior body surface against the vertical grid device and the second image with the posterior body surface against the vertical grid device.

Digestive System: Salivary Glands, Alimentary Canal, and Biliary System

⚑ AP OR PA PROJECTION
Right lateral decubitus position

Image receptor + grid: Positioned by manufacturer or department protocol for proper anatomy display orientation; CR plate: 14 × 17 inches (35 × 43 cm) lengthwise.

Position of patient
- Place the patient on the right side with the back or abdomen in contact with the vertical grid device.
- *Exercise care* to ensure that the patient does not fall from the cart or table; if a cart is used, *lock all wheels* securely.

Position of part
- With the patient lying on an elevated radiolucent support, center the MSP to the grid.
- Adjust the center of the IR to the level of the iliac crests (Fig. 15.136).
- *Shield gonads.*
- *Respiration*: Suspend.

Central ray
- *Horizontal* and perpendicular to the IR to enter the midline of the body at the level of the iliac crests.

Collimation
- Adjust the radiation field to no larger than 14 × 17 inches (35 × 43 cm). For smaller patients, collimate to within 1 inch (2.5 cm) of shadow of the abdomen flanks. Place side marker in the collimated exposure field.

Fig. 15.136 AP large intestine, right lateral decubitus position.

Structures shown

The right lateral decubitus position shows an AP or PA projection of the contrast-filled colon. This position best shows the "up" medial side of the ascending colon and the lateral side of the descending colon when the colon is inflated with air (Figs. 15.137 and 15.138).

The following should be clearly seen:
- Evidence of proper collimation and presence of side marker placed clear of anatomy of interest
- Area from the left colic flexure to the rectum
- No rotation of the patient, as demonstrated by symmetry of the ribs and pelvis

- For single-contrast examinations, adequate penetration of the barium; for double-contrast examinations, the air-inflated portion of the colon is of primary importance and should not be overpenetrated

◤ COMPENSATING FILTER

Image quality can be improved on larger patients with the use of a special decubitus filter.

Fig. 15.137 Double-contrast AP large intestine, right lateral decubitus position.

Fig. 15.138 Double-contrast AP large intestine, right lateral decubitus position.

Left colic flexure

Sigmoid

Transverse colon

Right colic flexure

⚕ PA OR AP PROJECTION
Left lateral decubitus position

Image receptor + grid: Positioned by manufacturer or department protocol for proper anatomy display orientation; CR plate: 14 × 17 inches (35 × 43 cm) lengthwise.

Position of patient
- Place the patient on the left side with the abdomen or back in contact with the vertical grid device.
- *Exercise care* to ensure that the patient does not fall from the cart or table; if a cart is used, *lock all wheels* securely in position.

Position of part
- With the patient lying on an elevated radiolucent support, center the MSP to the grid.
- Adjust the center of the IR at the level of the iliac crests (Fig. 15.139).
- *Shield gonads.*
- *Respiration*: Suspend.

Central ray
- *Horizontal* and perpendicular to the IR to enter the midline of the body at the level of the iliac crests.

Collimation
- Adjust the radiation field to no larger than 14 × 17 inches (35 × 43 cm). For smaller patients, collimate to within 1 inch (2.5 cm) of shadow of the abdomen flanks. Place side marker in the collimated exposure field.

Fig. 15.139 PA large intestine, left lateral decubitus position.

Structures shown

The left lateral decubitus position shows a PA or AP projection of the contrast-filled colon. This position best shows the "up" lateral side of the ascending colon and the medial side of the descending colon when the colon is inflated with air (Figs. 15.140 and 15.141).

The following should be clearly seen:
- Evidence of proper collimation and presence of side marker placed clear of anatomy of interest
- Area from the left colic flexure to the rectum
- No rotation of the patient, as demonstrated by symmetry of the ribs and pelvis
- For single-contrast examinations, adequate penetration of the barium; for double-contrast examinations, the air-inflated portion of the colon is of primary importance and should not be overpenetrated

Fig. 15.140 Double-contrast PA large intestine, left lateral decubitus position.

Fig. 15.141 Double-contrast PA large intestine, left lateral decubitus position.

Large Intestine

LATERAL PROJECTION
Right or left ventral decubitus position

Image receptor + grid: Positioned by manufacturer or department protocol for proper anatomy display orientation; CR plate: 14 × 17 inches (35 × 43 cm) lengthwise.

Position of patient
- Place the patient in the prone position with the right side or the left side against the vertical grid device.

Position of part
- Elevate the patient on a radiolucent support, and center the midcoronal plane to the grid.
- Adjust the center of the IR at the level of the iliac crests (Fig. 15.142A).
- *Shield gonads.*
- *Respiration:* Suspend.

Central ray
- *Horizontal* and perpendicular to the IR to enter the midcoronal plane of the body at the level of the iliac crests.

Collimation
- Adjust the radiation field to no larger than 14 × 17 inches (35 × 43 cm). For smaller patients, collimate to within 1 inch (2.5 cm) of shadow of the skin. Place side marker in the collimated exposure field.

Structures shown
The ventral decubitus position shows a lateral projection of the contrast-filled colon. This position best shows the "up" posterior portions of the colon and is most valuable in double-contrast examinations (see Fig. 15.142B).

The following should be clearly seen:
- Evidence of proper collimation and presence of side marker placed clear of anatomy of interest
- Area from the flexures to the rectum
- No rotation of the patient
- For single-contrast examinations, adequate penetration of the barium; for double-contrast examinations, the air-inflated portion of the colon is of primary importance and should not be overpenetrated
- Enema tip removed for an unobstructed image of the rectum (see Fig. 15.142C)

Left colic flexure
Rectum
Descending colon

Sigmoid
Right colic flexure
Transverse colon

Transverse colon
Ascending colon

xtable

200 mm

Fig. 15.142 (A) Patient in position for lateral projection, ventral decubitus position. (B) Left lateral large intestine, ventral decubitus position. (C) Lateral rectum, ventral decubitus position (enema tip removed).

AP, PA, OBLIQUE, AND LATERAL PROJECTIONS

Upright position

Upright AP, PA, oblique, and lateral projections may be taken as requested. The positioning and evaluation criteria for upright images are identical to criteria required for the recumbent positions. The IR is placed at a lower level, however, to compensate for the drop of the bowel caused by the effect of gravity (Figs. 15.143 through 15.145).

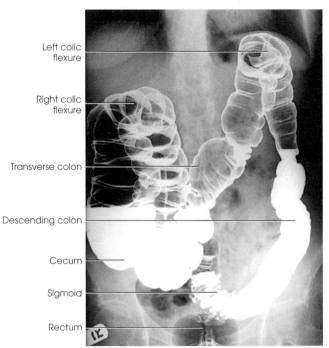

Left colic flexure
Right colic flexure
Transverse colon
Descending colon
Cecum
Sigmoid
Rectum

Fig. 15.143 Upright double-contrast AP large intestine.

Fig. 15.144 Upright double-contrast PA large intestine.

Fig. 15.145 Upright double-contrast AP oblique large intestine, RPO position.

COLOSTOMY STUDIES

Enterostomy (Greek *enteron,* "intestine" + *stoma,* "opening") is the general term applied to the surgical procedure of forming an artificial opening to the intestine, usually through the abdominal wall, for fecal passage. The regional terms are *colostomy, cecostomy, ileostomy,* and *jejunostomy.*

The colon is the most common site of disease in the large intestine, and surgical procedures are often performed on this structure. Loop colostomy is sometimes performed to divert the fecal column, temporarily or permanently, from areas of diverticulitis or ulcerative colitis. Most colostomies are performed because of malignancies of the lower bowel and rectum. When a tumor is present, the lower carcinomatous part of the bowel is resected, and the end of the remaining part of the bowel is brought to the surface through the abdominal wall. This passage, or *stoma,* has no sphincter.

Preparation of intestinal tract

Postoperative contrast enema studies are performed at suitable intervals to allow the clinician to determine the efficacy of treatment in a patient with diverticulitis or ulcerative colitis and to detect new or recurrent lesions in a patient who has had a tumor. Adequate cleansing of the bowel, which is as important in the presence of a colostomy as otherwise, is crucial to show polyps and other intraluminal lesions. In a patient with a colostomy, the usual preparation is irrigation of the stoma the night before the study and again on the morning of the examination.

Colostomy enema equipment

Although equipment must be scrupulously clean, and nondisposable items must be sterilized after each use, sterile technique is not required because the stoma is part of the intestinal tract. Except for a suitable device to prevent stomal leakage of contrast material, the equipment used in a patient with a colostomy is the same as that used in routine contrast enema studies. The same barium sulfate formula is used, and gas studies are made. Opaque and double-contrast studies can be performed in a single-stage examination with use of a disposable enema kit.

A device must be used to prevent spillage of contrast enema material in a patient with a colostomy. Otherwise, because of the absence of sphincter control, the contrast enema may escape through the colostomy almost as rapidly as it is injected. If this happens, bowel filling is unsatisfactory, and shadows cast by barium soilage of the abdominal wall and the examining table obscure areas of interest. Abdominal stomas must be effectively occluded for studies made by retrograde injection, and leakage around the stomal catheter must be prevented for studies made by injection into an abdominal or a perineal colostomy. Numerous devices are available for this purpose.

DIAGNOSTIC ENEMA

Diagnostic enemas may be given through a colostomy stoma with the use of tips and adhesive disks designed for the patient's use in irrigating the colostomy (Fig. 15.146). These tips are available in four sizes to accommodate the usual sizes of colostomy stomas. The tips usually have a flange to prevent them from slipping through the colostomy opening. An adhesive disk is placed over the flange to minimize reflux soilage. The enema tubing is attached directly to the tip, which the patient holds in position to prevent the weight of the tubing from displacing the tip to an angled position. In addition to keeping a set of Laird tips on hand, it is recommended that the patient be asked to bring an irrigation device.

Retention catheters or Foley catheters are also used in colostomy studies. Some radiologists use them alone, and others insert them through a device to prevent slipping and to collect leakage. Colostomy stomas are fragile and are subject to perforation by any undue pressure or trauma. Perforations have occurred during insertion of an inflated bulb into a blind pouch and as the result of overdistention of the stoma.

Fig. 15.146 Colostomy irrigation system with tip and stoma adhesive disk.

Preparation of patient

If the patient uses a special dressing, colostomy pouch, or stomal seal, he or she should be advised to bring a change for use after the examination. When fecal emission is such that a pouch is required, the patient should be given a suitable dressing to place over the stoma after the device has been removed.

The radiographer observes the following steps:

- Clothe the patient in a kimono type of gown that opens in front or back, depending on the location of the colostomy.

- Place the patient on the examining table in the supine position if he or she has an abdominal colostomy and in the prone position if he or she has a perineal colostomy.

- Before taking the preliminary image and while wearing disposable gloves, remove and discard any dressing.

- Cleanse the skin around the stoma appropriately.

- Place a gauze dressing over the stoma to absorb any seepage until the physician is ready to start the examination.

- Lubricate the stomal catheter or tube well (but not excessively) with a water-soluble lubricant. The catheter should be inserted by the physician or the patient. If a catheter is forced through a stoma, the colon may be perforated.

Spot images are taken during the examination. Postfluoroscopy images are taken as needed. The projections requested depend on the location of the stoma and the anatomy to be shown (Figs. 15.147 through 15.150).

Fig. 15.147 Opaque colon via perineal colostomy.

Fig. 15.148 Opaque colon via abdominal colostomy.

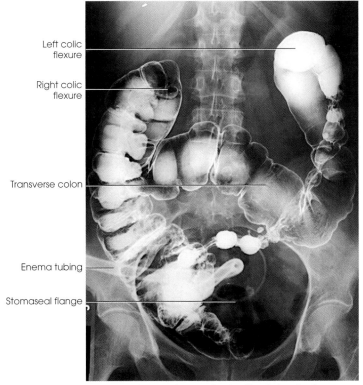

Left colic flexure

Right colic flexure

Transverse colon

Enema tubing

Stomaseal flange

Fig. 15.149 Double-contrast colon in a patient with abdominal colostomy.

Fig. 15.150 Double-contrast AP oblique colon via abdominal colostomy.

Large Intestine

DEFECOGRAPHY

Defecography, evacuation proctography, or *dynamic rectal examination* is a radiologic procedure performed on patients with defecation dysfunction. No preparation of the patient is necessary, and cleansing enemas are not recommended because water remaining in the rectum dilutes the contrast medium.

Early investigators[22] mixed a diluted suspension of barium sulfate, heated it, and added potato starch to form a smooth barium paste that was semisolid and malleable.[23,24] Barium manufacturers now package prepared barium products (100% weight/volume barium sulfate paste) with a special injector mechanism to instill barium directly into the rectum. In addition, viscous barium may be introduced into the vagina and the bladder filled with aqueous iodinated contrast media.

After the contrast medium is instilled, the patient is usually seated in the lateral position on a commercially available radiolucent commode in front of a fluoroscopic unit. A special commode chair is recommended so that the anorectal junction and the zone of interest on the image are not overexposed. Lateral projections are obtained during defecation by spot imaging at the approximate rate of 1 to 2 frames per second. Video recording of the defecation process may be used, but the special equipment necessary to interpret the images is not always available, and a hard copy of the images is unavailable.[25] The resulting images are then evaluated (Fig. 15.151). This evaluation includes measurements of the anorectal angle and the angle between the long axes of the anal canal and rectum. These measurements are compared with normal values. In addition, changes in proximity of the rectum to the vagina and bladder during defecation are assessed when these structures have been filled with contrast media (Fig. 15.152).

Fig. 15.151 Defecography. Lateral anus and rectum spot image showing long axis of anal canal *(line A-B)* and long axis of rectal canal *(line B-C)* in a patient with anorectal angle of 114 degrees. Anterior rectocele *(arrow)* also is shown.

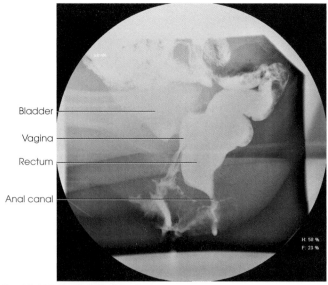

Fig. 15.152 Defecography. Lateral anal canal and rectum, vagina, and urinary bladder shown during patient straining.

(Courtesy Michelle Alting, AS, RT(R).)

Several techniques can be used to examine the gallbladder and the biliary ductal system. In many institutions, sonography is the modality of choice. This section of the atlas discusses the radiographic techniques currently available.

Table 15.1 lists some of the prefixes associated with the biliary system. *Cholegraphy* is the general term for a radiographic study of the biliary system. More specific terms can be used to describe the portion of the biliary system under investigation. *Cholecystography* is the radiographic investigation of the gallbladder, and *cholangiography* is the radiographic study of the biliary ducts.

Advances in sonography, CT, MRI, and nuclear medicine have reduced the radiographic examination of the biliary tract primarily to direct injection procedures including percutaneous transhepatic cholangiography (PTC), postoperative (T-tube) cholangiography, and endoscopic retrograde cholangiopancreatography (ERCP). The contrast agent selected for use in direct-injection techniques may be any one of the water-soluble iodinated compounds employed for intravenous urography.

TABLE 15.1

Biliary system combining forms

Root forms	Meaning
Chole-	Relationship with bile
Cysto-	Bag or sac
Choledocho-	Common bile duct
Cholangio-	Bile ducts
Cholecyst-	Gallbladder

Fig. 15.153 PTC with Chiba needle *(arrow)* in position, showing dilated biliary ducts.

Percutaneous Transhepatic Cholangiography

PTC[26] is another technique employed for preoperative radiologic examination of the biliary tract. This technique is used for patients with jaundice when the ductal system has been shown to be dilated by CT or sonography, but the cause of the obstruction is unclear. Performance of this examination has greatly increased because of the availability of the Chiba ("skinny") needle. In addition, PTC is often used to place a drainage catheter for treatment of obstructive jaundice. When a drainage catheter is used, diagnostic and drainage techniques are performed at the same time.

Fig. 15.154 PTC showing obstruction stone at ampulla *(arrow)*.

Fig. 15.155 PTC showing stenosis *(arrow)* of common hepatic duct caused by trauma.

PTC is performed by placing the patient on the radiographic table in the supine position. The patient's right side is surgically prepared and appropriately draped. After a local anesthetic is administered, the Chiba needle is held parallel to the floor and inserted through the right lateral intercostal space and advanced toward the liver hilum. The stylet of the needle is withdrawn, and a syringe filled with contrast medium is attached to the needle. Under fluoroscopic control, the needle is slowly withdrawn until contrast medium is seen to fill the biliary ducts. In most instances, the biliary tree is readily located because the ducts are generally dilated. After the biliary ducts are filled, the needle is completely withdrawn, and serial or spot AP projections of the biliary area are taken (Figs. 15.153 through 15.155).

BILIARY DRAINAGE PROCEDURE AND STONE EXTRACTION

If dilated biliary ducts are identified by CT, PTC, or sonography, the radiologist, after consultation with the referring physician, may elect to place a drainage catheter in the biliary duct.[27,28] A needle larger than the Chiba needle used in the PTC procedure is inserted through the lateral abdominal wall and into the biliary duct. A guidewire is passed through the lumen of the needle, and the needle is removed. After the catheter is passed over the guidewire, the wire is removed, leaving the catheter in place.

The catheter can be left in place for prolonged drainage, or it can be used for attempts to extract retained stones if they are identified. Retained stones are extracted using a wire basket and a small balloon catheter under fluoroscopic control. This extraction procedure is usually attempted after the catheter has been in place for some time (Figs. 15.156 and 15.157).

Right hepatic duct

Catheter

Drainage catheter in common bile duct

Contrast "spill" into duodenum

Tip of catheter

Fig. 15.156 PTC with drainage catheter in place.

Fig. 15.157 Post-PTC image showing wire basket *(arrow)* around retained stone.

Postoperative (T-Tube) Cholangiography

Postoperative, delayed, and *T-tube cholangiography* are radiologic terms applied to the biliary tract examination that is performed via a T-shaped or pigtail-shaped catheter left in the common hepatic and common bile ducts for postoperative drainage (Fig. 15.158). A pigtail catheter is required for laparoscopic biliary procedures because it can be placed percutaneously. The T-tube catheter can be placed only during an open surgical procedure. This examination is performed to show the caliber and patency of the ducts, the status of the sphincter of the hepatopancreatic ampulla, and the presence of residual or previously undetected stones or other pathologic conditions.

Postoperative cholangiography is performed in the radiology department. Preliminary preparation usually consists of the following:

1. The drainage tube is clamped the day before the examination to let the tube fill with bile as a preventive measure against air bubbles entering the ducts, where they would simulate cholesterol stones.
2. The preceding meal is withheld.
3. When indicated, a cleansing enema is administered about 1 hour before the examination. Premedication is not required.

The contrast agent used is one of the water-soluble iodinated contrast media. The density of the contrast medium used in postoperative cholangiograms is recommended to be no greater than 25% to 30% because small stones may be obscured with a higher concentration.

After a preliminary image of the abdomen has been obtained, the patient is adjusted in the RPO position (AP oblique projection) with the RUQ of the abdomen centered to the midline of the grid (Fig. 15.159).

Right hepatic duct

Hepatic duct

T-tube

Common bile duct

Pancreatic duct

Contrast medium in duodenum

Fig. 15.158 (A) Postoperative cholangiogram with T-tube catheter. (B) Postoperative cholangiogram with pigtail catheter.

With universal precautions employed, the contrast medium is injected under fluoroscopic control, and spot and conventional images are made as indicated. Otherwise, 10- × 12-inch (24- × 30-cm) exposure field or CR plates are exposed serially after each of several fractional injections of the medium and then at specified intervals until most of the contrast solution has entered the duodenum.

Stern et al.[29] stressed the importance of obtaining a lateral projection to show anatomic branching of the hepatic ducts in this plane and to detect any abnormality not otherwise shown (Fig. 15.160). The clamp generally is not removed from the T-tube before the examination is completed. The patient may be turned onto the right side for this study.

Fig. 15.159 AP oblique postoperative cholangiogram, RPO position, showing multiple stones in common bile duct *(arrows)*.

Fig. 15.160 Right lateral cholangiogram showing AP location of T-tube *(dots)*, common bile duct *(arrow)*, and hepatopancreatic ampulla (duct of Vater) *(arrowhead)*.

Biliary Tract and Pancreatic Duct

Endoscopic Retrograde Cholangiopancreatography

ERCP is a procedure used to diagnose biliary and pancreatic pathologic conditions. ERCP is a useful diagnostic method when the biliary ducts are not dilated and when no obstruction exists at the ampulla.

ERCP is performed by passing a fiberoptic endoscope through the mouth into the duodenum under fluoroscopic control. To ease passage of the endoscope, the patient's throat is sprayed with a local anesthetic. Because this causes temporary pharyngeal paresis, food and drink are usually prohibited for at least 1 hour after the examination. Food may be withheld for 10 hours after the procedure to minimize irritation to the stomach and small bowel.

After the endoscopist locates the hepatopancreatic ampulla (ampulla of Vater), a small cannula is passed through the endoscope and directed into the ampulla (Fig. 15.161). When the cannula is properly placed, a water-soluble, iodinated contrast medium is injected into the common bile duct. The patient may then be moved, fluoroscopy performed, and spot images taken (Figs. 15.162 and 15.163). Oblique spot images may be taken to prevent overlap of the common bile duct and the pancreatic duct. Because the injected contrast material should drain from normal ducts within approximately 5 minutes, images must be exposed immediately.

The contrast medium that is used depends on the preference of the radiologist or gastroenterologist. Dense contrast agents opacify small ducts well, but they may obscure small stones. If small stones are suspected, use of a more dilute contrast medium is suggested.[30] A history of patient sensitivity to an iodinated contrast medium in another examination (e.g., intravenous urography) does not contraindicate its use for ERCP. The patient must be watched carefully, however, for a reaction to the contrast medium during ERCP.

ERCP is often indicated when clinical and radiographic findings indicate abnormalities in the biliary system or pancreas. Sonography of the upper part of the abdomen before endoscopy is often recommended to assure the physician that no pancreatic pseudocysts are present. This step is important because contrast medium injected into pseudocysts may lead to inflammation or rupture.

Fig. 15.161 Cannulation procedure. Procedure is begun with the patient in left lateral position. This schematic diagram gives an overview of location of the examiner and position of scope and its relationship to various internal organs. *Inset:* Magnified view of tip of scope with cannula in papilla.

(From Stewart ET, Vennes JA, Geenen JE. *Atlas of endoscopic retrograde cholangiopancreatography.* St Louis: Mosby; 1977.)

Common hepatic duct

Pancreatic duct

Cystic stump

Common bile duct

Endoscope

Fig. 15.162 ERCP spot image, PA projection.

Pancreatic duct

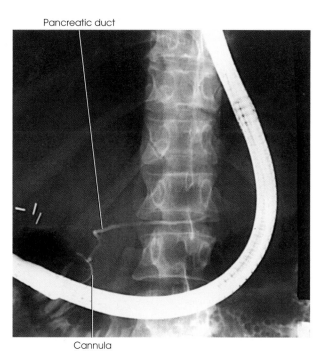

Cannula

Fig. 15.163 ERCP spot image, PA projection.

To show radiographically the origin and extent of fistulae (abnormal passages, usually between two internal organs) and sinuses (abnormal channels leading to abscesses), the following steps are taken:

- Fill the tract with a radiopaque contrast medium, usually under fluoroscopic control.
- Obtain right-angle projections. Oblique projections are occasionally required to show the full extent of a sinus tract.
- To explore fistulae and sinuses in the abdominal region, have the intestinal tract as free of gas and fecal material as possible.
- Unless the injection is made under fluoroscopic control, take a scout image of the abdomen to check the condition of the intestinal tract before beginning the examination.
- When more than one sinus opening is present, occlude each accessory opening with sterile gauze packing to prevent reflux of the contrast substance and to identify every opening with a specific lead marker placed over the dressing (Figs. 15.164 through 15.166).
- Dress and identify the primary sinus opening in a similar manner if the catheter is removed after the injection.

- When reflux of contrast medium occurs, cleanse the skin thoroughly before making an exposure.
- When fluoroscopy is not employed, place the patient in position for the first projection before the injection to prevent drainage of the opaque substance by unnecessary movement. An initial image is taken and evaluated before the examination is started or the patient's position is changed.

To show a fistula involving the colon, barium is instilled by enema. If a fistula involving the small bowel is suspected, the patient ingests a thin barium suspension, which is followed by fluoroscopy or radiography until it reaches the suspected region. The bladder is filled with iodinated contrast media when involvement of this structure is evaluated. Cutaneous fistulae and sinus tracts are opacified by introduction of an iodinated contrast medium through a small-diameter catheter. The procedures are performed using fluoroscopic observation, with images taken as indicated.

Fig. 15.164 AP abdomen showing contrast media–filled sinus tract with lead circular ring on body surface.

Fig. 15.165 Lateral abdomen showing sinus tract with lead circular ring on body surface.

Fig. 15.166 Oblique abdomen, LPO position, showing fistula (arrow).

References

1. Lee LIT, Pawar RR, Whitley D, et al. Incidence of different causes of benign obstruction of the salivary glands: retrospective analysis of 493 cases using fluoroscopy and digital subtraction sialography. *Br J Oral Maxillofac Surg.* 2015;53:54–57.
2. Iglauer S. A simple maneuver to increase the visibility of a salivary calculus in the roentgenogram. *Radiology.* 1933;21:297.
3. *ARRT Radiography Examination Content Specifications*; 2017.
4. *ACR Appropriateness Criteria®: Dysphagia*; 2013.
5. American College of Radiology. ACR practice parameter for the performance of esophagrams and upper gastrointestinal examinations in adults; 2013. Available at: https://www.acr.org/~/media/5223A3 FBC92E40378DF6E55FB8E6134B.pdf. (Accessed September 23, 2017.)
6. Hunter TB, Taljanovic MS. Foreign bodies, *Radiographics.* 2003;23(3):731–757.
7. Cockerill EM, et al. Optimal visualization of esophageal varices. *AJR Am J Roentgenol.* 1976;126:512.
8. ACR Manual on Contrast Media, v.10.3, 2017, p. 59.
9. Maglinte DD, Caudill LD, Krol KL, et al. The minimum effective dose of glucagon in upper gastrointestinal radiography. *Gastrointest Radiol.* 1982;7(2):119–122.
10. Gugliantini P. Utilitá delle incidenze oblique caudocraniali nello studio radiologico della stenosi congenita ipertrofica del piloro, *Ann Radiol Diagn.* 34:56, 1961. Abstract. *AJR Am J Roentgenol.* 1962;87:623.
11. Gordon SS. The angled posteroanterior projection of the stomach: an attempt at better visualization of the high transverse stomach. *Radiology.* 1957;69:393.
12. Wolf BS, Guglielmo J. Method for the roentgen demonstration of minimal hiatal herniation. *J Mt Sinai Hosp N Y.* 1956;23(738):741.
13. Wolf BS, Guglielmo J. The roentgen demonstration of minimal hiatus hernia. *Med Radiogr Photogr.* 1957;33:90.
14. Fitch D. The small-bowel see-through: an improved method of radiographic small bowel visualization. *Can J Med Radiat Technol.* 1995;26:167.
15. Miller RE. Complete reflux small bowel examination. *Radiology.* 1965;84:457.
16. Miller RE. Localization of the small bowel hemorrhage: complete reflux small bowel examination. *Am J Dig Dis.* 1972;17:1019.
17. American College of Radiology. ACR practice parameter for the performance of fluoroscopic contrast enema examination in adults; 2013. Available at: https://www.acr.org/~/media/17B62BAE4AAA4DEC8 75CF4544FDCF457.pdf. (Accessed September 23, 2017.)
18. ACR Manual on Contrast Media, v.10.3, 2017, p. 59.
19. Welin S. Modern trends in diagnostic roentgenology of the colon. *Br J Radiol.* 1958;31:453.
20. Miller RE. Barium pneumocolon: technologist-performed "7-pump" method. *AJR Am J Roentgenol.* 1982;139:1230.
21. American College of Radiology. ACR practice parameter for the performance of fluoroscopic contrast enema examination in adults; 2013. (Available at: https://www.acr.org/~/media/17B62BAE4AAA4 DEC875CF4544FDCF457.pdf. (Accessed September 23, 2017.)
22. Burhenne HJ. Intestinal evacuation study: a new roentgenologic technique. *Radiol Clin (Basel).* 1964;33:79.
23. Mahieu P, et al. Defecography: I. Description of a new procedure and results in normal patients. *Gastrointest Radiol.* 1984;9:247.
24. Mahieu P, et al. Defecography: II. Contribution to the diagnosis of defecation disorders. *Gastrointest Radiol.* 1984;9:253.
25. Mahieu PHG. Defecography. In Margulis AR, Burhenne H, eds. *Alimentary tract radiology.* vol 1. ed 4. St Louis: Mosby; 1989.
26. Evans JA, et al. Percutaneous transhepatic cholangiography. *Radiology.* 1962;78:362.
27. Molnar W, Stockum AE. Relief of obstructive jaundice through percutaneous transhepatic catheter—a new therapeutic method. *AJR Am J Roentgenol.* 1974;122:356.
28. Hardy CH, et al. Percutaneous transhepatic biliary drainage. *Radiol Technol.* 1984;56:8.
29. Stern WZ, et al. The significance of the lateral view in T-tube cholangiography. *AJR Am J Roentgenol.* 1962;87:764.
30. Cotton P, William C. *Practical gastrointestinal endoscopy.* Oxford, England: Blackwell; 1980.

16

URINARY SYSTEM AND VENIPUNCTURE

SUMMARY OF PROJECTIONS

PROJECTIONS, POSITIONS, AND METHODS

Page	Essential	Anatomy	Projection	Position	Method
304	⚜	Urinary system	AP		
306	⚜	Urinary system	AP oblique	RPO and LPO	
307	⚜	Urinary system	Lateral	R or L	
308	⚜	Urinary system	Lateral	Dorsal decubitus	
309		Renal parenchyma	AP		
312	⚜	Pelvicaliceal system and ureters: *Retrograde urography*	AP		
316	⚜	Urinary bladder	AP axial or PA axial		
318	⚜	Urinary bladder	AP oblique	RPO or LPO	
320	⚜	Urinary bladder	Lateral	R or L	
321	⚜	Male cystourethrography	AP oblique	RPO or LPO	
322		Female cystourethrography	AP		INJECTION

Icons in the Essential column indicate projections frequently performed in the United States and Canada. Students should be competent in these projections.
AP, Anteroposterior; *L,* left; *LPO,* left posterior oblique; *PA,* posteroanterior; *R,* right; *RPO,* right posterior oblique.

Urinary System

The *urinary system* includes two *kidneys*, two *ureters*, one *urinary bladder*, and one *urethra* (Figs. 16.1 and 16.2). The functions of the kidneys include removing waste products from the blood, maintaining fluid and electrolyte balance, and secreting substances that affect blood pressure and other important body functions. The kidneys normally excrete 1 to 2 L of urine per day. Urine is expelled from the body via the *excretory system*, as the urinary system is often called. The excretory system consists of the following:

- A variable number of urine-draining branches in the kidney called the *calyces* and an expanded portion called the *renal pelvis*, which together are known as the *pelvicaliceal system*
- Two long tubes called *ureters*, with one ureter extending from the pelvis of each kidney
- A saclike portion, the *urinary bladder*, which receives the distal portion of the ureters and serves as a reservoir
- A third and smaller tubular portion, the *urethra*, which conveys the urine to the exterior of the body

Suprarenal Glands

Closely associated with the urinary system are the two *suprarenal*, or *adrenal*, *glands*. These ductless endocrine glands have no functional relationship with the urinary system but are included in this chapter because of their anatomic relationship with the kidneys. Each suprarenal gland consists of a small, flattened body composed of an internal *medullary portion* and an outer *cortical portion*. Each gland is enclosed in a fibrous sheath and is situated in the retroperitoneal tissue in close contact with the fatty capsule overlying the medial and superior aspects of the upper pole of the kidney. The suprarenal glands furnish two important substances: (1) epinephrine, which is secreted by the medulla; and (2) cortical hormones, which are secreted by the cortex. These glands are subject to malfunction and numerous diseases. They are not usually shown on preliminary images but are delineated when computed tomography (CT) is used. The suprarenal circulation may be shown by selective catheterization of a suprarenal artery or vein in angiographic procedures.

A

B

C

Fig. 16.1 Anterior aspect of urinary system in relation to surrounding structures. (A) Abdominal structures. (B) Bony structures. (C) Three-dimensional CT image of urinary system in relation to bony structures.

Kidneys

The *kidneys* are bean-shaped bodies. The lateral border of each kidney is convex, and the medial border is concave. They have slightly convex anterior and posterior surfaces, and they are arbitrarily divided into upper and lower poles. The kidneys are approximately 4½ inches (11.5 cm) long, 2 to 3 inches (5 to 7.6 cm) wide, and about 1¼ inches (3 cm) thick. The left kidney usually is slightly longer and narrower than the right kidney.

The kidneys are situated behind the peritoneum (retroperitoneal) and are in contact with the posterior wall of the abdominal cavity, one kidney lying on each side of and in the same coronal plane with L3. The superior aspect of the kidney lies more posterior than the inferior aspect (see Fig. 16.2). Each kidney lies in an oblique plane and is rotated about 30 degrees anteriorly toward the aorta, which lies on top of the vertebral body (Fig. 16.3). This natural anatomic position is the basis for the 30-degree rotation of the AP oblique projections (RPO and LPO positions). In AP oblique projections, the elevated kidney is demonstrated without distortion, as the 30-degree rotation orients the upper kidney parallel to the IR plane. The dependent kidney is positioned almost perpendicular to the IR plane, so the lower kidney is oriented to demonstrate the anterior and posterior surfaces in the oblique positions.

The kidneys normally extend from the level of the superior border of T12 to the level of the transverse processes of L3 in sthenic individuals; they are higher in individuals with a hypersthenic habitus and lower in persons with an asthenic habitus. Because of the large space occupied by the liver, the right kidney is slightly lower than, or caudal to, the left kidney.

The outer covering of the kidney is called the *renal capsule*. The capsule is a semitransparent membrane that is continuous with the outer coat of the ureter. Each kidney is embedded in a mass of fatty tissue called the *adipose capsule*. The capsule and kidney are enveloped in a sheath of superficial fascia, the *renal fascia*, which is attached to the diaphragm, lumbar vertebrae, peritoneum, and other adjacent structures. The kidneys are supported in a fairly fixed position, partially through the fascial attachments and partially by the surrounding organs. They have respiratory movement of approximately 1 inch (2.5 cm) and normally drop no more than 2 inches (5 cm) in the change from the supine to the upright position.

The concave medial border of each kidney has a longitudinal slit, or *hilum*, for transmission of the blood and lymphatic vessels, nerves, and ureter (Fig. 16.4). The hilum expands into the body of the kidney to form a central cavity called the *renal sinus*. The renal sinus is a fat-filled space surrounding the renal pelvis and vessels.

Fig. 16.2 Lateral aspect of male urinary system in relation to surrounding structures.

Right kidney
Right ureter
Urinary bladder
Rectum
Prostate
Anal canal

Fig. 16.3 CT of kidneys with contrast, excretory phase, illustrates 30-degree anterior angulation of kidneys. Note carcinoma in left kidney, upper pole.

(From Haaga J, Boll D. *CT and MRI of the Whole Body.* 6th ed. Philadelphia: Elsevier; 2017.)

Each kidney has an outer renal cortex and an inner *renal medulla*. The renal medulla, composed mainly of the collecting tubules that give it a striated appearance, consists of 8 to 15 cone-shaped segments called the *renal pyramids*. The apices of the segments converge toward the renal sinus to drain into the pelvicaliceal system. The more compact renal cortex lies between the periphery of the organ and the bases of the medullary segments and extends medially between the pyramids to the renal sinus. These extensions of the cortex are called *renal columns*.

The essential microscopic components of the parenchyma of the kidney are called *nephrons* (Fig. 16.5). Each kidney contains approximately 1 million of these tubular structures. The individual nephron is composed of a *renal corpuscle* and a *renal tubule*. The renal corpuscle consists of a double-walled membranous cup called the *glomerular capsule* (Bowman capsule) and a cluster of blood capillaries called the *glomerulus*. The glomerulus is formed by a minute branch of the renal artery entering the capsule and dividing into capillaries. The capillaries turn back

and, as they ascend, unite to form a single vessel leaving the capsule.

The vessel entering the capsule is called the *afferent arteriole*, and the one leaving the capsule is termed the *efferent arteriole*. After exiting the glomerular capsules, the efferent arterioles form the capillary network surrounding the straight and convoluted tubules, and these capillaries reunite and continue on to communicate with the renal veins.

The thin inner wall of the capsule closely adheres to the capillary coils and is separated by a comparatively wide space from the outer layer, which is continuous with the beginning of a renal tubule. The glomerulus serves as a filter for the blood, permitting water and finely dissolved substances to pass through the walls of the capillaries into the capsule. The change from filtrate to urine is caused in part by the water and the usable dissolved substances being absorbed through the epithelial lining of the tubules into the surrounding capillary network.

Each renal *tubule* continues from a glomerular capsule in the cortex of the kidney and then travels a circuitous path through

the cortical and medullary substances, becoming the *proximal convoluted tubule*, the *nephron loop* (loop of Henle), and the *distal convoluted tubule*. The distal convoluted tubule opens into the collecting ducts that begin in the cortex. The *collecting ducts* converge toward the renal pelvis and unite along their course so that each group within the pyramid forms a central tubule that opens at a *renal papilla* and drains its tributaries into the minor calyx.

The *calyces* are cup-shaped stems arising at the sides of the papilla of each renal pyramid. Each calyx encloses one or more papillae so that there are usually fewer calyces than pyramids. The beginning branches are called the *minor calyces* (numbering from 4 to 13), and they unite to form two or three larger tubes called the *major calyces*. The major calyces unite to form the expanded, funnel-shaped renal pelvis. The wide upper portion of the *renal pelvis* lies within the hilum, and its tapering lower part passes through the hilum to become continuous with the ureter. This area where the renal pelvis transitions to the ureter is called the *ureteropelvic junction* (UPJ).

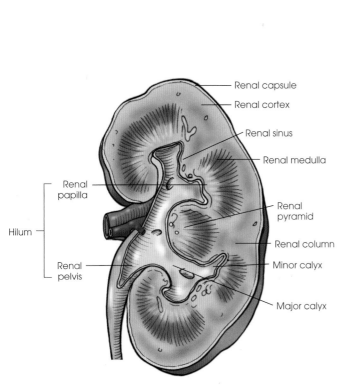

Fig. 16.4 Midcoronal section of kidney.

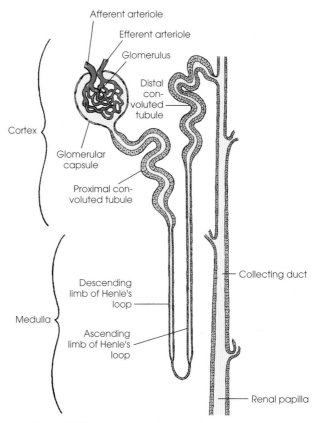

Fig. 16.5 Diagram of nephron and collecting duct.

Ureters

Each *ureter* is 10 to 12 inches (25 to 30 cm) long. The ureters descend behind the peritoneum and in front of the psoas muscle and the transverse processes of the lumbar vertebrae, pass inferiorly and posteriorly in front of the sacral wing, and then curve anteriorly and medially to enter the posterolateral surface of the urinary bladder at approximately the level of the ischial spine. The ureters convey the urine from the renal pelves to the bladder by slow, rhythmic peristaltic contractions.

Urinary Bladder

The *urinary bladder* is a musculomembranous sac that serves as a reservoir for urine. The bladder is situated immediately posterior and superior to the pubic symphysis and is directly anterior to the rectum in the male and anterior to the vaginal canal in the female. The *apex* of the bladder is at the anterosuperior aspect and is adjacent to the superior aspect of the pubic symphysis. The most fixed part of the bladder is the neck, which rests on the prostate in the male and on the pelvic diaphragm in the female.

The bladder varies in size, shape, and position according to its content. It is freely movable and is held in position by folds of the peritoneum. When empty, the bladder is located in the pelvic cavity. As the bladder fills, it gradually assumes an oval shape while expanding superiorly and anteriorly into the abdominal cavity. The adult bladder can hold approximately 500 mL of fluid when completely full. The urge for *micturition* (urination) occurs when about 250 mL of urine is in the bladder.

The ureters enter the posterior wall of the bladder at the lateral margins of the superior part of its *base* and pass obliquely through the wall to their respective internal orifices (Fig. 16.6). This portion of each ureter, where it joins the bladder, is called the *ureterovesical junction* (UVJ). These two openings are about 1 inch (2.5 cm) apart when the bladder is empty and about 2 inches (5 cm) apart when the bladder is distended. The openings are equidistant from the internal urethral orifice, which is situated at the neck (lowest part) of the bladder. The triangular area between the three orifices is called the *trigone*. The mucosa over the trigone is always smooth, whereas the remainder of the lining contains folds, called *rugae*, when the bladder is empty.

Fig. 16.6 (A) Anterior view of urinary bladder. (B) Axial CT image of pelvis showing contrast medium–filled bladder *(bl)*. (C) Sagittal MRI of female pelvis showing contrast medium–filled bladder *(bl)* and relationship to uterus *(ut)* and pubis *(pub)*.

Urethra

The *urethra*, which conveys the urine out of the body, is a narrow, musculomembranous tube with a sphincter type of muscle at the neck of the bladder. The urethra arises at the internal urethral orifice in the urinary bladder and extends about 1½ inches (3.8 cm) in the female and 7 to 8 inches (17.8 to 20 cm) in the male.

The female urethra passes along the thick anterior wall of the vagina to the external urethral orifice, which is located in the vestibule about 1 inch (2.5 cm) anterior to the vaginal opening (see Fig. 16.6). The male urethra extends from the bladder to the end of the penis and is divided into *prostatic*, *membranous*, and *spongy* portions (Fig. 16.7). The prostatic portion is about 1 inch (2.5 cm) long, reaches from the bladder to the floor of the pelvis, and is completely surrounded by the prostate. The membranous portion of the canal passes through the urogenital diaphragm; it is slightly constricted and about ½ inch (1.3 cm) long. The spongy portion passes through the shaft of the penis, extending from the floor of the pelvis to the external urethral orifice. The distal prostatic, membranous, and spongy parts of the male urethra also serve as the excretory canal of the reproductive system.

Prostate

The *prostate*, a small glandular body surrounding the proximal part of the male urethra, is situated just posterior to the inferior portion of the pubic symphysis. The prostate is considered part of the male reproductive system, but because of its close proximity to the bladder, it is commonly described with the urinary system. The conical base of the prostate is attached to the inferior surface of the urinary bladder, and its apex is in contact with the pelvic diaphragm. The prostate measures about 1½ inches (3.8 cm) transversely and ¼ inch (1.9 cm) anteroposteriorly at its base; vertically, the prostate is approximately 1 inch (2.5 cm) long. The prostate gland secretes a milky fluid that combines with semen from the seminal vesicles and vas deferens. These secretions enter the urethra via ducts in the prostatic urethra.

SUMMARY OF ANATOMY

Urinary system (excretory system)
Kidneys (R and L)
Ureters (R and L)
Urinary bladder
Urethra

Suprarenal glands (adrenal glands)
Medullary portion
Cortical portion

Kidneys
Adipose capsule
Renal fascia
Hilum
Renal capsule
Renal sinus
Renal cortex
  Renal columns
Renal medulla
  Renal pyramids
Nephrons
  Renal corpuscle
    Glomerular capsule (Bowman capsule)
    Glomerulus
    Afferent arteriole
    Efferent arteriole
  Renal tubule
    Proximal convoluted tubule
    Nephron loop (loop of Henle)
    Distal convoluted tubule
    Collecting ducts
    Renal papilla
Calyces
  Minor calyces
  Major calyces
  Renal pelvis

Urinary bladder
Apex
Base
Neck
Trigone
Rugae

Urethra
Male urethra
Prostatic
Membranous
Spongy

Prostate

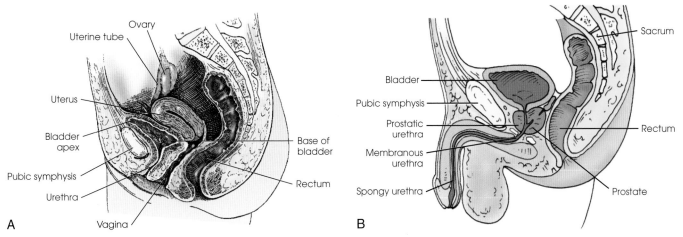

Fig. 16.7 (A) Midsagittal section through female pelvis. (B) Male pelvis.

SUMMARY OF PATHOLOGY

Condition	Definition
Benign prostatic hyperplasia (BPH)	Enlargement of prostate
Calculus	Abnormal concretion of mineral salts, often called a stone
Carcinoma	Malignant new growth composed of epithelial cells
Bladder	Carcinoma located in the bladder
Renal cell	Carcinoma located in the kidney
Congenital anomaly	Abnormality present at birth
Duplicate collecting system	Two renal pelves or ureters from the same kidney
Horseshoe kidney	Fusion of the kidneys, usually at the lower poles
Pelvic kidney	Kidney that fails to ascend and remains in the pelvis
Cystitis	Inflammation of the bladder
Fistula	Abnormal connection between two internal organs or between an organ and the body surface
Glomerulonephritis	Inflammation of the capillary loops in the glomeruli of the kidney
Hydronephrosis	Distention of renal pelvis and calyces with urine
Nephroptosis	Excessive inferior displacement of the kidneys or kidney prolapse
Phleboliths	Pelvic vein calcifications
Polycystic kidney	Massive enlargement of the kidney with the formation of many cysts
Pyelonephritis	Inflammation of the kidney and renal pelvis
Renal hypertension	Increased blood pressure to the kidneys
Renal obstruction	Condition preventing normal flow of urine through the urinary system
Stenosis	Narrowing or contraction of a passage
Tumor	New tissue growth where cell proliferation is uncontrolled
Wilms	Most common pediatric abdominal neoplasm affecting the kidney
Ureterocele	Ballooning of the lower end of the ureter into the bladder
Vesicoureteral reflux	Backward flow of urine from the bladder into the ureters

Eponymous (named) pathologies are listed in nonpossessive form to conform to the *AMA Manual of Style: A Guide for Authors and Editors.* 10th ed. Oxford: Oxford University Press; 2009.

SAMPLE EXPOSURE TECHNIQUE CHART ESSENTIAL PROJECTIONS

These techniques were accurate for the equipment used to produce each exposure. However, use caution when applying them in your department because "there is considerable variability in image receptor response owing to varying scatter sensitivity, the use of grids with different grid ratios, collimation, beam filtration, the choice of kilovoltage, source-to-image distance, and image receptor size."[1]

This chart was created in collaboration with Dennis Bowman, AS, RT(R), Clinical Instructor, Community Hospital of the Monterey Peninsula, Monterey, CA. http://digitalradiographysolutions.com/.

URINARY SYSTEM

Part	cm	kVp[a]	SID[b]	Collimation	CR[c] mAs	CR[c] Dose (mGy)[e]	DR[d] mAs	DR[d] Dose (mGy)[e]
Urinary system (urography)								
AP[f]	21	80	40"	14" × 17" (35 × 43 cm)	40[g]	5.480	16[g]	2.168
AP oblique[f]	24	80	40"	14" × 17" (35 × 43 cm)	56[g]	8.250	25[g]	3.660
Lateral[f]	27	80	40"	12" × 17" (30 × 43 cm)	100[g]	15.89	40[g]	6.320
Urinary bladder								
AP and PA axial[f]	16	80	40"	9" × 9" (23 × 23 cm)	56[g]	6.790	22[g]	2.670
AP oblique[f]	21	80	40"	9" × 9" (23 × 23 cm)	65[g]	8.510	28[g]	3.660
Lateral[f]	31	85	40"	8" × 9" (20 × 23 cm)	110[g]	20.41	45[g]	8.300

[1]ACR-AAPM-SIMM Practice Parameter for Digital Radiography, revised 2017.
[a]kVp values are for a high-frequency generator.
[b]40 inches minimum; 44–48 inches recommended to improve spatial resolution (mAs increase needed, but no increase in patient dose will result).
[c]AGFA CR MD 4.0 General IP, CR 75.0 reader, 400 speed class, with 6:1 (178LPI) grid when needed.
[d]GE Definium 8000, with 13:1 grid when needed.
[e]All doses are skin entrance for an average adult (160–200 pound male, 150–190 pound female) at part thickness indicated.
[f]Bucky/Grid.
[g]Large focal spot.

ABBREVIATIONS USED IN CHAPTER 16

ACR	American College of Radiology
ASRT	American Society of Radiologic Technologists
BPH	Benign prostatic hyperplasia
BUN	Blood urea nitrogen
CDC	US Centers for Disease Control and Prevention
EU	Excretory urogram
GFR	Glomerular filtration rate
IV	Intravenous
IVP	Intravenous pyelogram
IVU	Intravenous urogram
UPJ	Ureteropelvic junction
VCUG	Voiding cystourethrogram

See Addendum B for a summary of all abbreviations used in Volume 2.

Overview

Radiographic examination of the urinary system involves the use of a water-soluble iodinated contrast medium to allow visualization of the pertinent anatomy and, frequently, to evaluate physiologic function. The role of radiography in the evaluation of the urinary system has changed because of the increased use of multiplanar imaging modalities such as CT, magnetic resonance imaging (MRI), and ultrasonography (US). Multidetector CT, with three-dimensional reconstruction capabilities, has improved the visualization of small pathologies that were difficult or impossible to see on radiographic images. Despite the decreased use of contrast urography, the American College of Radiology (ACR) specifies that excretory urography is particularly useful in demonstrating the collecting system and ureters and in evaluating ureteral obstruction, compression, and displacement. In addition, contrast urography can be tailored to provide diagnostic information at a lower radiation dose than can be provided by helical multidetector CT.[1]

The specialized radiography procedures are preceded by a plain, or scout, image of the abdominopelvic areas for detection of abnormalities that can be shown on plain radiography. The preliminary examination may consist of only a KUB. Oblique or lateral projections, or both, may be obtained to localize calcifications, such as urinary calculi or phleboliths, and tumor masses. An upright position may be used to show the mobility of the kidneys to demonstrate nephroptosis and for the detection of low-grade obstruction.[2]

Preliminary radiography can usually show the position and mobility of the kidneys and usually their size and shape because of the contrast furnished by the radiolucent fatty capsule surrounding the kidneys. In addition, properly selected CT soft tissue windows can show the renal parenchyma without contrast media (Fig. 16.8). Visualization of the thin-walled drainage, or collecting, system (calyces and pelves, ureters, urinary bladder, and urethra) requires that the canals be filled with a contrast medium. The urinary bladder is outlined when it is filled with urine, but it is not adequately shown. The ureters and the urethra cannot be distinguished on preliminary images. A CT "stone protocol" without a contrast medium can clearly show calcified renal stones (Fig. 16.9).

IMAGING OF THE KIDNEYS

Cysts and tumor masses situated within the kidney are usually imaged using contrast-enhanced CT (Fig. 16.10) or US (Fig. 16.11). Angiographic procedures are used to investigate the blood vessels of the kidneys and the suprarenal glands (see Chapter 27, Volume 3). An example of the direct injection of contrast medium into the renal artery is shown in Fig. 16.12.

Radiologic investigations of the renal drainage, or collecting, system are performed by various procedures classified under the general term *urography*. This term embraces two regularly used techniques for filling the urinary canals with a contrast medium. Imaging of cutaneous urinary diversions has been described by Long.[3]

Fig. 16.8 CT of abdomen without contrast media showing parenchyma and renal pelvis of both kidneys *(arrows).*

(Courtesy Karl Mockler, RT(R).)

Fig. 16.9 CT "stone protocol" without contrast media showing renal calculus in left distal ureter *(arrow).*

(Courtesy Karl Mockler, RT(R).)

Antegrade filling

Antegrade filling techniques allow the contrast medium to enter the kidney in the normal direction of blood flow. In selective patients, this is done by introducing the contrast material directly into the kidney through a percutaneous puncture of the renal pelvis—a technique called *percutaneous antegrade urography*. Much more commonly used is the physiologic technique, in which the contrast agent is generally administered intravenously. This technique is called *excretory* or *intravenous urography* (EU or IVU) and is shown in Fig. 16.13.

IVU is used in examinations of the upper urinary tract in infants and children and is generally considered to be the preferred technique in adults unless the use of the retrograde technique is definitely indicated. Because the contrast medium is administered intravenously and all parts of the urinary system are normally shown, the excretory technique is correctly referred to as IVU. The term *pyelography* refers to the radiographic demonstration of the renal pelves and calyces. This examination has been erroneously called an intravenous pyelogram (IVP).

After the opaque contrast medium enters the bloodstream, it is conveyed to the renal glomeruli and is discharged into the capsules with the glomerular filtrate, which is excreted as urine. With the reabsorption of water, the contrast material becomes sufficiently concentrated to render the urinary canals radiopaque. The urinary bladder is well outlined by this technique, and satisfactory voiding urethrograms may be obtained.

Fig. 16.10 CT image of abdomen with contrast media showing early filling of both kidneys *(arrows).*

Fig. 16.11 US image of normal right kidney in the sagittal plane.

Fig. 16.12 Selective right renal arteriogram.

Fig. 16.13 Excretory urogram.

Fig. 16.14 Retrograde urogram.

Fig. 16.15 Voiding study after routine injection intravenous urogram (IVU). Dilation of proximal urethra *(arrows)* is the result of urethral stricture.

Fig. 16.16 Voiding studies of same patient as in Fig. 16.15 after infusion nephrourography. Note increase in opacification of contrast medium–filled cavities by this method and bladder diverticulum *(arrows)*.

Contrast-filled bladder

Catheter in urethra

Fig. 16.17 Cystogram.

Retrograde filling

In some procedures involving the urinary system, the contrast material is introduced against the normal flow. This is called *retrograde urography* (Fig. 16.14). The contrast medium is injected directly into the canals via ureteral catheterization for contrast filling of the upper urinary tract and via urethral catheterization for contrast filling of the lower part of the urinary tract. Cystoscopy is required to localize the vesicoureteral orifices for the passage of ureteral catheters.

Retrograde urographic examination of the proximal urinary tract is primarily a urologic procedure. Catheterization and contrast filling of the urinary canals are performed by the attending urologist in conjunction with a physical or endoscopic examination. This technique enables the urologist to obtain catheterized specimens of urine directly from each renal pelvis. Because the canals can be fully distended by direct injection of the contrast agent, the retrograde urographic examination sometimes provides more information about the anatomy of the different parts of the collecting system than can be obtained by the excretory technique. For the retrograde procedure, an evaluation of kidney function depends on an intravenously administered dye substance to stain the color of the urine that subsequently trickles through the respective ureteral catheters.

The antegrade and retrograde techniques of examination are occasionally required for a complete urologic study.

Investigations of the lower urinary tract—bladder, lower ureters, and urethra—are usually done by the retrograde technique, which requires no instrumentation beyond the passage of a urethral catheter. Investigations may also be done by the physiologic technique (Figs. 16.15 and 16.16). Bladder examinations are usually denoted by the general term *cystography* (Fig. 16.17). A procedure that includes inspection of the lower ureters is *cystoureterography* (Fig. 16.18), and a procedure that includes inspection of the urethra is *cystourethrography* (Fig. 16.19).

Fig. 16.18 Cystoureterogram: AP bladder showing distal ureters.

Fig. 16.19 Injection cystourethrogram showing urethra in a male patient.

293

Contrast media

Retrograde urography (Figs. 16.20 and 16.21) was first performed in 1904 with the introduction of air into the urinary bladder. In 1906, retrograde urography and cystography were performed with the first opaque medium, a colloidal silver preparation that is no longer used. Silver iodide, which is a nontoxic inorganic compound, was introduced in 1911. Sodium iodide and sodium bromide, also inorganic compounds, were first used for retrograde urography in 1918. The bromides and iodides are no longer widely used for examinations of the renal pelves and ureters because they irritate the mucosa and commonly cause considerable patient discomfort.

Because a large quantity of solution is required to fill the urinary bladder, iodinated salts in concentrations of 30% or less are used in cystography. A large selection of commercially available contrast media may be used for all types of radiographic examinations of the urinary system. It is important to review the product insert packaged with every contrast agent.

Excretory urography (Figs. 16.22 and 16.23) was first reported by Rowntree et al. in 1923.[4] These investigators used a 10% solution of chemically pure sodium iodide as the contrast medium. This agent was excreted too slowly, however, to show the renal pelves and ureters satisfactorily, and it proved too toxic for functional distribution. Early in 1929, Roseno and Jepkins[5] introduced a compound containing sodium iodide and urea. The latter constituent, which is one of the nitrogenous substances removed from the blood and eliminated by the kidneys, served to accelerate excretion and to fill the renal pelves with opacified urine quickly. Although satisfactory renal images were obtained with this compound, patients experienced considerable distress as a result of its toxicity.

In 1929, Swick developed the organic compound Uroselectan, which had an iodine content of 42%. Present-day ionic contrast media for excretory urography are the result of extensive research by many investigators. These media are available under various trade names in concentrations ranging from approximately 50% to 70%. Sterile solutions of the media are supplied in dose-size ampules or vials.

In the early 1970s, research was initiated to develop nonionic contrast media. Development progressed, and several nonionic contrast agents are currently available for urographic, vascular, and intrathecal injection. Although nonionic contrast media are less likely to cause a reaction in the patient, they are more expensive than ionic agents. Despite this cost, nonionics are most commonly used because of the increase in patient safety and comfort.

Fig. 16.20 Retrograde urogram with contrast medium–filled right renal pelvis and catheter in left renal pelvis.

Fig. 16.21 Retrograde urogram.

Fig. 16.22 Excretory urogram, 10 minutes after injection of contrast medium.

Fig. 16.23 Excretory urogram on same patient as in Fig. 16.22, 25 minutes after contrast medium injection.

Adverse reactions to iodinated media

The iodinated organic preparations that are compounded for urologic examinations are of low toxicity. Consequently, adverse reactions are usually mild and of short duration. Common reactions include a feeling of warmth and flushing. Occasionally nausea, vomiting, a few hives, and edema of the respiratory mucous membrane result. Severe and serious reactions occur only rarely but are always a possibility. The clinical history of each patient must be carefully checked, and the patient must be kept under careful observation for any sign of systemic reactions. According to the 2017 version of the ACR Manual on Contrast Media, "nearly all life-threatening contrast reactions occur within the first 20 minutes after contrast medium injection." The patient should not be left unattended during this time period. Emergency equipment and medication (diphenhydramine, epinephrine) to treat adverse reactions must be readily available. The ACR additionally states that the radiologist, or his or her qualified designee, who is on-site during the procedure must be prepared and able to treat these reactions.

Preparation of intestinal tract

Although unobstructed visualization of the urinary tracts requires that the intestinal tract be free of gas and solid fecal material (Fig. 16.24), bowel preparation is not attempted in infants and children. The use of cleansing measures in adults depends on the condition of the patient. Gas (particularly swallowed air, which is quickly dispersed through the small bowel) rather than fecal material usually interferes with the examination.

Hope and Campoy[6] recommended that infants and children be given a carbonated soft drink to distend the stomach with gas. By this maneuver, the gas-containing intestinal loops are usually pushed inferiorly, and the upper urinary tracts, particularly on the left side of the body, are clearly visualized through the outline of the gas-filled stomach. Hope and Campoy stated that the aerated drink should be given in an amount adequate to inflate the stomach fully: at least 2 oz. is required for a newborn infant, and 12 oz. is required for a 7-year-old child. In conjunction with the carbonated drink, Hope and Campoy recommended using a highly concentrated contrast medium. A gas-distended stomach is shown in Fig. 16.25.

Fig. 16.24 Preliminary AP abdomen for urogram.

Renal calyces

Renal pelvis

Abdominal ureter

Pelvic ureter

Urinary bladder

Fig. 16.25 Supine urogram at 15-minute interval with gas-filled stomach.

Berdon et al.[7] stated that the prone position resolves the problem of obscuring gas in most patients (Figs. 16.26 and 16.27). It is unnecessary to inflate the stomach with air alone or with air as part of an aerated drink. By exerting pressure on the abdomen, the prone position moves the gas laterally away from the pelvicaliceal structures. Gas in the antral portion of the stomach is displaced into its fundic portion, gas in the transverse colon shifts into the ascending and descending segments, and gas in the sigmoid colon shifts into the descending colon and rectum. These investigators noted, however, that the prone position occasionally fails to produce the desired result in small infants when the small intestine is dilated. Gastric inflation also fails in these patients because the dilated small intestine merely elevates the gas-filled stomach and does not improve visualization. They recommended examination of such infants *after* the intestinal gas has passed.

Preparation of patient

Medical opinion concerning patient preparation varies widely. With modifications as required, the following procedure seems to be in general use:

- When time permits, have the patient follow a low-residue diet for 1 to 2 days to prevent gas formation caused by excessive fermentation of the intestinal contents.
- Have the patient eat a light evening meal on the day before the examination.
- When indicated by costive bowel action, administer a non-gas-forming laxative the evening before the examination.
- Have the patient take nothing by mouth after midnight on the day of the examination. The patient should not be dehydrated, however. Patients with multiple myeloma, high uric acid levels, or diabetes must be well hydrated before IVU is performed; these patients are at increased risk for contrast medium-induced renal failure if they are dehydrated.
- In preparation for *retrograde urography*, have the patient drink a large amount of water (4 or 5 cups) several hours before the examination to ensure the excretion of urine in an amount sufficient for bilateral catheterized specimens and renal function tests.
- No patient preparation is usually necessary for the examination of the lower urinary tract.

Outpatients should be given explicit directions regarding any order from the physician pertaining to diet, fluid intake, and laxatives or other medication. The patient should also be given a suitable explanation for each preparative measure to ensure cooperation.

Fig. 16.26 Urogram: supine position. Intestinal gas obscuring left kidney.

Fig. 16.27 Urogram: prone position, in the same patient as in Fig. 16.26. Visualization of left kidney and ureter is markedly improved.

EQUIPMENT

Any standard radiographic table is suitable to perform preliminary excretory urography and most retrograde studies of the bladder and urethra. A combination cystoscopic-radiographic unit facilitates retrograde urographic procedures requiring cystoscopy. The cystoscopic unit is also used for IVU and retrograde bladder and urethra studies; however, for the patient's comfort, the table should have an extensible leg rest.

Infusion nephrourography requires a table equipped with tomographic apparatus. Tomography should be performed when intestinal gas obscures some of the underlying structures, or when hypersthenic patients are being examined (Fig. 16.28).

For the patient's comfort and to prevent delays during the examination, all preparations for the examination should be completed before the patient is placed on the table. In addition to an identification and side marker, excretory urographic studies require a time interval marker for each postinjection study. Body position markers (supine, prone, upright or semi-upright, Trendelenburg, decubitus) should also be used.

Some institutions perform excretory urograms (proximal urinary tract studies) using a 10 × 12-inch (24 × 30-cm) crosswise radiation field or CR plate, but these studies can also be made using a 14 × 17-inch (35 × 43-cm) lengthwise exposure field or CR plate (Figs. 16.29 and 16.30). The upright study is made using a lengthwise 14 × 17-inch (35 × 43-cm) radiation field or CR plate because it is taken to show the mobility of the kidneys, to demonstrate nephroptosis, and to outline the lower ureters and bladder. Studies of the bladder before and after voiding are usually taken using a crosswise 10 × 12-inch (24 × 30-cm) radiation field or CR plate.

The following guidelines are observed in preparing additional equipment for the examination:

- Have an emergency cart fully equipped and conveniently placed.
- Arrange the instruments for injection of the contrast agent on a small, movable table or on a tray.
- Have frequently used sterile items readily available. Disposable syringes and needles are available in standard sizes and are widely used in this procedure.
- Have required nonsterile items available: a tourniquet, a small waste basin, an emesis basin, general disposable wipes, one or two bottles of contrast medium, and a small prepared dressing for application to the puncture site.
- Have iodine or alcohol wipes available.
- Provide a folded towel or a small pillow that can be placed under the patient's elbow to relieve pressure during the injection.

Fig. 16.28 Urogram: AP projection using tomography.

Fig. 16.29 Urogram: AP projection of kidneys and proximal ureters, 10 × 12-inch (24 × 30-cm) radiation field.

(Courtesy St. Bernard's Medical Center, Jonesboro, AR.)

PROCEDURE

Image quality and exposure technique

Urograms should have the same contrast as abdominal images and are exposed with kVp sufficient to penetrate the iodinated contrast medium. The images must show a sharply defined outline of the kidneys, lower border of the liver, and lateral margin of the psoas muscles. The amount of bone detail visible in these studies varies according to the thickness of the abdomen (Fig. 16.31).

Motion control

The elimination of motion in urographic examinations depends on exposure time and on securing the full cooperation of the patient.

The examination procedure should be explained so that the adult patient is prepared for any transitory distress caused by an injection of contrast solution or by the cystoscopic procedure. The patient should be assured that everything possible will be done for the patient's comfort. The success of the examination depends in large part on the ability of the radiographer to gain the confidence of the patient.

Fig. 16.30 Urogram: AP projection using 14 × 17-inch (35- × 43-cm) radiation field.

(Courtesy St. Bernard's Medical Center, Jonesboro, AR.)

Fig. 16.31 AP abdomen showing margins of kidney *(dots)*, liver *(dashes)*, and psoas muscles *(dot-dash lines)*.

Fig. 16.32 Ureteral compression device in place for urogram.

Ureteral compression device

R

Fig. 16.33 Urogram showing ureteral compression device in proper position over distal ureters.

Ureteral compression

In excretory urography, compression is sometimes applied over the distal ends of the ureters. This compression is applied to retard the flow of the opacified urine into the bladder and to ensure adequate filling of the renal pelves and calyces. If compression is used, it must be placed so that the pressure over the distal ends of the ureters is centered at the level of the anterior superior iliac spine (ASIS). As much pressure as the patient can comfortably tolerate is applied with the immobilization band (Figs. 16.32 and 16.33). This pressure should be released slowly when the compression device is removed to reduce pain caused by rapid changes in intra-abdominal pressure. Compression is generally contraindicated if a patient has urinary stones, an abdominal mass or aneurysm, a colostomy, a suprapubic catheter, traumatic injury, or recent abdominal surgery.

As a result of improvements in contrast agents, ureteral compression is not routinely used in most health care facilities. With the increased doses of contrast medium now employed, most of the ureteral area is usually shown over a series of images. In addition, a prone image is an adequate substitute for ureteral compression for filling the pyelocaliceal system and mid-ureters.

Respiration

For purposes of comparison, all exposures are made at the end of the same phase of breathing—at the *end of expiration* unless otherwise requested. Because the normal respiratory excursion of the kidneys varies from ½ to 1½ inches (1.3 to 3.8 cm), it is occasionally possible to differentiate renal shadows from other shadows by making an exposure at a different phase of arrested respiration. When an exposure is made at a respiratory phase different from what is usually used, the image should be so marked.

PRELIMINARY EXAMINATION

A preliminary examination of the abdomen is made before a specialized investigation of the urinary tract is conducted. This examination sometimes reveals extrarenal lesions that are responsible for the symptoms attributed to the urinary tract and renders the urographic procedure unnecessary. An upright AP projection may also be required to show the mobility of the kidneys. An oblique or lateral projection, or both, in the dorsal decubitus position may be required to localize a tumor mass or to differentiate renal stones from gallstones or calcified mesenteric nodes.

The scout image—an AP projection with the patient recumbent—shows the contour of the kidneys; their location in the supine position; and the presence of renal calculi or calcifications outside the renal collecting system, such as phleboliths, which are small calcifications in the wall of pelvic veins (see Fig. 16.31). This image also serves to check the preparation of the gastrointestinal tract and to enable the radiographer to make any necessary alterations to exposure factors.

Radiation Protection

As with all radiographic procedures, it is the responsibility of the radiographer to minimize radiation exposure to the patient by
- Applying a gonadal shield if it does not overlap the area under investigation. For most projections in this chapter, females generally cannot be shielded without obscuring a portion of the urinary system.
- Restricting radiation to the area of interest by close collimation.
- Working carefully so that repeat exposures are unnecessary.

Intravenous Urography

IVU shows the function and structure of the urinary system. *Function* is shown by the ability of the kidneys to filter contrast medium from the blood and concentrate it with the urine. Anatomic *structures* are usually visualized as the contrast material follows the excretion route of the urine. The primary application of IVU is to evaluate the suspected or continued presence of ureteral obstruction.

The *ACR Practice Guideline for the Performance of Excretory Urography* (2014) emphasizes that an evaluation of the merits and availability of cross-sectional imaging modalities should be performed before IVU is performed. Indications for IVU include, but are not limited to, the following:
- Evaluation of known or suspected ureteral obstruction
- Recurrent urolithiasis—follow-up with limited images for recurrent calculi or stones of the kidneys or urinary tract to decrease patient's total radiation exposure compared to CT studies
- Assessment of suspected congenital abnormalities
- Evaluation of upper urinary tract to investigate abnormalities that increase infection risks
- Assessment of upper urinary tract lesions that may explain hematuria
- Assessment of the effects of trauma and therapeutic interventions

The most common contraindications for IVU relate to (1) the ability of the kidneys to filter contrast medium from the blood and (2) the patient's allergic history. Some contraindications can be overcome by the use of nonionic contrast agents. Patients with conditions in which the kidneys are unable to filter waste or excrete urine (renal failure, anuria) should have the kidneys evaluated by some technique other than excretory urography. Older patients and patients with any of the following risk factors are strong candidates to receive a nonionic contrast medium or should be examined using another modality: asthma, previous contrast media reaction, circulatory or cardiovascular disease, elevated creatinine level, sickle cell disease, diabetes mellitus, or multiple myeloma.

RADIOGRAPHIC PROCEDURE

Before the procedure begins, the patient should be instructed to empty the bladder and change into an appropriate radiolucent gown. Emptying the bladder prevents dilution of the contrast medium with urine. The patient's clinical history, allergic history, and blood creatinine levels should be reviewed. The normal creatinine level is 0.5 to 1.2 mg/100 mL. The glomerular filtration rate (GFR), a calculation that uses the creatinine level (plus age, race, gender, and body size), is the best overall index of kidney function. The National Kidney Foundation considers a normal GFR range to be 90 to 120 mL/min/1.73 m² and a value of 90 mL/min or less as an indicator of renal dysfunction; however, this is an age-related value, as GFR decreases with age. A below-normal GFR should be reviewed by the radiologist or the physician before the contrast media procedure is continued. The radiographer then takes the following steps:

- Place the patient on the table in the supine position, and adjust the patient to center the MSP of the body to the midline of the grid.
- Place a support under the patient's knees to reduce the lordotic curvature of the lumbar spine and to provide greater comfort for the patient (Fig. 16.34).

- Attach the footboard in preparation for a possible upright or semiupright position.
- If the head of the table is to be lowered farther to enhance pelvicaliceal filling, attach the shoulder support and adjust it to the patient's height.
- When ureteric compression is to be used, place the compression device so that it is ready for immediate application at the specified time.
- Obtain a preliminary, or scout, image of the abdomen. Then, prepare for the first postinjection exposure before the contrast medium is injected.
- Place CR plates in the Bucky tray, and for DR equipment, ensure the grid is engaged; position identification, side, and time interval markers; and make any change in centering or exposure technique as indicated by the scout image.
- Have ready a folded towel or other suitable support and the tourniquet for placement under the selected elbow.
- Prepare the contrast medium for injection using an aseptic technique.
- According to the preference of the examining physician, administer 30 to 100 mL of the contrast medium to an adult patient of average size. The dose administered to infants and children is regulated according to age and weight.
- Produce images at specified intervals from the time of *completion of the injection* of contrast medium. (This may depend on the protocol of the department.) These time intervals must be included on each image. Depending on the patient's hydration status and the speed of the injection, the contrast agent normally begins to appear in the pelvicaliceal system within 2 to 8 minutes.

Uptake of contrast medium is seen in the nephrons of the kidney if an image is exposed as the kidneys start to filter the contrast medium from the blood. The initial contrast "blush" of the kidney is termed the *nephrogram phase*. Nephrotomography, if a component of the routine IVU procedure, is usually performed during the nephrogram phase. As the kidneys continue to filter and concentrate the contrast medium, it is directed to the pelvicaliceal system. The greatest concentration of contrast medium in the kidneys normally occurs 15 to 20 minutes after injection. Typically, each image is reviewed immediately to determine, according to the kidney function of the individual patient, the time intervals at which the most intense kidney image can be obtained.

Fig. 16.34 Patient in supine position for urogram, AP projection. Note support under knees.

Fig. 16.35 Urogram at 3 minutes.

The most commonly recommended radiographic images for IVU are AP projections at time intervals ranging from 3 to 20 minutes (Figs. 16.35–16.37). Some physicians prefer bolus injection of the contrast medium followed by a 30-second image to obtain a nephrogram. AP oblique projections (30-degree) may be taken at 5- to 10-minute intervals. In some patients, supplemental images are required to show better all parts of the urinary system and to differentiate normal anatomy from pathologic conditions. These may include an AP projection with the patient in the Trendelenburg or upright position, oblique or lateral projections, or a lateral projection with the patient in the dorsal or ventral decubitus position.

Unless further study of the bladder is indicated or voiding urethrograms are to be made, the patient is sent to the lavatory to void. A postvoid image of the bladder (Figs. 16.38 and 16.39) may be taken to detect, by the presence of residual urine, conditions such as small tumor masses or enlargement of the prostate gland in men. When all necessary images have been obtained, the patient is released from the imaging department. Any contrast medium remaining in the body is filtered from the blood by the kidneys and eventually is excreted in the urine. Some physicians suggest having the patient drink extra fluids for a few days to help flush out the contrast medium.

Fig. 16.36 Urogram at 6 minutes.

Fig. 16.37 Urogram at 9 minutes.

Fig. 16.38 Prevoiding filled bladder.

Fig. 16.39 Postvoiding emptied bladder.

⚜ AP PROJECTION

Image receptor + grid: Positioned by manufacturer or department protocol for proper anatomy display orientation; CR plate: 14 × 17 inches (35 × 43 cm) lengthwise.

Position of patient
- Place the patient supine on the radiographic table for the AP projection of the urinary system. Preliminary (scout) and postinjection images are most commonly obtained with the patient supine (Fig. 16.40).
- Place a support under the patient's knees to relieve strain on the back.
- Place the patient in an upright or a semiupright position for an AP projection to show the opacified bladder and the mobility of the kidneys (Fig. 16.41).

- To show the lower ends of the ureters, it may be helpful to use the Trendelenburg position and an AP projection with the head of the table lowered 15 to 20 degrees and the central ray directed perpendicular to the IR. In this angled position, the weight of the contained fluid stretches the bladder fundus superiorly, providing an unobstructed image of the lower ureters and the vesicoureteral orifice areas.
- If needed, apply ureteral compression (see Fig. 16.32).

Position of part
- Center the MSP of the patient's body to the midline of the grid device.
- Place the patient's arms out of the collimated field.
- Center the IR at the level of the iliac crests. If the patient is too tall to include the entire urinary system, take a second exposure on a 10 × 12-inch (24 × 30-cm) radiation field (CR plate) centered to the bladder. The 10 × 12-inch (24 × 30-cm) exposure field or CR plate is crosswise and centered 2 to 3 inches (5 to 7.6 cm) above the upper border of the pubic symphysis.
- *Shield gonads.*
- *Respiration:* Suspend at the end of expiration.

Central ray
- Perpendicular to the IR at the level of the iliac crests

Collimation
- Adjust the radiation field to no larger than 14 × 17 inches (35 × 43 cm) lengthwise or 10 × 12 inches (24 × 30 cm) crosswise for the additional bladder image (if needed). For smaller patients, collimate to within 1 inch (2.5 cm) of the shadow of the abdomen flanks. Place the correct side marker in the collimated exposure field.

Structures shown
AP projection of the urinary system shows the kidneys, ureters, and bladder filled with contrast medium (Figs. 16.42 through 16.44).

NOTE: The prone position may be recommended to show the ureteropelvic region and to fill the obstructed ureter in the presence of hydronephrosis. The ureters fill better in the prone position, which reverses the curve of their inferior course. The kidneys are situated obliquely, slanting anteriorly in the transverse plane, so the opacified urine tends to collect in and distend the dependent part of the pelvicaliceal system. The supine position allows the more posteriorly placed upper calyces to fill more readily, and the anterior and inferior parts of the pelvicaliceal system fill more easily in the prone position.

Fig. 16.40 Supine urogram: AP projection.

Fig. 16.41 Upright urogram: AP projection.

EVALUATION CRITERIA

The following should be clearly seen:
- Evidence of proper collimation and presence of side marker placed clear of the anatomy of interest

AP and PA projections
- Entire renal outlines
- Bladder and pubic symphysis (a separate image of the bladder area is needed if the bladder was not included)
- No motion
- Contrast medium in the renal area, ureters, and bladder
- Surrounding anatomy
- Compression devices, if used, centered over the upper sacrum and resulting in good renal filling
- Vertebral column centered on the image
- No artifacts from elastic in the patient's underclothing
- Prostatic region inferior to the pubic symphysis on older male patients
- Time marker
- PA projection showing the lower kidneys and entire ureters (bladder included if patient size permits)
- Superimposing intestinal gas in the AP projection moved for the PA projection

AP bladder
- Bladder
- No rotation of the pelvis
- Prostate area in male patients
- Postvoid images clearly labeled and showing only residual contrast medium

Renal pelvis

Left kidney

Bladder

Fig. 16.42 Semiupright urogram: AP projection. Note mobility of kidneys.

Fig. 16.43 Supine urogram: AP projection.

Fig. 16.44 Trendelenburg position urogram: AP projection.

♠ AP OBLIQUE PROJECTION
RPO and LPO positions

Image receptor + grid: Positioned by manufacturer or department protocol for proper anatomy display orientation; CR plate: 14 × 17 inches (35 × 43 cm) lengthwise.

Position of patient
- Place the patient supine on the radiographic table for oblique projections of the urinary system. The kidneys are situated obliquely, slanting anteriorly in the transverse plane.
- When performing AP oblique projections, remember that the kidney closer to the IR is *perpendicular* to the plane of the IR and the kidney farther from the IR is *parallel* with this plane.

Position of part
- Turn the patient so that the midcoronal plane forms an angle of 30 degrees from the IR plane.
- Adjust the patient's shoulders and hips so that they are in the same plane, and place suitable supports under the elevated side as needed.
- Place the arms so that they are not superimposed on the urinary system.
- Center the spine to the grid (Fig. 16.45).
- Center the IR at the level of the iliac crests.
- *Shield gonads.*
- *Respiration:* Suspend at the end of expiration.

Central ray
- Perpendicular to the center of the IR at the level of the iliac crests, entering approximately 2 inches (5 cm) lateral to the midline on the elevated side

Collimation
- Adjust the radiation field to no larger than 14 × 17 inches (35 × 43 cm) lengthwise. For smaller patients, collimate to within 1 inch (2.5 cm) of the shadow of the abdomen flanks. Place the correct side marker in the collimated exposure field.

Structures shown
An AP oblique projection of the urinary system shows the kidneys, ureters, and bladder filled with contrast medium. The elevated kidney is parallel with the IR, and the downside kidney is perpendicular to the IR (Fig. 16.46).

The following should be clearly seen:
- Evidence of proper collimation and presence of side marker placed clear of the anatomy of interest
- Patient rotated approximately 30 degrees
- No superimposition of the kidney remote from the IR on the vertebrae
- Entire downside kidney
- Bladder and lower ureters on 14 × 17-inch (35 × 43-cm) exposure field if patient size permits
- Contrast medium in the kidneys, ureters, and bladder
- Surrounding anatomy
- Time marker

Fig. 16.45 Urogram: AP oblique projection, 30-degree RPO position.

Renal pelvis

Gas in colon
Ureter

Ureteral compression devices

R

Fig. 16.46 Urogram at 10 minutes: AP oblique projection, RPO position.

🌟 LATERAL PROJECTION
Right or left position

Image receptor + grid: Positioned by manufacturer or department protocol for proper anatomy display orientation; CR plate: 14 × 17 inches (35 × 43 cm) lengthwise.

Position of patient

- Turn the patient to a lateral recumbent position on the right or left side, as indicated.

Position of part

- Flex the patient's knees to a comfortable position, and adjust the body so that the midcoronal plane is centered to the midline of the grid.
- Place supports between the patient's knees and ankles.
- Flex the patient's elbows, and place the hands under the patient's head (Fig. 16.47).
- Center the IR at the level of the iliac crests.
- *Shield gonads.*
- *Respiration:* Suspend at the end of expiration.

Central ray

- Perpendicular to the IR, entering the midcoronal plane at the level of the iliac crest

Collimation

- Adjust the radiation field to no larger than 14 × 17 inches (35 × 43 cm) lengthwise. For smaller patients, collimate to within 1 inch (2.5 cm) of the anterior and posterior shadows of the abdomen. Place the correct side marker in the collimated exposure field.

Structures shown

A lateral projection of the abdomen shows the kidneys, ureters, and bladder filled with contrast material. Lateral projections are used to show conditions such as rotation or pressure displacement of a kidney and to localize calcareous areas and tumor masses (Fig. 16.48).

Fig. 16.47 Urogram: lateral projection.

Fig. 16.48 Urogram: lateral projection.

♠ LATERAL PROJECTION
Dorsal decubitus position

Image receptor + grid: Positioned by manufacturer or department protocol for proper anatomy display orientation; CR plate: 14 × 17 inches (35 × 43 cm) lengthwise.

Position of patient
- Place the patient in the supine position on a radiographic cart with the side in question in contact with the vertical grid device. Ensure that the wheels are *locked.*
- Place the patient's arms across the upper chest to ensure that they are not projected over any abdominal contents, or place them behind the head.
- Flex the patient's knees slightly to relieve strain on the back.

Position of part
- Adjust the height of the vertical grid device so that the long axis of the IR is centered to the midcoronal plane of the patient's body.
- Position the patient so that a point approximately at the level of the iliac crests is centered to the IR (Fig. 16.49).
- Adjust the patient to ensure that no rotation from the supine or prone position is present.
- *Shield gonads.*
- *Respiration:* Suspend at the end of expiration.

Central ray
- *Horizontal* and perpendicular to the center of the IR, entering the midcoronal plane at the level of the iliac crests

Collimation
- Adjust the radiation field to no larger than 14 × 17 inches (35 × 43 cm) lengthwise. For smaller patients, collimate to within 1 inch (2.5 cm) of skin shadow. Place the correct side marker in the collimated exposure field.

Structures shown
Rolleston and Reay[8] recommended the ventral decubitus position to show the UPJ in the presence of hydronephrosis. Cook et al.[9] advocated this position to determine whether an extrarenal mass in the flank is intraperitoneal or extraperitoneal, and they stated that the position makes it easy to screen kidneys and ureters for abnormal anterior displacement (Fig. 16.50).

Fig. 16.49 Urogram: lateral projection, dorsal decubitus position.

Fig. 16.50 Urogram: lateral projection, dorsal decubitus position.

Nephrotomography
AP PROJECTION

The renal parenchyma (nephrons and collecting tubes) is best visualized by performing tomography immediately after the introduction of the contrast medium. Evans et al.,[10,11] who introduced nephrotomography, found that by using tomography rather than stationary projections, they could eliminate superimpositions of intestinal contents and more clearly define small intrarenal lesions.

Indications and contraindications

The use of nephrotomography has dramatically declined because of the availability of sectional imaging modalities with greater specificity for renal disease. The ACR states that "nephrotomography may be useful to help distinguish renal calculi from intestinal contents."[12] Contraindications are mainly related to renal failure and contrast media sensitivity, as noted for IVU.

Examination procedure

After a contrast medium has been injected for IVU, the first AP projection of the abdomen is performed during the arterial phase of opacification (Fig. 16.51), and multiple tomograms of the upper abdomen are obtained during the nephrographic phase after the renal parenchyma becomes opacified—hence the term *nephrotomography* (Fig. 16.52). The nephrotic phase normally occurs within 5 minutes after the completion of injection or infusion.

Fig. 16.51 Urogram: AP projection, arterial phase.

Renal margin

Renal pelvis

Minor calyx

Fig. 16.52 Nephrotomogram: (A and B) AP projection at a level of 9 cm (A) and 10 cm (B) in the same patient as in Fig. 16.51.

US of the kidney has practically eliminated the need for percutaneous renal puncture. Cysts are easily differentiated from solid masses on US images (Fig. 16.53). Most masses that are clearly diagnosed as cystic by ultrasound examination are not surgically managed (Fig. 16.54).

Fig. 16.53 US image of normal kidney.

(Courtesy NEA Baptist Memorial Hospital, Jonesboro, AR.)

Fig. 16.54 US image of kidney with cyst. Note measurement markers in image.

(Courtesy NEA Baptist Memorial Hospital, Jonesboro, AR.)

The renal pelvis is entered percutaneously for direct contrast filling of the pelvicaliceal system in selected patients with hydronephrosis.[13-15] This procedure is commonly called a *nephrostogram* because the contrast media injection is frequently made through a percutaneous nephrostomy catheter under fluoroscopic guidance in an interventional radiology suite (Fig. 16.55). Another term for this procedure is *percutaneous antegrade pyelography*[15] to distinguish it from the retrograde technique of direct pelvicaliceal filling; this is usually restricted to the investigation of patients with marked hydronephrosis and patients with suspected hydronephrosis, for whom conclusive information is not gained by excretory or retrograde urography.

Fig. 16.55 Nephrostogram image obtained in interventional radiology suite. Note marked hydronephrosis.

(Courtesy John Youngman, RT(R) and Spencer Haywood, RT(R)(CT), NEA Baptist Memorial Hospital, Jonesboro, AR.)

Retrograde Urography
⚕ AP PROJECTION

Retrograde urography requires that the ureters be catheterized so that a contrast agent can be injected directly into the pelvicaliceal system. This technique provides improved opacification of the renal collecting system but little physiologic information about the urinary system.

Indications and contraindications

Retrograde urography is indicated for evaluation of the collecting system in patients who have renal insufficiency or who are allergic to iodinated contrast media. Because the contrast medium is not introduced into the circulatory system, the incidence of reactions is reduced.

Examination procedure

Similar to all examinations requiring instrumentation, retrograde urography is classified as an operative procedure. This combined urologic-radiologic examination is performed under careful aseptic conditions by the attending urologist with the assistance of a nurse and radiographer. The procedure is performed in a specially equipped cystoscopic-radiographic examining room, which, because of its collaborative nature, may be located in the urology department or the radiology department. A nurse is responsible for the preparation of the instruments and for the care and draping of the patient. A responsibility of the radiographer is to ensure that overhead parts of the radiographic equipment are free of dust for the protection of the operative field and the sterile layout.

The radiographer positions the patient on the cystoscopic table with knees flexed over the stirrups of the adjustable leg supports (Fig. 16.56). This is a modified lithotomy position; the true lithotomy position requires acute flexion of the hips and knees.

If a general anesthetic is not used, the radiographer explains the breathing procedure to the patient and checks the patient's position on the table. The kidneys and the full extent of the ureters in patients of average height are included on a lengthwise 14 × 17-inch (35 × 43-cm) exposure field or CR plate when the third lumbar vertebra is centered to the grid.

If the elevation of the thighs does not reduce the lumbar curve, a pillow is adjusted under the patient's head and shoulders so that the back is in contact with the table. Most cystoscopic-radiographic tables are equipped with an adjustable leg rest to permit extension of the patient's legs for certain radiographic studies.

The urologist performs catheterization of the ureters through a ureterocystoscope, which is a cystoscope with an arrangement that aids insertion of the catheters into the vesicoureteral orifices. After the endoscopic examination, the urologist passes a ureteral catheter well into one or both ureters (Fig. 16.57) and, while leaving the catheters in position, usually withdraws the cystoscope.

Fig. 16.56 Patient positioned on table for retrograde urography, modified lithotomy position.

Fig. 16.57 Retrograde urogram with catheters in proximal ureters: AP projection.

After taking two catheterized specimens of urine from each kidney for laboratory tests—one specimen for culture and one for microscopic examination—the urologist tests kidney function. For this test, a color dye is injected intravenously, and the function of each kidney is determined by the specified time required for the dye substance to appear in the urine as it trickles through the respective catheters.

Immediately after the kidney function test, the radiographer rechecks the position of the patient and exposes the preliminary image (if this has not been done previously) so that the images are ready for inspection by the time the kidney function test has been completed. After reviewing the image, the urologist injects contrast medium and proceeds with the urographic examination. When a bilateral examination is to be performed, both sides are filled simultaneously to avoid subjecting the patient to unnecessary radiation exposure. Additional studies in which only one side is refilled may be performed as indicated.

The most commonly used retrograde urographic series usually consists of three AP projections: the preliminary image showing the ureteral catheters in position (see Fig. 16.57), the pyelogram, and the ureterogram. Some urologists recommend that the head of the table be lowered 10 to 15 degrees for the pyelogram to prevent the contrast solution from escaping into the ureters. Other urologists recommend that pressure be maintained on the syringe during the pyelographic exposure to ensure complete filling of the pelvicaliceal system. The head of the table may be elevated 35 to 40 degrees for the ureterogram to show any tortuosity of the ureters and mobility of the kidneys.

Filling of the average normal renal pelvis requires 3 to 5 mL of contrast solution; however, a larger quantity is required when the structure is dilated. The best index of complete filling, and the one most commonly used, is an indication from the patient as soon as a sense of fullness is felt in the back.

When both sides are to be filled, the urologist injects the contrast solution through the catheters in an amount sufficient to fill the renal pelves and calyces. When signaled by the physician, the patient suspends respiration at the end of expiration, and the exposure for the pyelogram is made (Fig. 16.58).

After the pyelographic exposure, the head of the table may be elevated in preparation for the ureterogram. For this exposure, the patient is instructed to inspire deeply and then to suspend respiration at the end of full expiration. Simultaneously with the breathing procedure, the catheters are slowly withdrawn to the lower ends of the ureters as the contrast solution is injected into the canals. At a signal from the urologist, the ureterographic exposure is made (Fig. 16.59).

Additional projections are sometimes required, such as AP oblique projections in the RPO and LPO positions. Occasionally, a lateral projection, with the patient turned onto the affected side, is performed to show anterior displacement of a kidney or ureter and to delineate a perinephric abscess. Lateral projections with the patient in the ventral or dorsal decubitus position (as required) are also useful, showing the ureteropelvic region in patients with hydronephrosis.

Fig. 16.58 Retrograde urogram with renal pelves filled: AP projection.

Fig. 16.59 Retrograde urogram showing renal pelves and contrast medium–filled ureters: AP projection.

Urinary Bladder, Lower Ureters, Urethra, and Prostate

With few exceptions, radiologic examinations of the lower urinary tract are performed with the retrograde technique of introducing contrast material. These examinations are identified according to the specific purpose of the investigation by the terms *cystography*, *cystoureterography*, *cystourethrography*, and *prostatography*. Most often, they are denoted by the general term *cystography*. Cystoscopy is not required before retrograde contrast filling of the lower urinary canals, but when both examinations are indicated, they are usually performed in a single-stage procedure to spare the patient preparation and instrumentation for separate examinations. When cystoscopy is not indicated, these examinations are best carried out on an all-purpose radiographic table unless the combination table is equipped with an extensible leg rest.

Indications and contraindications

Retrograde studies of the lower urinary tract are indicated for vesicoureteral reflux, recurrent lower urinary tract infection, neurogenic bladder, bladder trauma, lower urinary tract fistulae, urethral stricture, and posterior urethral valves. Contraindications to lower urinary tract studies are related to catheterization of the urethra.

Contrast media

The contrast agents used for contrast studies of the lower urinary tracts are the same nonionic organic compounds used for IVU, but their concentration is reduced, usually to 30%, for retrograde urography.

Injection equipment

Examinations are performed under careful aseptic conditions. Infants, children, and usually adults may be catheterized before they are brought to the radiology department. When the patient is to be catheterized in the radiology department, a sterile catheterization tray must be set up to specifications. Because of the danger of contamination in transferring a sterile liquid from one container to another, the use of commercially available premixed contrast solutions is recommended.

Preliminary preparations

The following guidelines are observed in preparing the patient for the examination:

- Protect the examination table from urine soilage with radiolucent plastic sheeting and disposable underpadding. Correctly arranged disposable padding does much to reduce soilage during voiding studies and consequently eliminates the need for extensive cleaning between patients. A suitable disposal receptacle should be available.
- A few minutes before the examination, accompany the patient to a lavatory. Give the patient supplies for perineal care, and instruct the patient to empty the bladder.
- When the patient is prepared, place the patient on the examination table for the catheterization procedure.

Patients are usually tense, primarily because of embarrassment. It is important that they be given as much privacy as possible. Only required personnel should be present during the examination, and patients should be properly draped and covered according to room temperature.

Contrast injection

For retrograde cystography (Figs. 16.60 and 16.61), cystourethrography, and voiding cystourethrography, the contrast material is introduced into the bladder by injection or infusion through a catheter passed into position via the urethral canal. A small, disposable Foley catheter is used to occlude the vesicourethral orifice in the examination of infants and children, and this catheter may be used in the examination of adults when interval studies are to be made for the detection of delayed ureteral reflux.

Studies are made during voiding to delineate the urethral canal and to detect ureteral reflux, which may occur only during urination (Fig. 16.62). When urethral studies are to be made during injection of contrast material, a soft rubber urethral-orifice acorn is fitted directly onto a contrast-loaded syringe for female patients and is usually fitted onto a cannula attached to a clamp device for male patients.

RETROGRADE CYSTOGRAPHY

Contrast injection technique

In preparing for this examination, the following steps are taken:

- With the urethral catheter in place, adjust the patient in the supine position for a preliminary image and the first cystogram.
- Usually take cystograms of adult patients on 10 × 12-inch (24 × 30-cm) exposure field or CR plate placed lengthwise.
- Center the IR at the level of the soft tissue depression just above the most prominent point of the greater trochanters. This centering coincides with the middle area of a filled bladder of average size. The 12-inch (30-cm) exposure field includes the region of the distal end of the ureters to show ureteral reflux and the prostate and proximal part of the male urethra.
- When ureteral reflux is shown, a larger exposure field may be requested. Some radiologists request studies during contrast filling of the bladder and during voiding.
- After the preliminary image is taken, the physician removes the catheter clamp, and the bladder is drained in preparation for the introduction of contrast material. After introducing the contrast agent, the physician clamps the catheter and tapes it to the thigh to keep it from being displaced during position changes.

The initial cystographic images generally consist of four projections: one AP, two AP obliques, and one lateral. Additional studies, including voiding cystourethrograms, are obtained as indicated.

Fig. 16.60 Retrograde cystogram after introduction of contrast medium: AP projection.

Fig. 16.61 Retrograde cystogram after introduction of air: AP projection.

Fig. 16.62 Serial (polygraphic) voiding cystourethrograms in an infant girl with bilateral ureteral reflux *(arrowheads)*. Urethra is normal. Vaginal reflux *(arrows)* is a normal finding.

AP AXIAL OR PA AXIAL PROJECTION

Image receptor + grid: Positioned by manufacturer or department protocol for proper anatomy display orientation; CR plate: 10 × 12 inches (24 × 30 cm) lengthwise.

Position of patient

- Place the patient supine on the radiographic table for the AP projection of the urinary bladder.

NOTE: Preliminary (scout) and postinjection images are most commonly obtained with the patient supine. The prone position is sometimes used to image areas of the bladder not clearly seen on the AP axial projection. An AP axial projection using the Trendelenburg position at 15 to 20 degrees and with the central ray directed vertically is sometimes used to show the distal ends of the ureters. In this angled position, the weight of the contained fluid stretches the bladder fundus superiorly, giving an unobstructed projection of the lower ureters and the vesicoureteral orifice areas.

Position of part

- Center the MSP of the patient's body to the midline of the grid device.
- Adjust the patient's shoulders and hips so that they are equidistant from the IR.
- Place the patient's arms where they do not cast shadows on the IR.
- If the patient is positioned for a supine image, have the patient's legs extended so that the lumbosacral area of the spine is arched enough to tilt the anterior pelvic bones inferiorly. In this position, the pubic bones can more easily be projected below the bladder neck and proximal urethra (Fig. 16.63).
- Center the IR 2 inches (5 cm) above the upper border of the pubic symphysis (or at the pubic symphysis for voiding studies).
- *Respiration:* Suspend at the end of expiration.

Central ray

AP axial

- Angled 10 to 15 degrees caudal to the center of the IR. The central ray should enter 2 inches (5 cm) above the upper border of the pubic symphysis. When the bladder neck and proximal urethra are the main areas of interest, 5-degree caudal angulation of the central ray is usually sufficient to project the pubic bones below them. More or less angulation may be necessary, depending on the amount of lordosis of the lumbar spine. With greater lordosis, less angulation may be needed (see Fig. 16.63).

PA axial

- When performing PA axial projections of the bladder, direct the central ray through the region of the bladder neck at an angle 10 to 15 degrees cephalad, entering about 1 inch (2.5 cm) distal to the tip of the coccyx and exiting a little above the superior border of the pubic symphysis. If the prostate is the area of interest, the central ray is directed 20 to 25 degrees cephalad to project it above the pubic bones. For PA axial projections, the IR is centered to the central ray.
- Perpendicular to the pubic symphysis for voiding studies.

Collimation

- Adjust the radiation field to 10 × 12 inches (24 × 30 cm) lengthwise. Place the correct side marker in the collimated exposure field.

Fig. 16.63 Retrograde cystogram. AP axial bladder with 15-degree caudal angulation of central ray.

Structures shown

AP axial and PA axial projections show the bladder filled with contrast medium (Figs. 16.64 and 16.65). If reflux is present, the distal ureters are also visualized.

The following should be clearly seen:

- Evidence of proper collimation and presence of side marker placed clear of the anatomy of interest
- Regions of the distal end of the ureters, bladder, and proximal portion of the urethra
- Pubic bones projected below the bladder neck and proximal urethra
- Contrast medium in the bladder, distal ureters, and proximal urethra
- Surrounding anatomy

Fig. 16.64 Excretory cystogram: AP axial projection.

Fig. 16.65 Retrograde cystogram: AP axial projection. Note catheter in bladder.

🡇 AP OBLIQUE PROJECTION
RPO or LPO position

Image receptor + grid: Positioned by manufacturer or department protocol for proper anatomy display orientation; CR plate: 10 × 12 inches (24 × 30 cm) lengthwise.

Position of patient

- Place the patient in the supine position on the radiographic table.

Position of part

- Rotate the patient 40 to 60 degrees RPO or LPO, according to the preference of the examining physician (Fig. 16.66).

- Adjust the patient so that the pubic arch closest to the table is aligned over the midline of the grid.
- Extend and abduct the uppermost thigh enough to prevent its superimposition on the bladder area.
- Center the IR 2 inches (5 cm) above the upper border of the pubic symphysis and approximately 2 inches (5 cm) medial to the upper ASIS (or at the pubic symphysis for voiding studies).
- *Respiration:* Suspend at the end of expiration.

Central ray

- Perpendicular to the center of the IR. The central ray enters 2 inches (5 cm) above the upper border of the pubic symphysis and 2 inches (5 cm) medial to the upper ASIS. When the bladder neck and proximal urethra are the main areas of interest, 10-degree caudal angulation of the central ray is usually sufficient to project the pubic bones below them.
- Perpendicular at the level of the pubic symphysis for voiding studies.

Collimation

- Adjust the radiation field to 10 × 12 inches (24 × 30 cm) lengthwise. Place the correct side marker in the collimated exposure field.

Structures shown

Oblique projections show the bladder filled with contrast medium. If reflux is present, the distal ureters are also visualized (Figs. 16.67 and 16.68).

Fig. 16.66 Retrograde cystogram: AP oblique bladder, RPO position.

EVALUATION CRITERIA

The following should be clearly seen:

- Evidence of proper collimation and presence of side marker placed clear of the anatomy of interest
- Regions of the distal ends of the ureters and bladder, and the proximal portion of the urethra
- Pubic bones projected below the bladder neck and the proximal urethra
- Contrast medium in the bladder, distal ureters, and proximal urethra
- Surrounding anatomy
- No superimposition of the bladder by the uppermost thigh

Voiding studies

- Entire urethra visible and filled with contrast medium
- Urethra overlapping the thigh on oblique projections for improved visibility
- Urethra lying posterior to the superimposed pubic and ischial rami on the side down in oblique projections

Fig. 16.67 Excretory cystogram: AP oblique bladder, RPO position.

Fig. 16.68 Retrograde cystogram with catheter in bladder.

⚹ LATERAL PROJECTION
Right or left position

Image receptor + grid: Positioned by manufacturer or department protocol for proper anatomy display orientation; CR plate: 10 × 12 inches (24 × 30 cm) lengthwise.

Position of patient
• Place the patient in the lateral recumbent position on the right or the left side, as indicated.

Position of part
• Slightly flex the patient's knees to a comfortable position and adjust the body so that the midcoronal plane is centered to the midline of the grid.
• Flex the patient's elbows, and place the hands under the head (Fig. 16.69).
• Center the IR 2 inches (5 cm) above the upper border of the pubic symphysis at the midcoronal plane.
• *Respiration:* Suspend at the end of expiration.

Central ray
• Perpendicular to the IR and 2 inches (5 cm) above the upper border of the pubic symphysis at the midcoronal plane

Collimation
• Adjust the radiation field to 10 × 12 inches (24 × 30 cm) lengthwise. Place the correct side marker in the collimated exposure field.

Structures shown
A lateral image shows the bladder filled with contrast medium. If reflux is present, the distal ureters are also visualized. Lateral projections show the anterior and posterior bladder walls and the base of the bladder (Fig. 16.70).

The following should be clearly seen:
■ Evidence of proper collimation and presence of side marker placed clear of the anatomy of interest
■ Regions of the distal end of the ureters, bladder, and proximal portion of the urethra
■ Contrast medium in the bladder, distal ureters, and proximal urethra
■ Bladder and distal ureters visible through the pelvis
■ Superimposed hips and femur

Fig. 16.69 Cystogram: lateral projection.

Fig. 16.70 Cystogram: lateral projection.

✦ AP OBLIQUE PROJECTION
RPO or LPO position

Male cystourethrography may be preceded by an endoscopic examination, after which the bladder is catheterized so that it can be drained just before contrast material is injected.

The following steps are taken:
- Use a 10 × 12-inch (24 × 30-cm) lengthwise radiation field or CR plate with a grid for male cystourethrograms.
- The patient is adjusted on the combination table so that the IR can be centered at the level of the superior border of the pubic symphysis. This centering coincides with the root of the penis, and a 12-inch (30-cm) radiation field includes the bladder and the external urethral orifice.
- After inspecting the preliminary image, the physician drains the bladder and withdraws the catheter.
- The supine patient is adjusted in an oblique position so that the bladder neck and the entire urethra are delineated as free of bony superimposition as possible. Rotate the patient's body 35 to 40 degrees and adjust it so that the elevated pubis is centered to the midline of the grid. The superimposed pubic and ischial rami of the downside and the body of the elevated pubis usually are projected anterior to the bladder neck, proximal urethra, and prostate (Fig. 16.71).

- The patient's lower knee is flexed only slightly to keep the soft tissues on the medial side of the thigh as near to the center of the IR as possible.
- The elevated thigh is extended and retracted enough to prevent overlapping.
- With the patient in the correct position, the physician inserts the contrast medium–loaded urethral syringe or the nozzle of a device such as the Brodney clamp into the urethral orifice. The physician extends the penis along the soft tissues of the medial side of the lower thigh to obtain a uniform density of the deep and cavernous portions of the urethral canal.

- At a signal from the physician, instruct the patient to hold still; make the exposure while injection of contrast material is continued to ensure filling of the entire urethra (Fig. 16.72).
- The bladder may be filled with a contrast material so that a voiding study can be performed (Fig. 16.73). This is usually done without changing the patient's position. When a standing-upright voiding study is required, the patient is adjusted before a vertical grid device and is supplied with a urinal. (Further information on positioning is provided on pp. 318-319 of this chapter.)

Fig. 16.71 Cystourethrogram: AP oblique projection, RPO position.

Bladder

Prostatic urethra

Membranous urethra

Spongy (cavernous) urethra

Fig. 16.72 Injection cystourethrogram: AP oblique urethra, RPO position.

Fig. 16.73 Voiding cystourethrogram: AP oblique urethra, LPO position.

AP PROJECTION

INJECTION METHOD

The female urethra averages 1½ inches (3.5 cm) in length. Its opening into the bladder is situated at the level of the superior border of the pubic symphysis. From this point, the vessel slants obliquely inferiorly and anteriorly to its termination in the vestibule of the vulva, about 1 inch (2.5 cm) anterior to the vaginal orifice. The female urethra is subject to conditions such as tumors, abscesses, diverticula, dilation, and strictures. It is also subject to urinary incontinence during the stress of increased intra-abdominal pressure, as occurs during sneezing or coughing. In the investigation of abnormalities other than stress incontinence, contrast studies are made during injection of contrast medium or during voiding.

Cystourethrography is usually preceded by an endoscopic examination. For this reason, it may be performed by the attending urologist or gynecologist with the assistance of a nurse and a radiographer.

The following steps are observed:

- After the physical examination, the cystoscope is removed, and a catheter is inserted into the bladder so that the bladder can be drained just before injection of the contrast solution.
- The patient is adjusted in the supine position on the table.
- A 10 × 12-inch (24 × 30-cm) lengthwise radiation field or CR plate is used with a grid and centered at the level of the superior border of the pubic symphysis.
- A 5-degree caudal angulation of the central ray is usually sufficient to free the bladder neck of superimposition.
- After inspecting the preliminary image, the physician drains the bladder and withdraws the catheter. The physician uses a syringe fitted with a blunt-nosed, soft rubber acorn, which is held firmly against the urethral orifice to prevent reflux as the contrast solution is injected during exposure.

- Oblique projections may be required in addition to the AP projection. For oblique projections, the patient is rotated 35 to 40 degrees so that the urethra is posterior to the pubic symphysis. The uppermost thigh is extended and abducted enough to prevent overlapping.
- Further information on positioning is provided on p. 316 of this chapter.
- The physician fills the bladder for each voiding study to be made.
- For an AP projection (Figs. 16.74 and 16.75), the patient is maintained in the supine position, or the head of the table is elevated enough to place the patient in a semi-seated position.
- A lateral voiding study of the female vesicourethral canal is performed with the patient recumbent or upright. In either case, the IR is centered at the level of the superior border of the pubic symphysis.

Fig. 16.74 Voiding cystourethrogram: AP projection.

Contrast-filled bladder

Urethra

Fig. 16.75 Serial voiding images showing four stages of bladder emptying.

Radiologic technologists may perform venipuncture and administer medications by physician order for specific indications in certain types of intravenous (IV) therapy related to radiographic procedures. Most commonly, this medication consists of some type of radiographic contrast medium.[16] For this reason, this chapter provides additional information on the professional and legal considerations of IV access and medication administration, common medications in the imaging department, patient education and assessment, infection control, venipuncture equipment and procedure, contrast reactions, and documentation.

Professional and Legal Considerations

Because of patient risk and legal liabilities, the radiologic technologist must follow professional recommendations, state regulations, and institutional policies for the administration of medications. The information presented in this section is meant to be an introduction to IV therapy. Competency in this area requires the completion of a formal course of instruction with supervised clinical practice and evaluation.

The American Society of Radiologic Technologists (ASRT) includes venipuncture and IV medication administration in the curriculum guidelines for educational opportunities offered to technologists. Additional support for the administration of medications and venipuncture as part of the technologist's scope of practice is found in the ACR's 2017 Resolution 5 and *Manual on Contrast Media* (2017).[17,18] These documents support the injection of contrast materials and diagnostic levels of radiopharmaceuticals within specific established guidelines by certified or licensed radiologic technologists. The ASRT Standards of Practice for Radiography also support the administration of medication by technologists.

Technologists who perform venipuncture and contrast media administration must be knowledgeable about the specific state regulations and facility policies that govern these activities. Technologists also are responsible for professional decisions and actions in their practice. Competency in the skills of venipuncture and contrast media administration are based on cognitive knowledge, proficiency in psychomotor skills, positive affective values, and validation in a clinical setting.

Medications

Medications for a specific procedure are prescribed by a physician, who is also responsible for obtaining informed consent for the procedure. A technologist may administer medications for radiographic procedures, which can require medications for sedation, pain management, contrast media administration, and emergencies.[19] Technologists must be knowledgeable of medications used in the radiology department. IV medications are administered into the body via the vascular system; when administered, they cannot be retrieved. Before administering any medication, the technologist must know the medication's name, dosages, indications, contraindications, and possible adverse reactions (Table 16.1).

Patient Education

The manner in which the technologist approaches the patient can have a direct influence on the patient's response to the procedure. Although the technologist may consider the procedure routine, the patient may be totally unfamiliar with its specifics. Apprehension experienced by the patient can cause vasoconstriction, making venipuncture more difficult and painful.[20] Careful explanation and a confident, sympathetic attitude can help the patient relax.

The technologist must provide information about the procedure in terms the patient can understand, including the steps, duration, and limitations or restrictions associated with the procedure. The patient's questions must be answered in "layman's" language. By explaining the details of the procedure, the technologist can help alleviate fears and solicit cooperation from the patient.

The technologist must tell the truth about the procedure, and attempt to provide accurate information regarding the degree of discomfort associated with a procedure. *The patient should never be told that insertion of the needle used in venipuncture does not hurt.* A miscommunication of this type violates patient trust.

TABLE 16.1

Medications commonly used in an imaging department

Generic Name	Brand NAME	Indications	Action	Adverse Reactions
Atropine sulfate	Atropine *How supplied:* injection, tablets	Symptomatic bradycardia, bradyarrhythmia	Inhibits acetylcholine at parasympathetic neuroeffector junction, enhancing and increasing heart rate	Bradycardia, headache, dry mouth, nausea, vomiting
Diphenhydramine hydrochloride	Benadryl *How supplied:* tablets, capsules, elixir, syrup, injection	Allergic reactions, sedation	Competes with histamine for special receptors on effector cells; prevents but does not reverse histamine-mediated responses	Seizures, sleepiness, insomnia, incoordination, restlessness, nausea, vomiting, diarrhea
Meperidine hydrochloride	Demerol *How supplied:* tablets, syrup, injection	Mild to moderate pain; adjunct to anesthesia	Binds with opiate receptors of CNS	Seizures, cardiac arrest, shock, respiratory depression
Dopamine hydrochloride	Dopamine *How supplied:* injection	Shock, increase cardiac output, correct hypotension	Stimulates dopaminergic and α and β receptors of sympathetic nervous system	Tachycardia, hypotension, nausea, vomiting, anaphylactic reactions
Adrenaline	Epinephrine *How supplied:* injection, inhaler	Restore cardiac rhythm in cardiac arrest; bronchospasm; anaphylaxis	Relaxes bronchial smooth muscle by stimulating β_2 receptors and α and β receptors in sympathetic nervous system	Palpations, ventricular fibrillation, shock, nervousness
Glucagon	Glucagon *How supplied:* injection	Slow peristalsis; prevent or decrease bowel spasm[a]	Increases blood glucose level by promoting catalytic depolymerization of hepatic glycogen to glucose	Bronchospasm, hypotension, nausea, vomiting
Morphine sulfate	Morphine *How supplied:* tablets, syrup, oral suspension, injection	Severe pain	Binds with opiate receptors of CNS	Bradycardia, shock, cardiac arrest, apnea, respiratory depression, respiratory arrest
Chloral hydrate	Noctec *How supplied:* capsules, syrup, suppositories	Sedation	Unknown, sedative effects may be caused by its primary metabolite	Drowsiness, nightmares, hallucinations, nausea, vomiting, diarrhea
Promethazine hydrochloride	Phenergan *How supplied:* tablets, syrup, injection, suppositories	Nausea, sedation	Competes with histamine for special receptors on effector cells; prevents but does not reverse histamine-mediated responses	Dry mouth
Diazepam	Valium *How supplied:* tablets, capsules, oral solutions, injections	Anxiety	Unknown; probably depresses CNS at limbic and subcortical levels	Cardiovascular collapse, bradycardia, respiratory depression, acute withdrawal syndrome
Midazolam hydrochloride	Versed *How supplied:* injection	Preoperative sedation (to induce sleepiness or drowsiness and relieve apprehension)	Unknown; thought to depress CNS at limbic and subcortical levels	Apnea, depressed respiratory rate, nausea, vomiting, hiccups, pain at injection site
Hydroxyzine hydrochloride	Vistaril *How supplied:* tablets, syrup, capsules, injection	Nausea and vomiting, anxiety, preoperative and postoperative adjunctive therapy	Unknown; actions may be due to suppression of activity in key regions of subcortical area of CNS	Dry mouth, dyspnea, wheezing, chest tightness

[a]*ACR Manual on Contrast Media*, v.10.3, 2017, p. 70.
Data from *Nursing 2006 drug handbook*. Ambler, PA: Lippincott Williams & Wilkins; 2006.

Interactions	Effects on Diagnostic Imaging Procedures	Contraindications	Patient Care Considerations
May increase anticholinergic drug effects; use together cautiously	None known	Patients with obstructive disease of gastrointestinal tract, paralytic ileus, toxic megacolon, tachycardia, myocardia or ischemia, or asthma	Watch for tachycardia in cardiac patients; may lead to ventricular fibrillation
Increased effects when used with other CNS depressants	None known	Hypersensitivity to drug during acute asthmatic attacks and in newborns or premature neonates and breastfeeding women	Use with extreme caution in patients with angle-closure glaucoma, asthma, COPD
May be incompatible when mixed in same IV container	None known	Patients with hypersensitivity to drug and patients who have received MAO inhibitors within past 14 days	Give slowly by direct IV injection; oral dose is less than half as effective as parenteral dose; compatible with most IV solutions
α and β blockers may antagonize effects	None known	Patients with uncorrected tachycardia, pheochromocytoma, or ventricular fibrillation	During infusion, frequently monitor ECG, blood pressure, cardiac output, central venous pressure, pulse rate, urine output, and color and temperature of limbs
Avoid using with α blockers (may cause hypotension)	None known	Patients with shock, organic brain damage, cardiac dilation, arrhythmias, coronary insufficiency, or cerebral arteriosclerosis	Drug of choice in emergency treatment of acute anaphylactic reactions; avoid IM use of parenteral suspension into buttocks
Inhibits glucagon-induced insulin release	None known	Patients with hypersensitivity to drug or with pheochromocytoma	Arouse patient from coma as quickly as possible and give additional carbohydrates orally to prevent secondary hypoglycemic reactions
In combination with other depressants and narcotics, use with extreme caution	None known	Patients with hypersensitivity to drug or conditions that would preclude administration of IV opioids	Use with extreme caution in patients with head injuries or increased intracranial pressure and in elderly patients
Alkaline solutions incompatible with aqueous solutions of chloral hydrate	None known	Patients with hepatic or renal impairment, severe cardiac disease, or hypersensitivity to drug	Note two strengths of oral liquid form; double-check dose, especially when administering to children
Increased effects when used with other CNS depressants	Discontinue drug 48 h before myelogram because of high risk of seizures	Patients with hypersensitivity to drug; intestinal obstruction, prostatic hyperplasias	Do not administer subcutaneously
Other CNS depressants	May cause minor changes in ECG patterns	Patients with hypersensitivity to drug or soy protein, shock, coma, or acute alcohol intoxication	Monitor respirations and have emergency resuscitation equipment available before administering
CNS depressants may increase risk of apnea	None known	Patients with hypersensitivity to drug, acute angle-closure glaucoma, shock, coma, or acute alcohol intoxication	Use cautiously in patients with uncompensated acute illness and in elderly patients; have emergency resuscitation equipment available before administering
Can increase CNS depression	None known	Hypersensitivity to drug, during pregnancy, and in breastfeeding women	If used in conjunction with other CNS medication, observe for oversedation

Patient Assessment

The patient must be assessed before any medication is administered. A thorough patient history must be obtained, including any allergies the individual may have specifically to medications, foods, or other environmental agents. A history of allergies, particularly a previous reaction to a medication or contrast media, is strongly correlated with the probability of an adverse reaction. This knowledge is essential for a technologist to be well prepared for a contrast administration.

Other assessment criteria include the patient's current medications. Knowledge of some common medication actions can help the radiologic technologist evaluate changes in a patient's condition during a procedure. Certain diabetic medications interact adversely with contrast media. The interaction of medications must be assessed before the procedure is performed.

During the physical evaluation, it is important to determine whether the patient has previously undergone surgical procedures that might affect site selection for venipuncture (e.g., a mastectomy with resultant compromised lymph nodes and vascular abnormalities, such as atrioventricular shunts). To determine the appropriate type and amount of medication to be administered, the physician requires information about the patient's past and current disease processes, such as hypertension and renal disease. Evaluation of the GFR (normal range 90 to 120 mL/min/1.73 m^2), blood urea nitrogen (BUN) level (average range 7 to 20 mg/dL), and creatinine level (average range 0.5 to 1.2 mg/dL) should be included among the assessment criteria.

Infection Control

Each time the body system is entered, the potential for contamination exists.[21] Strict aseptic techniques and universal precautions must always be used when medications are administered with a needle.[22] If a medication is injected incorrectly, a microorganism may enter the body and cause an infection or other complications. The US Centers for Disease Control and Prevention (CDC) has developed specific guidelines to prevent the transmission of infection during the preparation and administration of medications. These guidelines are part of the standard precautions used by every health care facility, and the technologist must strictly adhere to the guidelines when performing radiologic procedures.

Studies using IV filters have shown a significant reduction in infusion phlebitis. Filters are devices located within the tubing used for IV administration. Filters prevent the injection of particulate and microbial matter into the circulatory system. The use of a filter for a bolus injection reduces the rate at which medication can be injected. In addition, the viscosity of a medication may determine whether a filter is used and the rate of injection. Although a filter helps in reducing the possibility of bacteria being introduced into the blood, its use creates additional factors of risks versus benefits. The physician or health care facility should have policies to address these issues.

Venipuncture Supplies and Equipment
NEEDLES AND SYRINGES

The technologist assembles the proper syringe and needle for the planned injection. The syringe may be glass or plastic. Plastic syringes are disposed of after only one use; glass syringes may be cleaned and must be sterilized before they are used again. The syringe has three parts: the *tip*, where the needle attaches to the syringe; the *barrel*, which includes the calibration markings; and the *plunger*, which fits snugly inside the barrel and allows the user to instill the medication (Fig. 16.76). The tip of the syringe for an IV injection has a locking device to hold the needle securely. The size of the syringe depends on the volume of material to be injected. The technologist should select a syringe one size larger than the volume desired. This larger syringe maximizes the accuracy of the dose by allowing the total amount of medication to be drawn into one syringe.

All needles used in venipuncture are disposable and are used only once. During preparation and administration of contrast media, the technologist may use several types of needles, including a hypodermic needle, a butterfly set, and an over-the-needle cannula (Fig. 16.77).

Fig. 16.76 Plastic disposable syringes.

Fig. 16.77 Types of needles: over-the-cannula needle, or angiocatheter *(bottom)*; hypodermic needle *(center)*; and metal butterfly needle *(top)*.

Hypodermic needles vary in gauge and length (see Fig. 16.77). Needle *gauge* refers to the *diameter* of the needle bore, with the gauge increasing as the diameter of the bore decreases. A 16-gauge needle is larger than a 22-gauge needle. As the bore of the needle increases, a given volume of fluid may be administered more rapidly. If the bore size is reduced and fluid volume and rate of administration remain constant, the pressure (force) of the injection increases. The *length* of a needle is measured in inches and may range from ½ inch (1.3 cm; used for intradermal injections) to 4½ inches (11.5 cm; used for intrathecal [spinal] injections). In general, needles 1 to 1½ inches (2.5 to 3.8 cm) long are most commonly used for IV injections. The needle has three parts: the *hub*, which is the part that attaches to the syringe; the *cannula* or *shaft*, which is the length of the needle; and the *bevel*, which is the slanted portion of the needle tip. Needles should be visually examined before and after use to determine whether any structural defects, such as nonbeveled points or bent shafts, are present.[23]

Butterfly sets or *angiocatheters* are preferable to a conventional hypodermic needle for most radiographic IV therapies. The butterfly set consists of a stainless steel needle with plastic appendages on either side and approximately 6 inches of plastic tubing that ends with a connector. The plastic appendages, often called wings, aid in inserting the needle and stabilizing the needle after venous patency has been confirmed.

The *over-the-needle cannula* is a device in which, after the venipuncture is made, the catheter is slipped off the needle into the vein and the steel needle is removed. This type of needle is recommended for long-term therapy or for rapid infusions, such as infusions that use an automated power injector. The choice of needle should be based on assessment of the patient, institutional policy, and technologist preference.

MEDICATION PREPARATION

Although IV drug administration offers the most immediate results in terms of effect, certain safety precautions must be followed. The technologist must identify the correct patient before medication is administered. During preparation and again before administration, the medication in the container also must be verified.

If medication is supplied in a bottle or vial, the preparation procedure has several variations. First, the solution must be evaluated for contamination. Discoloration and dissolution are the most common signs of contamination. If either of those is observed, the solution should not be used. Then, the protective cap is removed, with care taken not to contaminate the underlying surface. Containers have rubber stoppers through which a hypodermic needle can be inserted. If a single-dose vial is being used, and no contamination has occurred, the rubber stopper requires no additional cleansing. Multiple-dose vial stoppers must be cleaned with an alcohol wipe.

Fig. 16.78 Place tip of needle above level of fluid before injection of air to decrease air bubbles in solution.

For a closed system to be maintained and to reduce the chance of possible infection, a volume of air equal to the amount of desired fluid must be injected into the bottle. The plunger of the syringe is pulled back to the level of the desired amount of medication. The shaft of the plunger must not be contaminated at any time during preparation of the medication. The needle on the syringe is inserted into the rubber stopper, all the way to the hub of the needle. Then, the vial is inverted by placing the end of the needle above the fluid level in the bottle (Fig. 16.78). Next, a small amount of air is *slowly* injected into the vial *above* the level of the fluid. This technique helps decrease air bubbles in the solution. After the air has been injected, the vial and syringe are held inverted and perpendicular to a horizontal plane, and the tip of the needle is pulled *below* the fluid level. The desired amount of medication is aspirated into the syringe by pulling down on the plunger of the syringe. This procedure may have to be repeated several times to expel all of the medication. If air bubbles cling to the syringe casing, the syringe may be lightly tapped to release them. A one-handed method is used to recap the syringe (Fig. 16.79).

Fig. 16.79 When recapping a syringe, use a one-handed method.

Preparation of an infusion from a glass bottle or plastic bag begins with identification and verification of the solution and its expiration date (Fig. 16.80). The solution should not contain any visible particles. The tubing used for the infusion is determined by the method of injection and the type of container. Electronic infusion devices require different tubing than gravity infusion devices. A glass container necessitates vented tubing (Fig. 16.81), whereas a plastic container requires nonvented tubing (Fig. 16.82).

To prepare for drip infusion of a medication, the technologist removes the tubing from the sterile package and closes the clamp (Fig. 16.83). Failure to close the clamp may result in loss of the vacuum in the solution container. The protective coverings are removed from the port of the solution and the tubing spike. Then, the fill chamber of the tubing is squeezed, and the spike is inserted into the solution. The solution is then inverted, and the chamber is released. The solution should fill the chamber to the measurement line. The tubing is primed by opening the clamp, which allows the solution to travel the length of the tubing, expelling any air. The tube is filled with solution, the clamp is closed, and the protective covering is secured. The solution is then ready for administration.

Procedure
SITE SELECTION

Selection of an appropriate vein for venipuncture is crucial. Finding the vein is sometimes difficult, and the most visible veins are not always the best choice.[24] Technologists administer IV medication and contrast media via the venous system. If a pulse is palpated during assessment for a puncture site, that vessel must *not* be used because it is an *artery*. The prime factors to consider in selecting a vein are (1) suitability of location, (2) condition of the vein, (3) purpose of the infusion, and (4) duration of therapy. The veins most often used in establishing IV access are the basilic or cephalic veins on the back of the hand; the basilic vein on the medial, anterior forearm, and elbow; and the cephalic vein on the lateral, anterior forearm, and elbow. The anterior surface of the elbow is also referred to as the *antecubital* space (Fig. 16.84).[25]

A general rule is to select the most distal site that can accept the desired-size needle and tolerate the injection rate and solution. Although the veins located at the antecubital space may be the most accessible, the largest, and the easiest to puncture, they may not be the best choice. Because of their convenient location, these sites may be overused and can become scarred or sclerotic. Antecubital accesses are located over an area of joint flexion; any motion can dislodge the cannula, causing infiltration or resulting in mechanical phlebitis. A flexible IV catheter is the needle of choice for the placement of a venous access in the antecubital space. The patient's arm should be immobilized to inhibit the ability to flex the elbow.

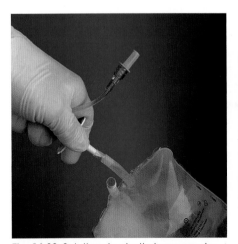

Fig. 16.80 Identify the correct solution and expiration date.

Fig. 16.81 Vented tubing is required for glass bottle containers.

Fig. 16.82 Solutions in plastic bags require nonvented tubing.

Fig. 16.83 Close tubing clamp before inserting spike into container of solution.

The condition of the vein must also be considered in the selection of an appropriate puncture site. The selected vein must be able to tolerate the needed or desired cannula size. The vein should have resilience qualities and be anchored by surrounding supportive tissues to prevent rolling.

Another consideration in vein selection is the rate of flow required for the procedure and the viscosity and amount of medication to be administered. Larger veins should be selected for infusions of large quantities or for rapid infusions. Large veins are also used for the infusion of highly viscous solutions or solutions that are irritating to vessels.[26]

The expected duration of the therapy and the patient's comfort are other factors that must be considered in selecting a venipuncture site. If a prolonged course of therapy is anticipated, areas over flexion joints should be avoided, and the dorsal surfaces of the upper limbs should be carefully examined. Venous access in these locations provides greater freedom and comfort to the patient.

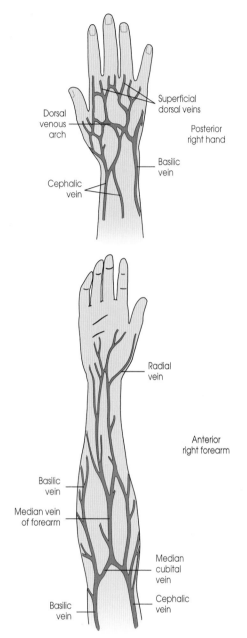

Fig. 16.84 Veins easily accessible for venipuncture.

SITE PREPARATION

The surface of the skin must be prepared and cleaned. If the area selected for venipuncture is hairy, the hair should be clipped to permit better cleansing of the skin and visualization of the vein; this also makes removal of the cannula less painful when the infusion is terminated. Shaving is not recommended. The skin is cleansed with an antiseptic, which should remain in contact with the skin for at least 30 seconds. The preferred solution is iodine tincture 1% to 2%. Isopropyl alcohol 70% is recommended if the patient is sensitive to iodine. The skin should be cleaned in a *circular motion from the center of the injection site* to approximately a 2-inch circle. When the swab has been placed on the skin, it should not be lifted from the surface until the cleansing process is complete (Fig. 16.85).

Many facilities have a policy that provides the patient an opportunity to request a local anesthetic for IV infusion catheter placement. This technique reduces the pain felt by the patient during the insertion of an angiocatheter or needle. The local anesthetic can be administered topically or by injection. Follow the facility protocol for local anesthetic administration. Typical guidelines are as follows:

First, 0.1 to 0.2 mL of 1% lidocaine without epinephrine or sterile saline is prepared in a tuberculin or insulin syringe with a 23- to 25-gauge needle. The site for injection is selected and prepared. Then, the anesthetic is injected subcutaneously (beneath the skin, into the soft tissue) or intradermally (immediately under the skin in the dermal layer) at the venipuncture site. Topical anesthesia is achieved by applying 5 g of eutectic mixture of local anesthetic cream and covering the area with an occlusive dressing. Maximal effects are achieved in 45 to 60 minutes.

The medication to be injected should already be prepared, and any tubing should be primed with the solution to prevent the injection of air into the vascular system.

VENIPUNCTURE

After the solution has been prepared, the site has been selected, and the type of syringe and the needle to be used have been determined, the technologist is ready to perform the venipuncture.

Techniques for venipuncture follow one of two courses: (1) the *direct*, or *one-step*, entry method or (2) the *indirect* method. The *direct*, or *one-step*, method is performed by thrusting the cannula through the skin and into the vein in one quick motion. The needle and cannula enter the skin directly over the vein. This technique is excellent as long as large veins are available.[27] The *indirect* method is a two-step technique. First, the over-the-needle cannula is inserted through the skin adjacent to or below the point where the vein is visible. The cannula is advanced and maneuvered to pierce the vein. For the actual venipuncture procedure, the technologist washes the hands. The patient is identified. Next, the technologist instructs the patient about the procedure. The technologist performs the following steps:

Fig. 16.85 Prepare site for venipuncture.

Fig. 16.86 Put on clean gloves.

Fig. 16.87 Apply tourniquet 6 to 8 inches above intended venipuncture site, with free end directed superiorly.

1. The technologist puts on gloves and cleans the area in accordance with facility protocol (Fig. 16.86).
2. A local anesthetic is administered according to facility policy (optional).
3. A tourniquet is placed 6 to 8 inches (15 to 20 cm) above the intended site of puncture. The tourniquet should be tight enough to distend the vessels but not occlude them. The loose ends of the tourniquet should be placed away from the injection site to prevent contamination of the aseptic area (Fig. 16.87).
4. The technologist holds the patient's limb with the nondominant hand, using that thumb to stabilize and anchor the selected vein. The best method of accessing the vein—direct or indirect technique—is determined.
5. Using the dominant hand, the technologist places the needle bevel up at a 45-degree angle to the skin's surface. The bevel-up position produces less trauma to the skin and vein (Fig. 16.88).
6. The technologist uses a quick, sharp darting motion to enter the skin with the needle. On entering the skin, the technologist decreases the angle of the needle to 15 degrees from the long axis of the vessel. Using an indirect method, the technologist slowly proceeds with a downward motion on the hub or wings of the needle; while raising the point of the needle, the technologist advances the needle parallel and then punctures the vein. The needle may have to be maneuvered slightly to facilitate actual venous puncture. If the direct method of access is used, the needle is placed on the skin directly over the vein, and entry into the vein is accomplished in one movement of the needle through the skin and vein. When the vein is entered, a backflow of blood may occur—this indicates a successful venipuncture.
7. After the vein is punctured and blood return is noted, the cannula is advanced cautiously up the lumen of the vessel for approximately ¾ inch (1.9 cm).
8. Release the tourniquet (Fig. 16.89).
9. If a backflow of blood does not occur, verify venous access before injecting the medication. Aspiration of blood directly into the syringe of medication verifies placement before injection. Another method of placement verification is to attach a syringe of normal saline to the hub of the needle before aspirating for blood. The advantage of this method is that only saline, an isotonic solution, is injected if the needle is not in place and extravasation occurs. A successful venipuncture does not guarantee a successful injection. If a bolus injection is desired, the tourniquet may not be released until the injection has been completed. If this technique is used, the protocol must be included in the facility's policies and procedures.
10. Anchor the needle with tape and a dressing, as required by policy (Fig. 16.90). Then administer the medication (Fig. 16.91).

Fig. 16.88 Stabilize vein and enter skin with needle at 45-degree angle.

Fig. 16.89 Release tourniquet after venous access has been obtained. Do not permit tourniquet to touch needle.

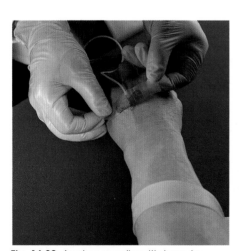

Fig. 16.90 Anchor needle with tape to secure placement.

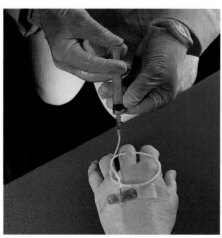

Fig. 16.91 Administer medication.

With experience, a technologist's fingers become sensitive to the sensation of the needle entering the vein—the resistance encountered as the needle penetrates the wall of the vein and the "pop" felt at the loss of resistance as the cannula enters the lumen. If both walls of the vein are punctured with a needle, the vessel develops a hematoma. The cannula should be removed immediately, and direct pressure should be applied to the puncture site. If a venipuncture attempt is unsuccessful with an over-the-needle cannula and the needle has been removed from the cannula, the needle should not be reinserted into the catheter. Reinserting the needle into the cannula can shear a portion of the catheter.

ADMINISTRATION

The technologist should administer the medication or contrast medium at the established rate. During the injection process, the injection site should be observed and palpated proximal to the puncture for signs of infiltration. An infiltration, or extravasation, is a process whereby fluid passes into the tissue instead of the vein.

A patient may have a venous access that was established before the radiologic procedure. Careful assessment of site and medication compatibility must be performed before the existing IV line can be used. (Compatibility is the ability of one medication to mix with another.) Special precautions should be taken with a patient who is currently receiving cardiac, blood pressure, heparin, or diabetes medications. The physician, nurse, or pharmacist should be consulted before medication is administered to such a patient. Verification must be obtained to ensure that the medication being infused through the established IV line is compatible with the *contrast medium* to be administered. Before the contrast medium is injected, the infusion should be stopped, and the line should be flushed with normal saline through the port nearest the insertion site. The *contrast medium* is then administered, and the line is flushed again with normal saline. The amount of normal saline used depends on the facility's policies and procedures. After the contrast medium has been administered, the IV infusion solution is restarted.

Heparin or saline locks allow intermittent injections through a port. The port is a small adapter with an access that is attached to an IV catheter when more than one injection is anticipated.[28] As determined by procedure criteria, the cannula is flushed with heparin and saline to maintain patency during dormant periods.

The patency (open, unobstructed flow) of the intermittent device is verified by aspirating blood and injecting normal saline without infiltration. Then, the medication is administered. Finally, the medication is flushed through the device with saline. Depending on protocols, the device may then be flushed with heparin or normal saline.

After the medication has been administered and the radiologic procedure has been completed, the venous access may be discontinued. The radiologic technologist should carefully remove any tape or protective dressing covering the puncture site. Using a 2 × 2-inch (6 × 6-cm) gauze pad at the injection site, the technologist removes the needle by pulling it straight from the vein. Direct pressure on the site is applied with the gauze only after the needle has been removed (Fig. 16.92). The technologist then puts the contaminated gloves, needles, and gauze in appropriate disposal containers (Fig. 16.93).

Fig. 16.92 Remove IV access.

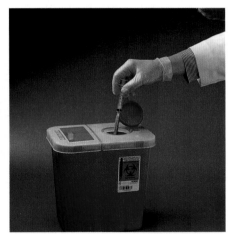

Fig. 16.93 Discard needles in puncture-resistant containers.

Reactions and Complications

Any *medication* has the potential to be harmful if it is not administered properly.[29] Technologists must be aware of possible untoward medication reactions and be able to recognize and report signs and symptoms of side effects as they occur.[30] The technologist who prepares a medication should also perform the administration.

Reactions can be mild, moderate, or severe. Mild reactions can include a sensation of warmth, a metallic taste, or sneezing. Moderate reactions can manifest as nausea, vomiting, or itching. Finally, a severe, or *anaphylactic*, reaction can cause a respiratory or cardiac crisis. The treatment for each category of reaction should be established in the procedures of each facility or department. The role of the radiologic technologist in the case of a reaction should also be defined in these documents. Competent professional standards of practice for the technologist include monitoring the patient's vital signs before, during, and after injection of a contrast medium or certain types of medications. The specific monitoring criteria should be established by institutional policy. If an untoward event should occur, responding personnel would have access to important information about the patient's condition before the event occurred.

Every health care provider should be familiar with emergency procedures in the work environment. Emergency crash carts contain many medications and pieces of equipment that require regular review. Proficiency in the operation of equipment and administration of medications must be maintained. The technologist must have the knowledge, proficiency, and confidence to manage crisis situations.

Infiltration, or *extravasation*, is another complication associated with the administration of contrast media or medications. This complication occurs when the medication or contrast material enters the soft tissue instead of the vein.[31] Signs include swelling, redness, burning, and pain. The most common cause of extravasation is needle displacement. If infiltration occurs, the procedure should be stopped immediately, and venous access should be discontinued. The physician must be notified, and specific treatment instructions must be requested. Although the ACR reports no clear consensus on the most effective treatment for extravasation, common therapies are (1) cold compress to alleviate pain at the injection site and (2) warm compress to increase blood flow to the site for more rapid absorption of the extravasated contrast.[31] The incident should be charted in the manner specified by department protocol.

Documentation

In the administration of any medication, the radiologic technologist should always observe five "rights of medication administration":
- The right patient
- The right medication
- The right route
- The right amount
- The right time

The *right patient* must receive the medication. The identity of the patient must be confirmed before the medication is administered. Methods of patient identification include checking the patient's wristband and asking the patient to restate his or her name. If the patient is unable to speak, seek assistance in identifying the patient from a family member or significant other. Ensuring that the *right medication* is administered requires that the name of the medication be verified at least three times: during the selection process, during preparation, and immediately before administration. The amount of medication is determined by the physician or by departmental protocols. The *right route*, *right amount*, and *right time* are determined by the physician, the type of medication, and the procedure.

Documentation of the five rights of medication administration should be included in every patient's permanent medical record. In addition to these five rights, the documentation should include the size, type, and location of the needle; the number of venipuncture attempts; and the identity of the health care personnel who performed the procedure. Information about how the patient responded to the procedure should also be documented. The following is an example of the correct documentation technique for a technologist performing venipuncture and administering a medication:

> *4-15-99 at 0900 a venous access on Mr. John Q Public was performed using an 18-gauge angiocatheter. The access was established in the dorsum of the left hand after one attempt. Then, 100 mL of [the specific name of the medication] was administered by IV push via the access. The patient tolerated the injection procedure and medication without complaints of pain or discomfort and with no unexpected side effects.*
>
> **Sandy R. Ray, RT**

The objective of medication therapy and administration is to provide maximal benefit to the patient with minimal harm. Medications are intended to help maintain health, treat or prevent disease, relieve symptoms, alter body processes, and diagnose disease. All medications are not ideal in their effects on the human body. It is important that health care providers understand their roles and responsibilities in the administration of medications. Because the medications used by the radiologic technologist are imperfect, caution for the patient's well-being and skill in the administration of medications are priorities. Patients have the right to expect that the personnel who administer medications are informed about dosages, actions, indications, adverse reactions, interactions, contraindications, and special considerations. Education, training, licensing, and experience are crucial in establishing competency in this area of practice.

References

1. American College of Radiology. *ACR Practice guideline for the performance of excretory urography*; 2009. revised.
2. American College of Radiology. *ACR–SAR practice parameter for the performance of excretory urography*; 2014.
3. Long BW. Radiography of cutaneous urinary diversions. *Radiol Technol*. 1988;60:109.
4. Rowntree LG, et al. Roentgenography of the urinary tract during excretion of sodium iodide. *JAMA*. 1923;8:368.
5. Roseno A, Jepkins H. Intravenous pyelography, *Fortschr Roentgenstr* 39:859, 1929, *AJR Am J Roentgenol*. 1929;22:685. Abstract.
6. Hope JW, Campoy F. The use of carbonated beverages in pediatric excretory urography. *Radiology*. 1955;64:66.
7. Berdon WE, et al. Prone radiography in intravenous pyelography in infants and children. *AJR Am J Roentgenol*. 1968;103:444.
8. Rolleston GL, Reay ER. The pelvi-ureteric junction. *Br J Radiol*. 1957;30:617.
9. Cook IK, et al. Determination of the normal position of the upper urinary tract in the lateral abdominal urogram. *Radiology*. 1971;99:499.
10. Evans JA, et al. Nephrotomography, *AJR Am J Roentgenol*. 1954;71:213.
11. Evans JA. Nephrotomography in the investigation of renal masses. *Radiology*. 1957;69:684.
12. ACR Appropriateness Criteria. Acute onset flank pain—suspicious of stone disease. Available at: https://acsearch.acr.org/docs/69362/narrative.
13. Wickbom I. Pyelography after direct puncture of the renal pelvis. *Acta Radiol*. 1954;41:505.
14. Weens HS, Florence TJ. The diagnosis of hydronephrosis by percutaneous renal puncture. *J Urol*. 1954;72:589.
15. Casey WC, Goodwin WE. Percutaneous antegrade pyelography and hydronephrosis. *J Urol*. 1955;74:164.
16. Tortorici M. *Administration of imaging pharmaceuticals*. Philadelphia: Saunders; 1996.
17. American College of Radiology. *ACR practice parameter for the use of intravascular contrast media*; 2017.
18. *ACR manual on contrast media,* v.10.3, 16, 2017.
19. Kowalczyk N, Donnett K. *Integrated patient care for the imaging professional*. St Louis: Mosby; 1996.
20. *Managing IV therapy: skillbuilders*. PA: Springhouse; 1991. Springhouse.
21. Smith S, et al. *Clinical nursing skills: basic to advanced skills*. ed 6. Stamford, CT: Appleton & Lange; 2003.
22. Adler AM, Carlton RR. *Introduction to radiography and patient care*. ed 4. Philadelphia: Saunders; 2007.
23. Strasinger S, DiLorenzo M. *Phlebotomy workbook for the multiskilled healthcare professional*. ed 2. Philadelphia: FA Davis; 2003.
24. Steele J. *Practical IV therapy*. Springhouse, PA: Springhouse; 1988.
25. Jensen S, Peppers M. *Pharmacology and drug administration for imaging technologists*. ed 2. St Louis: Elsevier/Mosby; 2006.
26. Adler AM, Carlton RR. *Introduction to radiologic sciences and patient care*. ed 5. St Louis: Elsevier/Saunders; 2012.
27. Weinstein SM. *Plumer's principles and practice of intravenous therapy*. ed 8. Little, Brown: Boston; 2006.
28. Ehrlich R, Coakes D. *Patient care in radiography*. ed 8. St Louis: Elsevier/Mosby; 2013.
29. Kowalczyk N, Donnett K. *Integrated patient care for the imaging professional*. St Louis: Mosby; 1996.
30. Adler AM, Carlton RR. *Introduction to radiography and patient care*. ed 3. Philadelphia: Saunders; 2003.
31. American College of Radiology, ACR Committee on Drugs and Contrast Media. *ACR manual on contrast media*. Reston, VA: American College of Radiology; 2013. version 9, 2013.

17

REPRODUCTIVE SYSTEM

SUMMARY OF PROJECTIONS

PROJECTIONS, POSITIONS, AND METHODS

Page	Essential	Anatomy	Projection	Position	Method
344		Hysterosalpingography	AP, lateral, axial, oblique		
351		Male reproductive system			ULTRASOUND

Female Reproductive System

The female reproductive system consists of an internal and an external group of organs connected by the vaginal canal. This chapter does not address the anatomy of the external genitalia because those structures do not require radiographic demonstration. The internal genital organs consist of the female gonads, or *ovaries,* which are two glandular bodies homologous to the male testes, and a system of canals composed of the *uterine tubes, uterus,* and *vagina.*

OVARIES

The two ovaries are small glandular organs with an internal secretion that controls the menstrual cycle and an external secretion containing the *ova,* or female reproductive cells (Fig. 17.1). Each ovary is shaped approximately like an almond. The ovaries lie one on each side, inferior and posterior to the uterine tube and near the lateral wall of the pelvis. They are attached to the posterior surface of the broad ligament of the uterus by the *mesovarium.*

The ovary has a core of vascular tissue, the *medulla,* and an outer portion of glandular tissue, the *cortex.* The cortex contains *ovarian follicles* in all stages of development, and each follicle contains one ovum. A fully developed ovarian follicle is referred to as a *graafian follicle.* As the minute ovum matures, the size of the follicle and its fluid content increase so that the wall of the follicle's sac approaches the surface of the ovary. In time it ruptures, liberating the ovum and follicular fluid into the peritoneal cavity. Extrusion of an ovum by the rupture of a follicle is called *ovulation,* and it usually occurs once during the menstrual cycle. When the ovum is in the pelvic cavity, it is drawn toward the uterine tube.

UTERINE TUBES

The two *uterine tubes,* or fallopian tubes, arise from the lateral angle of the uterus, pass laterally above the ovaries, and open into the peritoneal cavity. These tubes collect ova released by the ovaries and convey the cells to the uterine cavity. Each tube is 3 to 5 inches (7.6 to 13 cm) long (Fig. 17.2) and has a small diameter at its uterine end, which opens into the cavity of the uterus by a minute orifice. The tube itself is divided into three parts: the isthmus, the ampulla, and the infundibulum. The *isthmus* is a short segment near the uterus. The *ampulla* comprises most of the tube and is wider than the isthmus. The terminal and lateral portion of the tube is the *infundibulum* and is flared in appearance. The infundibulum ends in a series of irregular prolonged processes called *fimbriae,* and one of the fimbriae is attached to or near the ovary.

The mucosal lining of the uterine tube contains hairlike projections called *cilia.* The lining is arranged in folds that increase in number and complexity as they approach the fimbriated extremity of the tube. The cilia draw the ovum into the tube, which then convey it to the uterine cavity by peristaltic movements. Passage of the ovum through the tube requires several days. Fertilization of the cell occurs in the outer part of the tube, and the fertilized ovum migrates to the uterus for implantation.

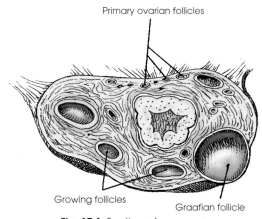

Primary ovarian follicles

Growing follicles

Graafian follicle

Fig. 17.1 Section of an ovary.

Cavity of uterus

Isthmus

Ampulla

Infundibulum

Round ligament

Fimbriae

Fig. 17.2 Section of left uterine tube.

UTERUS

The *uterus* is a pear-shaped, muscular organ (Figs. 17.3 and 17.4). Its primary functions are to receive and retain the fertilized ovum until development of the fetus is complete and, when the fetus is mature, to expel it during birth.

The uterus consists of four parts: fundus, body, isthmus, and cervix. The *fundus* is the bluntly rounded, superiormost portion of the uterus. The *body* narrows from the fundus to the isthmus and is the point of attachment for the ligaments that secure the uterus within the pelvis. The *isthmus* (superior part of the cervix), a constricted area between the body and the cervix, is approximately ½ inch (1.3 cm) long. The *cervix,* the cylindric vaginal end of the uterus, is approximately 1 inch (2.5 cm) long. The vagina is attached around the circumference of the cervix.

The *nulliparous* uterus (i.e., the uterus of a woman who has not given birth) is approximately 3 inches (7.6 cm) in length, almost half of which represents the length of the cervix, which is approximately 3/4 inch (1.9 cm) in diameter. During pregnancy, the body of the uterus gradually expands into the abdominal cavity, reaching the epigastric region in the eighth month. After parturition, the organ shrinks to almost its original size but undergoes characteristic changes in shape.

The uterus is situated in the central part of the pelvic cavity, where it lies posterior and superior to the urinary bladder and anterior to the rectal ampulla. The long axis, which is slightly concave anteriorly, is directed inferiorly and posteriorly at a near right angle to the axis of the vaginal canal, into which the lower end of the cervix projects.

The cavity of the body of the uterus, or the uterine cavity proper, is triangular in shape when viewed in the frontal plane. The canal of the cervix is dilated in the center and constricted at each extremity, and the proximal end of the canal is continuous with the canal of the isthmus. The distal orifice is called the *uterine ostium.*

The mucosal lining of the uterine cavity is called the *endometrium.* This lining undergoes cyclic changes, called the *menstrual cycle,* at about 4-week intervals from puberty to menopause. During each premenstrual period, the endometrium is prepared for implantation and nutrition of the fertilized ovum. If fertilization has not occurred, the menstrual flow of blood and necrosed particles of uterine mucosa ensues.

VAGINA

The *vagina* is a muscular structure with walls and a canal lying posterior to the urinary bladder and urethra, and anterior to the rectum. Averaging about 3 inches (7.6 cm) in length, the vagina extends inferiorly and anteriorly from the uterus to the exterior. The *mucosa* of the vagina is continuous with that of the uterus. The space between the labia minora, which is known as the *vaginal vestibule,* contains the *vaginal orifice* and the *urethral orifice.*

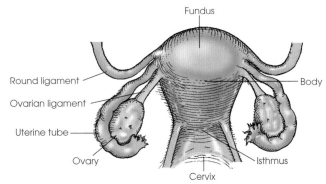

Fig. 17.3 Superoposterior view of uterus, ovaries, and uterine tubes.

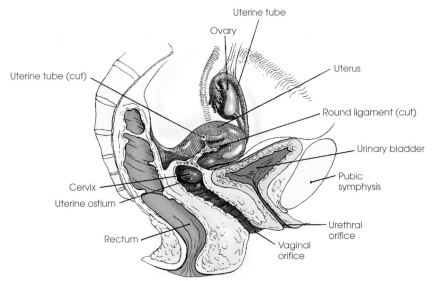

Fig. 17.4 Sagittal section showing relation of internal genitalia to surrounding structures.

FETAL DEVELOPMENT

During the *implantation* process, the fertilized ovum, called a *zygote,* is passed from the uterine tube into the uterine cavity, where it adheres to and becomes embedded in the uterine lining. About 2 weeks after fertilization of the ovum, the *embryo* begins to appear. The embryo becomes a fetus 9 weeks after fertilization and then assumes a human appearance (Fig. 17.5).

During the first 2 weeks of embryonic development, the growing fertilized ovum is primarily concerned with establishing its nutritive and protective covering, the *chorion* and the *amnion*. As the chorion develops, it forms (1) the outer layer of the protective membranes enclosing the embryo, and (2) the embryonic portion of the *placenta,* by which the umbilical cord is attached to the mother's uterus and through which food is supplied to and waste is removed from the fetus. The amnion, often referred to as the "bag of water" by the laity, forms the inner layer of the fetal membranes and contains amniotic fluid, in which the fetus floats. After birth, the uterine lining is expelled with the fetal membranes and the placenta, constituting the afterbirth. A new endometrium is then regenerated.

The fertilized ovum usually becomes embedded near the fundus of the uterine cavity, most frequently on the anterior or posterior wall. Implantation occasionally occurs so low, however, that the fully developed placenta encroaches on or obstructs the cervical canal. This condition results in premature separation of the placenta, termed *placenta previa* (Fig. 17.6).

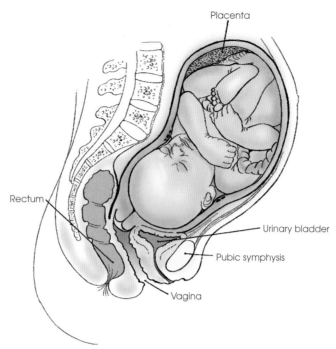

Fig. 17.5 Sagittal section showing fetus of about 7 months of age.

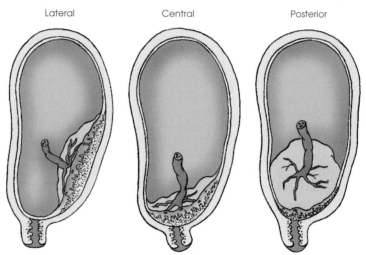

Fig. 17.6 Schematic drawings of several placental sites in low implantation.

Male Reproductive System

The male genital system consists of a pair of male *gonads,* the *testes,* which produce spermatozoa, two excretory channels, the *ductus deferens* (vas deferens). the *prostate,* the ejaculatory ducts, the *seminal vesicles,* and a pair of *bulbourethral glands,* which produce secretions that are added to the secretions of the testes and ductal mucosa to constitute the final product of seminal fluid. The *penis,* the *scrotum,* and the structures enclosed by the scrotal sac (testes, epididymides, spermatic cords, and part of the ductus deferens) are the external genital organs.

TESTES

The *testes* are ovoid bodies, averaging 1½ inches (3.8 cm) in length and about 1 inch (2.5 cm) in width and depth (Fig. 17.7). Each testis is divided into 200 to 300 partial compartments that constitute the glandular substance of the testis. Each compartment houses one or more convoluted, germ cell–producing tubules; these tubules converge and unite to form 15 to 20 ductules, which emerge from the testis to enter the head of the epididymis.

The *epididymis* is an oblong structure that is attached to the superior and lateroposterior aspects of the testis. The ductules leading out of the testis enter the head of the epididymis to become continuous with the coiled and convoluted ductules that make up this structure. As the ductules pass inferiorly, they progressively unite to form the main duct, which is continuous with the ductus deferens.

DUCTUS DEFERENS

The *ductus deferens* is 16 to 18 inches (40 to 45 cm) long and extends from the tail of the epididymis to the posteroinferior surface of the urinary bladder. Only its first part is convoluted. From its beginning, the ductus deferens ascends along the medial side of the epididymis on the posterior surface of the testis to join the other constituents of the spermatic cord, with which it emerges from the scrotal sac and passes into the pelvic cavity through the inguinal canal (Fig. 17.8). Near its termination, the duct expands into an *ampulla* for storage of seminal fluid and ends by uniting with the duct of the seminal vesicle.

SEMINAL VESICLES

The two *seminal vesicles* are sacculated structures about 2 inches (5 cm) long (Fig. 17.9). They are situated obliquely on the lateroposterior surface of the bladder, where, from the level of the ureterocystic junction, each slants inferiorly and medially to the base of the prostate. Each ampulla of the ductus deferens lies along the medial border of the seminal vesicle to form the ejaculatory duct.

EJACULATORY DUCTS

Each *ejaculatory duct* is formed by the union of the ductus deferens and the duct of the seminal vesicle. The ejaculatory ducts average about ½ inch (1.3 cm) in length and originate behind the neck of the bladder. The two ducts enter the base of the prostate and, passing obliquely inferiorly through the substance of the gland, open into the prostatic urethra at the lateral margins of the prostatic utricle. These ducts eject sperm into the urethra before ejaculation.

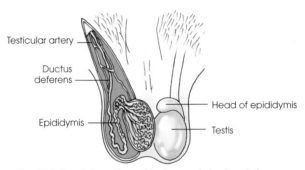

Fig. 17.7 Frontal section of testes and ductus deferens.

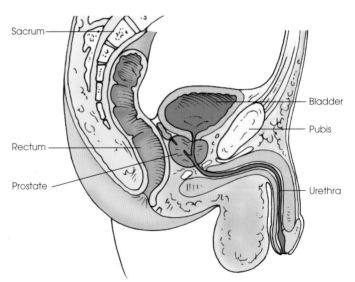

Fig. 17.8 Sagittal section showing male genital system.

PROSTATE

The *prostate,* an accessory genital organ, is a cone-shaped organ that averages 1 ¼ inches (3.2 cm) in length. The prostate encircles the proximal portion of the male urethra and, extending from the bladder neck to the pelvic floor, lies in front of the rectal ampulla approximately 1 inch (2.5 cm) posterior to the lower two-thirds of the pubic symphysis (see Fig. 17.9). The prostate comprises muscular and glandular tissue. The ducts of the prostate open into the prostatic portion of the urethra.

Because of advances in diagnostic ultrasound imaging, radiographic examinations of the male reproductive system are performed less often than in the past. The prostate can be ultrasonically imaged through the urine-filled bladder or by using a special rectal transducer, and the seminal ducts can be imaged when the rectum is filled with an ultrasound gel and a special rectal transducer is used. Testicular ultrasonic scans are performed to evaluate a palpable mass or an enlarged testis and to check for metastasis. Most testicular scans are performed because of a palpable mass or an enlarged testis.

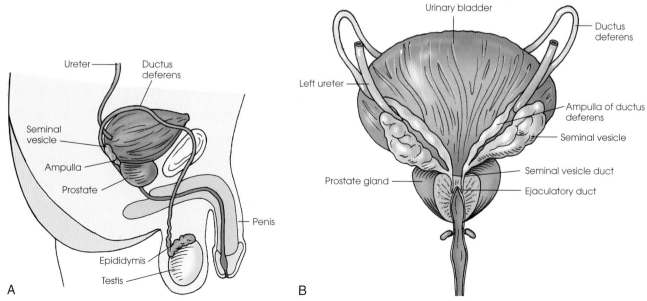

Fig. 17.9 (A) Sagittal section through male pelvis. (B) Posterior view of male reproductive organs.

SUMMARY OF ANATOMY

Female reproductive system
Ovaries
Uterine tubes
Uterus
Vagina

Ovaries
Ova
Mesovarium
Medulla
Cortex
Ovarian follicles
Graafian follicle
Ovulation

Uterine tubes (fallopian tubes)
Isthmus
Ampulla
Infundibulum
Fimbriae
Cilia

Uterus
Fundus
Body
Isthmus
Cervix
Uterine ostium
Endometrium

Vagina
Mucosa
Vaginal vestibule
Vaginal orifice
Urethral orifice

Fetal development
Zygote
Embryo
Fetus
Placenta

Male reproductive system
Testes
Ductus deferens (vas deferens)
Prostate
Ejaculatory ducts
Seminal vesicles
Bulbourethral glands
Penis
Scrotum

Testes
Epididymis

Ductus deferens
Ampulla

SUMMARY OF PATHOLOGY

Condition	Definition
Adhesion	Union of two surfaces that are normally separate
Cryptorchidism	Condition of undescended testis
Endometrial polyp	Growth or mass protruding from endometrium
Epididymitis	Inflammation of the epididymis
Uterine tube obstruction	Condition preventing normal flow through uterine tube
Fistula	Abnormal connection between two internal organs or between an organ and the body surface
Testicular torsion	Twisting of the testis at its base, causing acute ischemia
Tumor	New tissue growth where cell proliferation is uncontrolled
Dermoid cyst	Tumor of the ovary filled with sebaceous material and hair
Prostate cancer	Second most common malignancy in men
Seminoma	Most common type of testicular tumor
Uterine fibroid	Smooth muscle tumor of the uterus

ABBREVIATIONS USED IN CHAPTER 17

HSG	Hysterosalpingography
IUD	Intrauterine device

See Addendum B for a summary of all abbreviations used in Volume 2.

Female Radiography
NONPREGNANT PATIENT

Radiologic investigations of the nonpregnant uterus, accessory organs, and vagina are denoted by the terms *hysterosalpingography* (HSG), *pelvic pneumography,* and *vaginography.* Each procedure requires the use of contrast medium and should be performed under aseptic conditions. *HSG* involves the introduction of a radiopaque contrast medium through a uterine cannula. The procedure is performed to determine the size, shape, and position of the uterus and uterine tubes, to delineate lesions such as polyps, submucous tumor masses, or fistulous tracts, and to investigate the patency of the uterine tubes in patients who have been unable to conceive (Fig. 17.10).

Pelvic pneumography, which requires the introduction of a gaseous contrast medium directly into the peritoneal cavity, is now rarely performed because of the development of ultrasound techniques for evaluating the pelvic cavity. *Vaginography* is performed to investigate congenital abnormalities, vaginal fistulas, and other pathologic conditions involving the vagina.

Contrast media

Various opaque media are used in examinations of the female genital passages; the water-soluble contrast media employed for intravenous urography are widely used for HSG and vaginography.

Preparation of intestinal tract

Preparation of the intestinal tract for any of these examinations usually consists of the following:

1. A non–gas-forming laxative is administered on the preceding evening if the patient is constipated.
2. Before reporting for the examination, the patient receives cleansing enemas until the return flow is clear.
3. The meal preceding the examination is withheld.

Appointment date and care of patient

Gynecologic examinations should be scheduled approximately 10 days after the onset of menstruation, as this is the interval during which the endometrium is least congested. More important, because this time interval is a few days before ovulation normally occurs, there is little danger of irradiating a recently fertilized ovum.

The relatively minor instrumentation required for the introduction of contrast medium in these examinations normally does not necessitate hospitalization or premedication. Some patients experience unpleasant but transitory aftereffects. The radiology department should have facilities in which an outpatient can rest in the recumbent position before returning home.

The patient is requested to empty her bladder completely immediately before the examination in order to prevent pressure displacement and superimposition of the bladder on the pelvic genitalia. In addition, the patient's vagina is irrigated just before the examination. At this time, the patient should be given the necessary supplies and instructed to cleanse the perineal region.

Radiation protection

To deliver the least possible amount of radiation to the gonads, the radiologist restricts fluoroscopy and imaging to the minimum required for a satisfactory examination.

Hysterosalpingography

HSG is performed by a physician, with spot images made while the patient is in the supine position on a fluoroscopy table. The examination may also be performed by the physician with conventional radiographic images obtained using an overhead tube. When fluoroscopy is used, spot images may be the only images obtained. Preparation of the patient for the examination includes the following steps:

- After irrigation of the vaginal canal, complete emptying of the bladder and perineal cleansing, and place the patient on the examining table.
- Adjust the patient in the lithotomy position, with the knees flexed over leg rests.
- When a combination table is used, adjust the patient's position to permit the IRs to be centered to a point 2 inches (5 cm) proximal to the pubic symphysis; lengthwise 10 × 12-inch (24 × 30-cm) IRs or collimated field sizes are used for all studies.

Fig. 17.10 HSG reveals bilateral hydrosalpinx of uterine tubes *(arrows).* Contrast medium–filled uterine cavity is normal *(arrowheads).*

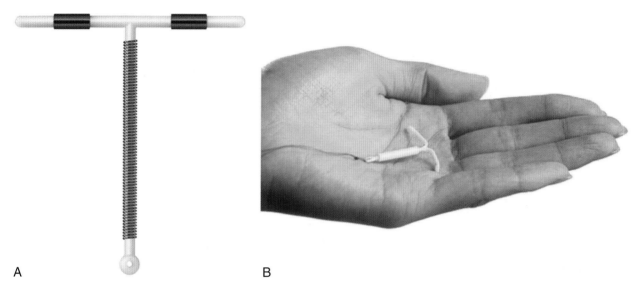

A   B

Fig. 17.15 Temporary intrauterine contraceptive device (IUD). (A) ParaGard (intrauterine copper contraceptive) manufactured by Teva Women's Health, Inc. Actual size is 32 × 36 mm. (B) Mirena (levonorgestrel-releasing intrauterine system) manufactured by Bayer Healthcare Pharmaceuticals.

Fig. 17.16 Permanent contraceptive IUD, Essure by Bayer Healthcare Pharmaceuticals.

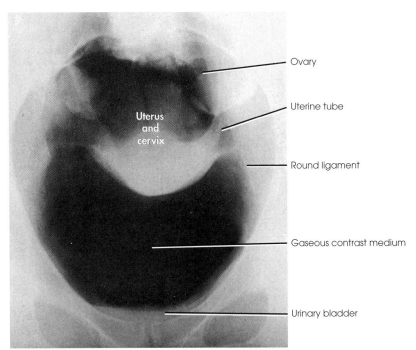

Fig. 17.17 Normal pelvic pneumogram. (See Fig. 17.3 for correlation with image.)

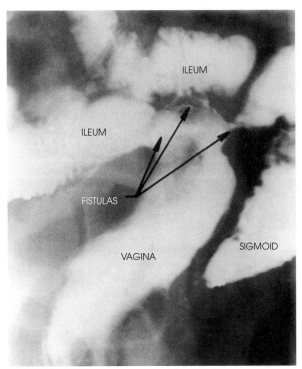

Fig. 17.18 Vaginogram, spot image, PA oblique projection, LAO position. Sigmoid fistula and two ileal fistulas are shown.

Pelvic pneumography

Pelvic pneumography, gynecography, and *pangynecography* are the terms used to denote radiologic examinations of the female pelvic organs via intraperitoneal gas insufflation (Fig. 17.17). These procedures have essentially been replaced by ultrasonography and other diagnostic techniques. (Pelvic pneumography is described in Volume 3 of the fourth edition of this atlas.)

Vaginography

Vaginography is used in the investigation of congenital malformations and pathologic conditions such as vesicovaginal and enterovaginal fistulas. The examination is performed by introducing a contrast medium into the vaginal canal. Lambie et al.[2] recommended using a thin barium sulfate mixture to investigate fistulous communications with the intestine. At the end of the examination, the patient is instructed to expel as much of the barium mixture as possible, and the canal is cleansed by vaginal irrigation. To investigate other conditions, Coe[3] advocated the use of an iodinated organic compound.

A rectal retention tube is employed to introduce the contrast medium so that a moderately inflated balloon can be used to prevent reflux. In one technique, the physician inserts only the tip of the tube into the vaginal orifice. The patient is then asked to extend her thighs and to hold them in close approximation to keep the inflated balloon pressed firmly against the vaginal entrance. In another technique, the tube is inserted far enough to place the deflated balloon within the distal end of the vagina and the balloon is inflated under fluoroscopic observation. The barium mixture is introduced with the usual enema equipment. The water-soluble medium is injected with a syringe.

Vaginography is performed on a combination fluoroscopy-radiography table. Contrast medium is injected under fluoroscopic control, and spot images are exposed as indicated during the filling (Fig. 17.18).

The images in Figs. 17.19 through 17.21 were taken with the central ray directed perpendicular to the midpoint of the IR. For localized studies, the central ray is centered at the level of the superior border of the pubic symphysis.

In each examination, the radiographic projections required are determined by the radiologist according to fluoroscopic findings. Low rectovaginal fistulas are best shown in the lateral projection, and fistulous communications with the sigmoid or ileum or both are best shown in oblique projections.

EVALUATION CRITERIA

The following should be clearly seen:
- Superior border of the pubic symphysis centered on the image
- Any fistulas in their entirety
- Pelvis on oblique projections not superimposed by the proximal thigh
- Superimposed hips and femora in the lateral image
- The vagina and any fistula

Fig. 17.19 Vaginogram, AP projection, showing small fistulous tract *(arrow)* projecting laterally from apex of vagina and ending in abscess.

Fig. 17.20 Vaginogram, AP oblique projection, RPO position. Fistulas to ileum and sigmoid are shown.

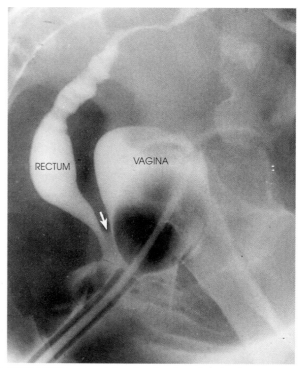

Fig. 17.21 Vaginogram, lateral projection, showing low rectovaginal fistula.

PREGNANT PATIENT

Ultrasonography provides visualization of the fetus and placenta with no apparent risk to the patient or fetus. Diagnostic sonography is the preferred diagnostic tool for examining a pregnant woman. For informational purposes, the following radiographic procedures are defined:

- *Fetography*—radiographic examination of the fetus in utero to detect suspected abnormalities of development, to confirm suspected fetal death, to determine the presentation and position of the fetus, and to determine whether the pregnancy is single or multiple (Fig. 17.22). This examination should be performed after the 18th week of gestation due to the danger of radiation-induced fetal malformations.
- *Pelvimetry*—radiographic examination to demonstrate the architecture of the maternal pelvis and the size of the fetal head so as to determine the necessity of a cesarean section.
- *Placentography*—radiographic examination to demonstrate the walls of the uterus for localization of the placenta in cases of suspected placenta previa.
- For more detailed information on these procedures, refer to the 12th and earlier editions of this atlas.

Radiation protection

Radiologic examinations of pregnant patients are performed only when the required information can be obtained in no other way. In addition to the danger of genetic changes that may result from reproductive cell irradiation is the danger of radiation-induced malformations of the developing fetus. When possible, radiation for any purpose is avoided during pregnancy, especially during the first trimester of gestation. If examination of the abdominopelvic region is necessary, it is restricted to the absolute minimum number of images. The radiographer's responsibility is to perform the work carefully and thoughtfully so that repeat exposures will not be unnecessary.

Fig. 17.22 Fetography, PA projection. Twin pregnancy showing two fetal heads *(arrows and arrowheads).*

Male Imaging

SEMINAL DUCTS

Imaging examinations of the seminal ducts are performed to investigate certain genitourinary abnormalities, such as cysts, abscesses, tumors, inflammation, and sterility. Ultrasound is the most commonly used modality for examination of the male reproductive organs.

Contrast studies of the seminal vesicles may be studied in the 13th and previous editions of this atlas.[4–6] Ultrasound now demonstrates the anatomy of the male reproductive system as well as the previously mentioned pathologies, as shown in Figs. 17.23 through 17.26.

Fig. 17.23 Ultrasound image of normal left testicle and epididymis, sagittal plane.

(Courtesy Nisa Hinklin, RT(R), RDMS(AB), NEA Baptist Memorial Hospital, Jonesboro, AR.)

Fig. 17.24 Ultrasound image, sagittal plane. Epididymitis and scrotal mass *(M)*. Note enlarged and patchy, mottled echogenicity, as compared with normal epididymis in Fig. 17.23.

(Courtesy Natalie Cox, RT(R), RDMS(AB)(OB), NEA Baptist Memorial Hospital, Jonesboro, AR.)

Fig. 17.25 Bilateral midline transverse images of testicles. Testicular torsion, right side. (A) Ultrasound image showing enlarged right testicle and patchy echogenicity (note homogeneous echogenicity of normal left testicle). (B) Color Doppler in same patient, same plane. Note lack of color in right testicle. Evidence of torsion.

(Courtesy Nisa Hinklin, RT(R), RDMS(AB), NEA Baptist Memorial Hospital, Jonesboro, AR.)

Fig. 17.26 Transrectal ultrasound image of normal seminal vesicles (long axis).

(From Curry R, Tempkin B. *Sonography: Introduction to normal structure and function.* ed 4. St. Louis: Elsevier; 2016.)

PROSTATE

Prostatography is a term applied to investigation of the prostate by radiographic, cystographic, or vesiculographic procedures. It is seldom performed today because of advances in diagnostic sonography (Fig. 17.27). Radiographic examination of the prostate gland is described in the 8th and earlier editions of this atlas.

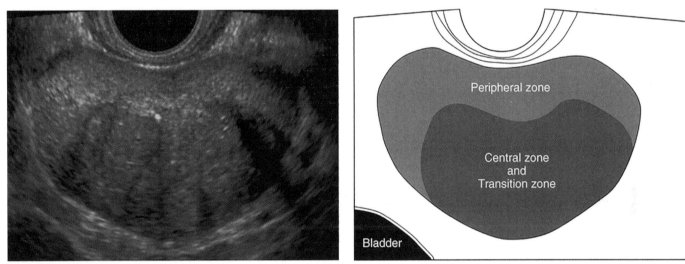

Fig. 17.27 Transrectal ultrasound image of normal prostate gland showing zonal anatomy.

(From Curry R, Tempkin B. *Sonography: Introduction to normal structure and function,* 4th ed. St. Louis: Elsevier; 2016.)

References

1. Wittmer MH, Famuvide AO, Creedon DJ, et al. Hysterosalpingography for assessing efficacy of essure microinsert permanent birth control device. *AJR Am J Roentgenol.* 2006;187:955–958.

2. Lambie RW, Rubin S, Dann DS. Demonstration of fistulae by vaginography. *AJR Am J Roentgenol.* 1963;90:717–720.

3. Coe FO. Vaginography. *AJR Am J Roentgenol Radium Ther Nucl Med.* 1963;90:721–722.

4. Boreau J, Jagailloux S, Vasselle B, et al. Epididymography. *Med Radiogr Photogr.* 1953;29:63–66.

5. Boreau J. *L'étude radiologique des voies séminales normales et pathologiques.* Paris: Masson & Cie; 1953.

6. Vasselle B. *Etude radiologique des voies séminales de l'homme.* Thesis. Paris, 1953.

18

MAMMOGRAPHY

HANEEN ZEIDAN

PROJECTIONS, POSITIONS, AND METHODS

Page	Essential	Anatomy	Projection	Method
400	♠	Breast	Craniocaudal (CC)	
402	♠	Breast	Mediolateral oblique (MLO)	
406	♠	Breast	Craniocaudal (CC)	IMPLANT
408	♠	Breast	Craniocaudal (CC ID)	IMPLANT DISPLACED
410	♠	Breast	Mediolateral oblique (MLO)	IMPLANT
411	♠	Breast	Mediolateral oblique (MLO ID)	IMPLANT DISPLACED
414		Breast	Variable (M)	MAGNIFICATION
415	♠	Breast	Variable	SPOT COMPRESSION
419	♠	Breast	Mediolateral (ML)	
421		Breast	Lateromedial (LM)	
423	♠	Breast	Exaggerated craniocaudal (XCCL)	
425		Breast	Craniocaudal (CV)	CLEAVAGE
427		Breast	Craniocaudal (RL)	ROLL LATERAL
427		Breast	Craniocaudal (RM)	ROLL MEDIAL
429		Breast	Tangential (TAN)	
431		Breast	Variable (CL)	CAPTURED LESION
434		Breast	Caudocranial (FB)	FROM BELOW
436		Breast	Mediolateral oblique (AT)	AXILLARY TAIL
440		Breast	Lateromedial oblique (LMO)	
442		Breast	Superolateral to inferomedial oblique (SIO)	

Icons in the Essential column indicate projections frequently performed in the United States and Canada. Students should be competent in these projections.

Principles of Mammography

INTRODUCTION AND HISTORICAL DEVELOPMENT

The worldwide incidence of breast cancer is increasing. In the United States, one in eight women who live to age 95 years develop breast cancer some time during their lifetime. Breast cancer is one of the most common malignancies diagnosed in women; only lung cancer has a greater overall mortality in women. Research has failed to reveal the precise etiology of breast cancer, and only a few major factors, such as family history, are known to increase a woman's risk of developing the disease. Most women who develop breast cancer have no family history of the disease, however.

Despite its frequency, breast cancer is one of the most treatable cancers. Because this malignancy is most treatable when it is detected early, efforts have been directed toward developing breast cancer screening and early detection methods. Death rates for breast cancer in the United States have declined by 38% since 1989,[1] with larger decreases in younger women; from 2005 to 2009, rates decreased 3.0% per year in women younger than 50 and 2.0% per year in women 50 and older.[2] The decrease in breast cancer death rates represents progress in earlier detection, improved treatment, and possibly decreased incidence as a result of declining use of menopausal hormone therapy (MHT).

Before the radical mastectomy was introduced by Halstead in 1898, breast cancer was considered a fatal disease. Less than 5% of patients survived 4 years after diagnosis, and the local recurrence rate for surgically treated breast cancer was >80%. Radical mastectomy increased the 4-year survival rate to 40% and reduced the rate of local recurrence to approximately 10%. No additional improvement in breast cancer survival rates occurred over the next 60 years. Some of the principles of breast cancer management were developed during this time, however, and these remain valid:
1. Patients in the early stage of the disease respond well to treatment.
2. Patients with advanced disease do poorly.
3. The earlier the diagnosis, the better the chance of survival.

Reflecting these principles, the theory of removing all palpable breast masses in hopes of finding earlier cancers was developed, and it was recognized that careful physical examination of the breast could lead to the detection of some early breast cancers. Most patients with breast cancer still were not diagnosed until their disease was advanced, however. This fact, coupled with the dismal breast cancer survival statistics, highlighted the need for a tool for the early detection of breast cancer. Mammography filled that need (Fig. 18.1).

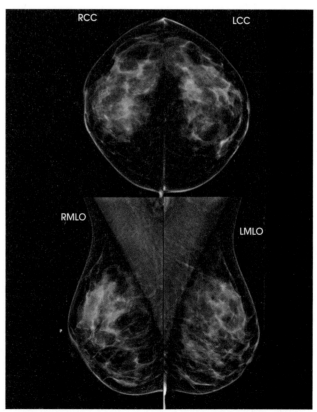

Fig. 18.1 Four-image, bilateral mammogram. Craniocaudal and mediolateral oblique projections show normal, symmetric, heterogeneously dense breast parenchyma.

Principles of Mammography

357

In 1913, Albert Soloman, a German physician, reported the radiographic appearance of breast cancers. Using radiographic studies of cancerous breasts removed at surgery, he described the mechanism of how breast cancer spread. Stafford Warren of Rochester, New York, noted in 1926 that he was able to see a reasonable image of the female breast during thoracic aortic fluoroscopy and published a report of 119 women, 48 with breast cancer.[3] The first published radiograph of a living person's breast, made by Otto Kleinschmidt, appeared in a 1927 German medical textbook on malignant tumors. Although publications on mammography appeared in South America, the United States, and Europe during the 1930s, the use of mammography for the diagnosis of breast cancer received little clinical interest. A few pioneers, including LeBorgne in Uruguay, Gershon-Cohen in the United States, and Gros in Germany, published excellent comparisons of mammographic and pathologic anatomy and developed some of the clinical techniques of mammography. At that time, the significance of breast microcalcifications was also well understood.

By the mid-1950s, mammography was considered a reliable clinical tool because of such refinements as low-kilovoltage x-ray tubes with molybdenum targets and high-detail, industrial-grade x-ray film. During this time, Egan in the United States and Gros in Germany popularized the use of mammography by utilizing industrial-grade x-ray film for diagnosing and evaluating breast cancer. Breast xerography was introduced in the 1960s and was popularized by Wolfe and Ruzicka. Xerography substantially reduced the radiation dose received by the patient compared with the dose received using industrial-grade x-ray film (Fig. 18.2). Because many physicians found xerographic images easier to understand and evaluate, xeromammography became widely used for evaluating breast disease. The first attempts at widespread population screening began at this time.

The combination of higher-resolution, faster x-ray film, and an intensifying screen was first introduced by the DuPont Company. As a result, radiation exposure to the patient was reduced even more. Improved screen-film combinations were developed by Kodak and DuPont in 1975. By this time, extremely high-quality mammography images could be produced with very low patient radiation exposure. After 1975, faster lower-dose films, the magnification technique, and grids for scatter reduction were introduced. These factors, along with improved positioning and clinical techniques, catapulted mammography into use as a mainstream diagnostic and screening tool for breast cancer.

Fig. 18.2 (A) Right lateral xeromammogram, circa 1981. (B) *Circled area* from (A) is photographically magnified, showing small area of microcalcifications. (C) Film-screen magnification study 10 years later shows same calcifications. This was proven to be ductal carcinoma in situ on biopsy.

EVOLUTION OF MAMMOGRAPHY SYSTEMS

Because the breast is composed of tissues with very similar densities and effective atomic numbers, little difference in attenuation is noticed when conventional x-ray equipment and techniques are used. Therefore, manufacturers have developed imaging systems that optimally and consistently produce images with high contrast and resolution.

Diligent research and development began in the 1960s, and the first dedicated mammography unit was introduced in 1967 by CGR (France) (Fig. 18.3). In the 1970s, increased awareness of the elevated radiation doses prevalent in mammography served as the catalyst for the rapid progression of imaging systems. In the 1970s and the early 1980s, xeromammography, named for the Xerox Corporation that developed it, was widely used (see Fig. 18.2). This method, which utilized charged selenium plates as an image receptor (IR), used much less radiation than the direct-exposure, silver-based films that were available. The charged plates were processed using a device that sprayed blue powder, which adhered to the plates according to the charged latent image. The powder was then transferred to paper, giving xerography its distinctive look.

Eventually, film manufacturers introduced several generations of mammography film-screen systems that used even less exposure and improved tissue visualization. Each subsequent new system showed improvement in contrast and resolution while minimizing patient dose.

In the 1980s, the American College of Radiology (ACR) accreditation program established quality standards for breast imaging to optimize mammographic equipment, processors, and screen-film systems to ensure the production of high-quality images. This program was expanded in the 1990s to include quality control and personnel qualifications and training. The voluntary ACR program became the model from which the Mammography Quality Standards Act of 1992 (MQSA) operates, and the ACR has been instrumental in designing clinical practice guidelines for quality mammography in the United States. The evolution of mammography has resulted in the implementation of radiographic systems designed specifically for breast imaging.

MAMMOGRAPHY EQUIPMENT

Over the years, equipment manufacturers have produced dedicated mammography units with high-frequency generators, various tube and filter materials, focal spot sizes that allow tissue magnification, specialized grids to help improve image quality, digital imaging capabilities, and streamlined designs with ergonomic patient positioning aids.

The high-frequency generators offer more precise control of kilovolt (peak) (kVp), milliamperes (mA), and exposure time. The linearity and reproducibility of radiographic exposures using high-frequency generators are uniformly excellent. The greatest benefit of these generators may be the efficient waveform output that produces a higher effective energy x-ray beam per set kVp and mA. High-frequency generators are not as bulky and can be installed within the single-standing mammography unit operating on single-phase incoming line power, facilitating installation and creating a less intimidating appearance (see Fig. 18.3).

Fig. 18.3 (A) First dedicated mammography system: Senographe by CGR (France). (B) Senographe DMR film-screen mammography unit by General Electric (Milwaukee, WI). (C) Dimensions 3D digital breast tomosynthesis unit by Hologic (Bedford, MA).

As manufacturers of dedicated mammography equipment have sought to improve image quality, they have tried many different combinations of tube and filter materials. The most widely accepted combinations used at this time are molybdenum target with molybdenum filter (Mo/Mo), molybdenum target with rhodium filter (Mo/Rh), rhodium target with rhodium filter (Rh/Rh), tungsten/rhodium (W/Rh), and tungsten/silver (W/Ag). The Mo/Rh and Rh/Rh combinations are most commonly used; W/Rh and W/Ag are used for better penetration of extremely dense, thick breasts.

Specialized grids were developed for mammography during the 1980s to reduce scatter radiation and increase image contrast in mammography. Many units employ moving linear focused grids, but other manufacturers have developed very specialized grids. The Hologic (Lorad) High Transmission Cellular (HTC) grid employs a honeycomb-pattern, multidirectional design.

All dedicated mammography units today, with the exception of slit-scan digital units, still employ grids.

Manufacturers also knew that technologists and physicians were interested in the comfort of their patients. They worked to make the examination more tolerable for patients, more ergonomically acceptable, and more efficient for the technologist performing the examination while developing positioning aids to increase visualization of the tissue. Some of these aids include rounded corners on breast platforms and compression paddles, automatic release of compression after exposure, and foot pedal controls.

The next logical step toward improved breast imaging has been the adoption of full-field digital mammography (FFDM), which was first approved by the FDA in 2000, and digital breast tomosynthesis (DBT), also referred to as 3D breast imaging, which was approved in 2011. To bring mammography into the digital world was no simple task. To achieve the resolution and detail necessary for breast imaging, entire systems, from acquisition to diagnostic review workstations, were developed by competing manufacturers. Each of these included proprietary components that made integration of the units into a current picture archiving and communication system (PACS) network difficult. Integrating the Healthcare Enterprise (IHE) has brought together manufacturers of the many components necessary in a FFDM system to work out problems of compatibility and language, allowing facilities the opportunity to transition more seamlessly into digital mammography. More work will be needed in this arena as structural (mammography, CT, DBT) and functional (MR, single photon emission computed tomography [SPECT], positron emission tomography [PET], molecular) imaging are combined.

Full-Field Digital Mammography

Mammography has been the last area in the field of radiography to take advantage of digital technology. In addition to the many technical issues associated with FFDM, the prohibitive cost of the equipment and its maintenance made digital mammography not practical for all facilities. Its many advantages in imaging dense breast tissue have provided the motive, however, for more than 98% of mammography facilities in the United States to transition to this technology over the past decade; 38% of these facilities have also moved forward into DBT.[4]

FFDM units allow radiologists to manipulate digital images electronically, potentially saving patients from undergoing additional projections and additional radiation. The ability to manipulate digital images improves the sensitivity of mammography, especially in women with dense breast tissue. Results of the American College of Radiology Imaging Network Digital Mammographic Imaging Screening Trial (ACRIN DMIST) study, a multifacility, multiunit study comparing film-screen mammography with digital mammography, were published in September 2005.[5] The authors of this study concluded that FFDM would benefit some patients, specifically women younger than age 50, premenopausal and perimenopausal women, and women of any age with dense breast tissue.

Digital breast imaging requires much finer resolution than other body imaging. FFDM images are extremely large files that require a great deal of archival space in PACS. Because of regulations safeguarding the image quality of mammography, the images cannot be interpreted on a traditional PACS workstation; they can be interpreted only on high-resolution 5-megapixel or better monitors.

Innovative solutions and approaches to FFDM continue to be developed. In 2011, the FDA approved DBT for clinical use, and since then, it has consistently proven advantageous. It is now considered the new standard of patient care in many practices.

Digital Breast Tomosynthesis

DBT is a three-dimensional imaging technology that acquires images of a stationary, compressed breast at multiple angles during a short scan. These images are reconstructed into thin, high-resolution slices that can be displayed individually or in a dynamic cine mode. With the ability to view each separate slice representing breast tissue as thin as 1 mm, DBT allows for improved image detail in mammography. While the positioning of the breast remains unchanged, each DBT unit differs in its acquisition of the images.

DBT utilizes the same mammographic positioning and compression used with conventional FFDM, but instead of taking one image perpendicular to the compressed breast, the x-ray tube arches over the patient, taking a series of low-dose images. Each manufacturer's machine differs in how the tomosynthesis image is acquired. These variations include tube angle range, movement of the tube as it acquires images, and a stationary versus arching detector.

As the x-ray unit begins taking tomosynthesis exposures, the tube shifts in one direction, then moves over the central pivot point of the breast to a corresponding angle from the opposite direction. This tube angular range can vary from 11 to 60 degrees depending on the manufacturer.

The number of images taken depends on the thickness of the breast; the thicker the breast, the more images or slices. Typically, each exam acquires between 7 and 30 low-dose tomosynthesis projections.

Different manufacturers' DBT machines also vary on the movement of the tube. One method is the sweep mode, which rotates the tube in a smooth, continuous manner from one point to the other as images are pulsed at the frame rate of the detector. With the step-and-shoot method, the tube stops at each angle or position to acquire an image while the tube is stationary. The tube then moves between each image either in an arch or sweeps across a linear path depending on a stationary or mobile detector. Tubes with a stationary detector arch over the compressed breast. In moving systems, the tube and receptor are synchronized as they sweep across a linear field.[6]

While each system varies on when and how the tomosynthesis images are taken, all DBT systems on the market have the same capabilities to acquire these images in numerous ways. Tomosynthesis views can be taken at any position or angle and with spot compression paddles, but not as magnified views.[7] Each unit can also take an FFDM image alone, a series of just DBT images, FFDM-DBT combination, or a DBT synthesized view. The DBT machines can simultaneously combine the two-dimensional FFDM and the additional exposures necessary to reconstruct a three-dimensional image while the patient is positioned and compressed once. Some machines include a procedure that takes only the series of tomographic low-dose images and processes them to form one two-dimensional image. This synthesized mammography image is essentially each tomographic slice put into focus through a mathematical algorithm. Research has proven that the quality of synthesized images is equivalent to FFDM images, while gaining the benefits of tomosynthesis views with the same patient dose as FFDM alone.[8]

Patient dose has been a concern since the introduction of DBT. For radiologists to assess changes in breast tissue, a two-dimensional image is needed to compare with prior images for evaluating if tissue abnormalities or microcalcification clusters are present in the breast.[8] The initial application of DBT in the clinical practice primarily used FFDM-DBT combination images. This nearly doubles the patient dose; however, the mean glandular dose is still below the limits approved by the FDA, which constitutes an acceptable risk.[9] By eliminating the FFDM and utilizing synthesized mammography, the mean glandular dose decreases by 40% to 50% compared to FFDM-DBT. This dose is equivalent to FFDM images, thus becoming the preferred modality.[8]

The benefits of DBT include increased visualization of breast abnormalities and decreased patient recall rates. Numerous studies have found an increased detection rate for invasive breast cancer with FFDM-DBT versus FFDM. A large study by Friedewald et al. accredited FFDM-DBT with a 41% increase in detection among the screening population.[9] With DBT, radiologists can better visualize areas of architectural distortion (AD), masses and focal asymmetries otherwise obscured by overlying tissue (Fig. 18.4). Microcalcification clusters can also be discerned from adjacent masses. DBT helps physicians determine mammographic extent of disease with a more precise assessment of tumor sizes. It also aids in localizing single-view abnormalities by determining where the lesion is located within the tomographic slices.[7]

As DBT imaging separates breast tissue with each slice, it reduces tissue overlap, thus considerably reducing recall rates.[8] Skin calcifications are easier to distinguish, and other benign findings such as lymph nodes are more evident.[7] These advantages have made DBT with synthetic mammography the current modality of choice for breast cancer screening.

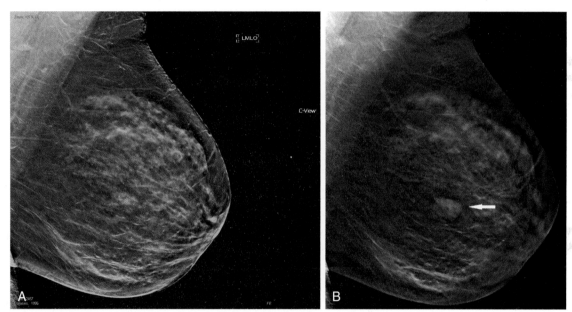

Fig. 18.4 (A) Digital breast tomosynthesis view utilizing synthesized mammography. (B) One of the tomosynthesis slices taken at the same time; note a mass *(arrow)* is better defined than in the two-dimensional view.

Computer-Aided Detection

When performing mammographic interpretation, the radiologist must locate any suspicious lesions (sensitivity) and then determine the probability that the lesion is malignant or benign (specificity). Even with high-quality mammography, some breast cancers are missed on initial interpretation. Double-reading of screening mammograms by a second radiologist can improve detection rates by approximately 10%.[10] It has also been found that double-reading plus the use of computer-aided detection (CAD) can increase detection rates by an additional 8%.[11] Efforts have been made to develop and apply a CAD system to achieve the same result as double-reading. The use of CAD with a single reader has shown a 17% increase in ductal carcinoma in situ (DCIS) diagnoses and a 6% increase in early-stage invasive cancer diagnoses. However, these results do come with an increase in false positive exams, leading to increased additional testing and biopsies.[12]

CAD is a method by which a radiologist can use computer analysis of digitally acquired images as a "second opinion" before making a final interpretation. CAD works similarly to a spell-check on a computer; an area is pointed out for the radiologist to check, but it is up to the radiologist to decide whether the area is suspicious enough to warrant additional procedures. CAD requires that the mammographic image exists in a digital format to facilitate computer input. The computer may detect lesions that are missed by the radiologist, minimizing the possibility of false-negative readings (Fig. 18.5). When a lesion is detected, the computer can be programmed with basic algorithms to estimate the likelihood of malignancy, increasing true-positive rates. Ultimately, the objective of this technology is to improve early detection rates and minimize the number of unnecessary breast biopsies. Another advantage of CAD is that computers are not subject to the bias, fatigue, or distractions to which a radiologist may be subject. Because of the high rates of sensitivity and specificity shown by CAD, it has been implemented in many mammography practices.

Fig. 18.5 Left mediolateral oblique (LMLO) and left craniocaudal (LCC) projections of extremely dense breast with CAD markers (arrows) indicating areas of suspicion that proved to be cancer.

BREAST CANCER SCREENING

It is now known that high-quality mammography, careful physical examination, and monthly breast self-examination (BSE) can result in the detection of breast cancer at an early stage—when it is most curable.

The 5-year relative survival rate for female invasive breast cancer patients has improved from 75% in the mid-1970s to 90% today. The 5-year relative survival for women diagnosed with localized breast cancer (cancer that has not spread to lymph nodes or other locations outside the breast) is 99%[13]; 61% of breast cancers are diagnosed at the localized stage.[14] If the cancer has spread to nearby lymph nodes (regional stage) or distant lymph nodes or organs (distant stage), the survival rate falls to 85% or 26%, respectively.[13]

Mammography must be performed well to be fully effective. The ACR had been a proponent of high standards in breast imaging since 1967 and implemented an optional Mammography Accreditation Program in 1989. In 1992, the MQSA was implemented to mandate the maintenance of high-quality breast cancer screening programs. In 1994, mammography became the only radiographic examination to be fully regulated by the federal government. MQSA requires formal training and continuing education for all members of the breast imaging team. In addition, imaging equipment must be inspected regularly, and all quality assurance activities must be documented. Facilities are also required to provide protocols documenting responsibility for communicating mammogram results to the patient and the referring physician, providing follow-up, tracking patients, and monitoring outcomes. The goal of MQSA is for high-quality mammography to be performed by individuals most qualified to do so and by individuals who are willing to accept full responsibility for providing that service with continuity of care.

RISK VERSUS BENEFIT

In the mid-1970s, the media-influenced public perception was that radiation exposure from diagnostic x-rays would induce more breast cancers than would be detected. Although radiation dosage during a mammography examination has decreased dramatically since the 1970s, fear of radiation exposure still causes some women to refuse mammography, and many women who undergo the examination are concerned about exposure levels and the resultant risk of carcinogenesis. To assuage these fears, the radiographer must understand the relationship between breast irradiation and breast cancer and the relative risks of mammography in light of the natural incidence of breast cancer and the potential benefit of the examination.[15] No direct evidence exists to suggest that the small doses of diagnostic x-rays used in mammography can induce breast cancer. It has been shown, however, that large radiation doses can increase the incidence of breast cancer, and that the risk is dose dependent. Evidence to support an increased risk of breast cancer from breast irradiation comes from studies of three groups of women in whom the incidence of breast cancer increased after they were exposed to large doses of radiation: (1) women exposed to the atomic bombs at Hiroshima and Nagasaki, (2) women with tuberculosis who received multiple fluoroscopic examinations of the chest, and (3) women who were treated with radiation for postpartum mastitis. The radiation dose received by these women (600 to 700 rads) was many times higher than the dose received from mammography.

An important observation in the previously mentioned population studies is that the breast tissue of young women in their teenage years to early 20s seems to be much more sensitive to radiation than the breast tissue of women older than 30 years. Because breast irradiation is a concern, radiologic examinations need to be performed with only the radiation dose that is necessary for providing accurate detection.

Screening versus diagnostic mammography

The frequency with which women should undergo screening mammography depends on their age and personal risk of developing breast cancer. Current recommendations from the American Cancer Society, the ACR, and the Society of Breast Imaging are that all women older than 40 years should undergo annual mammography and should continue yearly mammography for as long as they are in reasonably good health otherwise. A baseline examination performed sometime before the onset of menopause is useful for comparison during subsequent evaluations. High-risk patients should consider beginning screening mammography at an earlier age.

The term *screening mammography* is applied to a procedure performed on an asymptomatic patient or a patient who presents without any known breast problems. For a procedure to be used as a screening method, it must meet the following criteria:
1. It must be simple.
2. It must be acceptable.
3. It must show high sensitivity.
4. It must show high specificity.
5. It must be reproducible.
6. It must be cost-effective.
7. It must have a low risk-to-benefit ratio.

Mammography is a relatively simple procedure that takes only about 15 minutes to complete. The acceptability of mammography has been confirmed in numerous studies. Mammography cannot detect all cancerous lesions, however. An annual clinical breast examination is recommended by the American Cancer Society. Many physicians also recommend that women perform monthly BSE. Even when mammography is performed properly, approximately 10% of cancers remain radiographically occult, particularly in dense breasts and augmented breasts. Even so, mammography has greater sensitivity and specificity for detecting breast tumors than any other currently available noninvasive diagnostic technique. When compared with magnetic resonance imaging (MRI) and ultrasonography, mammography is more cost-effective and more reproducible when quality control standards are maintained. Mammography must be performed properly to maintain these characteristics, however. As with other imaging modalities, high-quality mammography requires an extremely dedicated staff with the appropriate training and expertise.

Breast cancer screening studies have shown that early detection is essential for reducing mortality and that the most effective approach is to combine clinical breast examination with mammography at directed intervals. Although massive screening efforts initially may seem cost-prohibitive, the actual cost of screening in the long term is much less than the expenses involved in caring for patients with advanced breast disease. To this end, screening patients at high risk for breast cancer with the addition of annual breast MRI has been added to screening recommendations.

The preceding paragraphs describe the screening of patients who do not have significant breast symptoms. All patients with clinical evidence of significant or potentially significant breast disease should undergo a *diagnostic mammogram* and subsequent work-up as necessary. Diagnostic mammograms are problem-solving examinations in which specific projections are obtained to rule out cancer or to get a better view of a suspicious area seen on routine screening projections. They are also indicated if a woman presents with a palpable mass or other symptoms. The area of interest may be better shown using image enhancement methods, such as spot compression and the magnification technique. Further work-up may be necessary if mammography does not show a correlative mass. Alternative imaging modalities such as ultrasonography are often used to complete a successful work-up. The radiologist and radiographer direct and conduct the diagnostic mammogram to facilitate an accurate interpretation.

Although most diagnostic mammograms conclude with probable benign findings, some women are asked to return for subsequent mammograms in 3 or 6 months to assess for interval changes. Other women must consult with a specialist or surgeon about possible options such as fine-needle aspiration biopsy (FNAB), core biopsy, or excisional biopsy.

Although it is an excellent tool for detecting breast cancer, mammography does *not* permit diagnosis of breast cancer.

Some lesions may appear consistent with malignant disease but turn out to be completely benign conditions. Breast cancer can be diagnosed only by a pathologist through evaluation of tissue extracted from the lesion. After interpreting the diagnostic work-up, the radiologist must carefully determine whether core biopsy and/or surgical intervention is warranted.

RISK FACTORS

Assessing a woman's risk for developing breast cancer is complicated. An accurate patient history must be elicited to identify potential individual risk factors. The radiologist considers these known risks after interpreting the mammogram. Other than gender, factors that are known to influence the development of breast cancer include age, hormonal history, and family history.

Besides being female, increasing age is the most important risk factor for breast cancer. Potentially modifiable risk factors include weight gain after age 18, being overweight or obese (for postmenopausal breast cancer), use of menopausal hormone therapy (combined estrogen and progestin), physical inactivity, and alcohol consumption. Medical findings that predict higher risk include high breast tissue density (a mammographic measure of the amount of glandular tissue relative to fatty tissue), high bone mineral density (women with low density are at increased risk for osteoporosis), and biopsy-confirmed hyperplasia (overgrowth of cells),

especially atypical hyperplasia (overgrowth of abnormal cells). High-dose radiation to the chest for cancer treatment also increases risk. Reproductive factors that increase risk include a long menstrual history (menstrual periods that start early and/or end later in life), recent use of oral contraceptives, never having children, and having one's first child after age 30.

Risk is also increased by a family history of breast cancer, particularly having one or more first-degree relatives with breast cancer (although most women with breast cancer do not have a family history of the disease). Inherited mutations (alterations) in breast cancer susceptibility genes account for approximately 5% to 10% of all female breast cancers and an estimated 4% to 40% of all male breast cancers but are very rare in the general population (much <1%).[16] Most of these mutations are located in *BRCA1* and *BRCA2* genes, although mutations in other known genes have also been identified. Individuals with a strong family history of breast and certain other cancers, such as ovarian and colon cancer, should consider counseling to determine whether genetic testing is appropriate. Prevention measures may be possible for individuals with breast cancer susceptibility mutations.[17] In *BRCA1* and *BRCA2* mutation carriers, studies suggest that prophylactic removal of the ovaries and/or breasts decreases the risk of breast cancer considerably, although not all women who choose this surgery would have developed breast cancer. Women who consider prophylactic surgery should undergo counseling before reaching a decision. The drugs tamoxifen and raloxifene have been approved to reduce breast cancer risk in women at high risk. Raloxifene appears to have a lower risk of certain side effects, such as uterine cancer and blood clots; however, it is approved only for use in postmenopausal women.

Limited but accumulating evidence suggests that long-term heavy smoking increases the risk of breast cancer, particularly among women who began smoking at an early age. The International Agency for Research on Cancer has concluded that limited evidence indicates that shift work, particularly at night, is also associated with an increased risk of breast cancer.[18]

Breast

The terms *breast* and *mammary gland* are often used synonymously. Anatomy textbooks tend to use the term *mammary gland*, whereas radiography textbooks tend to use the term *breast*. The breasts (mammary glands) are lobulated glandular structures located within the *superficial fascia* of the anterolateral surface of the thorax of both males and females. The mammary glands divide the superficial fascia into anterior and posterior components. The mammary tissue is completely surrounded by fascia and is enveloped between the anterior and posterior layers of the superficial fascia. In females, the breasts are secondary sex characteristics and function as accessory glands to the reproductive system by producing and secreting milk during lactation. In males, the breasts are rudimentary and without function. Male breasts are subject to abnormalities such as neoplasms that require radiologic evaluation; however, this occurs more rarely than in female breasts.

Female breasts vary considerably in size and shape, depending on the amount of fat and glandular tissue and the condition of the suspensory ligaments. Each breast is usually cone-shaped, with the base or posterior surface of the breast overlying the *pectoralis major* and *serratus anterior* muscles. These muscles extend from the second or third rib inferiorly to the sixth or seventh rib, and from near the lateral margin of the sternum laterally toward the anterior axillary plane. An additional portion of breast tissue, the *axillary prolongation* or *axillary tail* (*AT*), extends from the upper lateral base of the breasts into the *axillary fossa* (Fig. 18.6).

The breast tapers anteriorly from the base, ending in the *nipple*, which is surrounded by a circular area of pigmented skin called the *areola*. The breasts are supported by *Cooper's ligaments*, suspensory ligaments that extend from the posterior layers of the superficial fascia through the anterior fascia into the subcutaneous tissue and skin. It is the condition of these ligaments—not the relative fat content—that gives the breasts their firmness or lack of firmness.

The adult female breast consists of 15 to 20 *lobes*, which are distributed such that more lobes are superior and lateral than inferior and medial. Each lobe is divided into many *lobules*, which are the basic structural units of the breast. The lobules contain the glandular elements, or *acini*. Each lobule consists of several acini, numerous draining ducts, and the interlobular stroma or connective tissue. These elements are part of the breast parenchyma and participate in hormonal changes. By the late teenage years to early 20s, each breast contains several hundred lobules. These lobules tend to decrease in size with increasing age, particularly after pregnancy—a normal process called *involution*.

The openings of each *acinus* join to form *lactiferous ductules* that drain the lobules, which join to form 15 to 20 lactiferous ducts, one for each lobe. Several lactiferous ducts may combine before emptying directly into the nipple. As a result, there are usually fewer duct openings on the nipple than there are breast ducts and lobes. The individual lobes are incompletely separated from each other by Cooper's ligaments. The space between the lobes contains fatty tissue and additional connective tissue. A layer of fatty tissue surrounds the gland, except in the area immediately under the areola and nipple (Fig. 18.7).

The lymphatic vessels of the breast drain laterally into the *axillary lymph nodes* and medially into the chain of *internal mammary lymph nodes* (Fig. 18.8). Approximately 75% of lymph drainage is toward the axilla, and 25% is toward the internal mammary chain. The number of axillary nodes varies from 12 to 30 (sometimes more). The axilla is occasionally radiographed during breast examinations so the axillary nodes can be evaluated. The internal mammary nodes are situated behind the sternum and manubrium and, if enlarged, are occasionally visible on a lateral chest radiograph.

The radiographer must take into account breast anatomy and patient body habitus to successfully image as much breast tissue as possible. The compression paddle size determines the size of the exposure field, so it must be appropriate for the breast being imaged. Smaller breasts should not be imaged using the larger compression paddle because other body structures may interfere with the compression device, resulting in an unacceptable image, and compression of more than the breast tissue often increases patient discomfort. Breasts that are larger than the image receptor device and the larger compression paddle must be carefully positioned and imaged in sections, termed *mosaic* or *tiling* imaging.

The natural mobility of the breast is another important consideration. The lateral and inferior aspects of the breast are mobile, whereas the medial and superior aspects are fixed. The breast is most effectively positioned by moving the mobile aspects toward the fixed tissues. Likewise, the radiographer should avoid moving the compression paddle against fixed tissues because this would cause less breast tissue to be imaged.

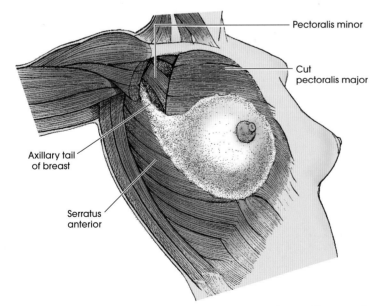

Fig. 18.6 Relationship of breast to chest wall. Note extension of breast tissue posteriorly into axilla.

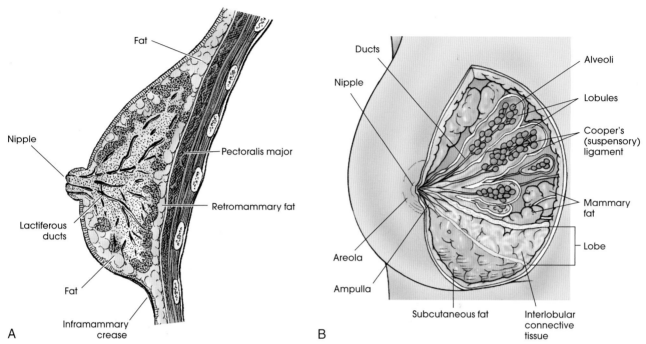

Fig. 18.7 (A) Sagittal section through female breast, illustrating structural anatomy. (B) Breast anterior view.

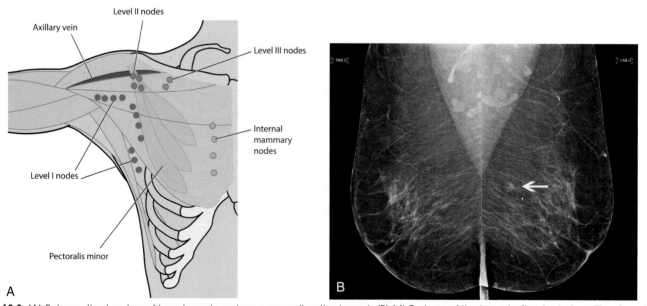

Fig. 18.8 (A) Schematic drawing of lymph node system surrounding the breast. (B) MLO views of the breast often include axillary lymph nodes; occasionally intramammary lymph nodes may also be seen *(arrow)*.

Tissue Variations

The *glandular* and *connective tissues* of the breasts are soft tissue-density structures. The ability to show radiographic detail within the breast depends on the fat within and between the breast lobules and the fat surrounding the breasts. The postpubertal adolescent breast contains primarily dense connective tissue and casts a relatively homogeneous radiographic image with little tissue differentiation. The development of glandular tissue decreases radiographic contrast. During pregnancy, significant hypertrophy of glands and ducts occurs within the breasts. This change causes the breasts to become extremely dense and opaque (Fig. 18.9). After the end of lactation, considerable involution of glandular and parenchymal tissues usually occurs, and these tissues are replaced with increased amounts of *fatty tissue*. Fat accumulation varies markedly among individuals. This normal fat accumulation significantly increases the natural radiographic contrast within the breasts. The breasts of patients with fibrocystic parenchymal conditions may not undergo this involution.

Fig. 18.9 CC and MLO projections of a nursing mother. During lactation, the breasts become very dense and opaque as the ducts and glands become hypertrophic and engorged with milk. If mammography must be performed on a nursing mother, it is best to have the patient nurse or pump her breasts immediately before imaging.

The glandular and connective tissue elements of the breast can regenerate as needed for subsequent pregnancies. After menopause, the glandular and stromal elements undergo gradual atrophy. External factors, such as surgical menopause and hormone replacement therapy (HRT) may inhibit this normal process. From puberty through menopause, mammotrophic hormones influence cyclic changes in the breasts. The glandular and connective tissues are in a state of constant change (Fig. 18.10).

Breast tissue density is the ratio of fatty to glandular tissue within the breast. The more glandular tissue, the denser the breast, meaning that it is more difficult for x-rays to penetrate the tissue. Breasts are classified into four density ranges: fatty, scattered, heterogeneously dense, and extremely dense (Fig. 18.11). Breast density has been brought to the forefront recently, with several states mandating that patients are told the composition of their personal breast density and the classification that the radiologist has reported.

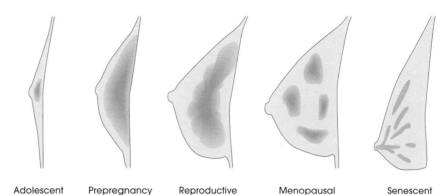

Adolescent   Prepregnancy   Reproductive   Menopausal   Senescent

Fig. 18.10 Diagrammatic profile drawings of breast, illustrating most likely variation and distribution of radiographic density *(shaded areas)* related to the normal life cycle from adolescence to senescence. This normal sequence may be altered by external factors, such as pregnancy, hormone medications, surgical menopause, and fibrocystic breast condition.

Fig. 18.11 When reading the mammogram, the radiologist classifies the tissue density into one of four categories based on the ratio of fatty to glandular tissue within the breast: (A) Fatty. (B) Scattered. (C) Heterogeneously dense. (D) Extremely dense.

PATHOLOGIC AND MAMMOGRAPHIC FINDINGS

Numerous radiographic findings, benign or malignant, can be evident within the breast tissue on any mammogram. Distinguishing the characteristics of a finding is the main function of the mammogram. From these characteristics, the radiologist can make a determination of the probability of malignancy. This helps the radiologist determine whether biopsy of the lesion is necessary, if the lesion is most likely benign, or if the area should be followed carefully for indications of change. Characterization of a finding helps the radiologist make these determinations, but it must be kept in mind that cancer is a very tricky disease, and sometimes even the most benign-appearing lesion can be found to be malignant. Therefore, sometimes biopsies are performed on probable benign lesions to ensure that they truly are benign.

Each breast is a symmetric mirror image of the other. Subtle variations may normally occur from one breast to the other, but an asymmetric variation that is new or enlarging can be cause for concern and can lead to a more thorough work-up. These variations generally present as a mass or density, calcifications within the tissue, or distortion within the architecture of the breast tissue. When these findings are noted on a screening mammogram, the radiologist will often request additional diagnostic mammography views or specialized imaging such as ultrasonography for a more clear view of the area of concern.

Masses

A mass is generally categorized by its shape, by the margins of the mass, and by its radiographic density.
- The *shape* of a lesion is described as round, oval, lobular, or irregular. A round or oval mass is more likely to indicate benign pathology such as a cyst (a fluid-filled pocket within the tissue) or a lymph node (depending on its location). An irregularly shaped mass can more likely indicate a malignancy, or it can be an indication of trauma to an area of breast tissue. This illustrates the importance of taking a thorough patient history.
- The *margins*, or borders, of the mass are described as circumscribed (meaning well defined or sharply defined), microlobulated (having small undulations throughout the contour, such as a blackberry), obscured (meaning that parts are hidden by superimposed tissue), indistinct or ill-defined, or spiculated (showing fine spicules, or lines, radiating from the center of the mass). Margin characteristics help the clinician to predict whether a mass is malignant or benign. A mass with a well-defined border is more likely to

Fig. 18.12 (A) Right CC projection of a patient who had previously undergone surgical biopsy for removal of a benign mass reveals an area of architectural distortion with spiculated borders *(thick arrow)*. (B) MLO projection reveals that the area coincides with the surgical scar. Note the radiopaque skin marker that the technologist placed over the site of the scar *(thin arrows)*.

be benign. Masses with obscured, ill-defined, indistinct margins are suspicious, and a spiculated mass is more worrisome. Microlobulated masses have a 50% chance of being malignant. Post-biopsy scarring may appear as a spiculated mass, and an accurate patient history revealing previous breast biopsies can prevent an unnecessary work-up (Fig. 18.12).

- Examples of benign stellate or spiculated lesions include radial scar, fat necrosis, breast abscess, and sclerosing adenosis. Examples of benign circumscribed masses include fibroadenoma (Fig. 18.13), cyst, intramammary lymph node, hematoma, and galactocele.

Fig. 18.13 Circumscribed masses are often benign. (A) TAN MAG projection of a fibroadenoma. (B) Magnified view of a retroareolar cyst. A mass is determined to be solid or cystic (fluid-filled) on ultrasound. (C) DBT slice of a microlobulated mass, which proved to be malignant on biopsy.

Tissue Variations

Fig. 18.14 Radiolucent masses include (A) oil cyst with a calcified rim. Oil cysts are formed when trauma or surgical intervention causes necrosis of fatty tissue. In time, a calcific rim is formed by the body to isolate the necrotic tissue. (B) Lipoma—a lesion consisting of fatty tissue. (C) Hamartoma—a lesion consisting of a mixture of fatty and fibrous tissue.

- *Density* may be described as high density, equal density or isodense, low density, or radiolucent. Breast cancer that forms a visible mass is more likely to be higher in density than the fibroglandular tissue surrounding it, but it can be of equal density. However, breast cancers never contain fatty tissue. Masses that are radiolucent contain fat and are overwhelmingly benign appearing. These include oil cysts, lipomas, galactoceles, and mixed tissue lesions such as hamartomas and fibroadenomas (Fig. 18.14).

The malignant or benign nature of a mass cannot be determined on the basis of *location*. Most cancers are detected in the upper outer quadrant (UOQ) of the breast; however, most breast lesions—both malignant and benign—are found in that quadrant. Cancer can occur in any region of the breast with a certain degree of probability. It is important to determine the location of a lesion for additional diagnostic procedures such as core biopsy or open surgical biopsy.

Interval change may increase the suspicion of malignancy. The radiologist carefully compares current images with previous ones and notes whether the mass is newly apparent, an interval enlargement is present, the borders have become nodular or ill defined, a mass has increased in density, or calcifications have appeared (Fig. 18.15).

Almost all (98%) of the axillary lymph nodes are located in the UOQ. These nodes are well circumscribed, may have a central or peripheral area of fat, and can be kidney bean-shaped (see Fig. 18.8). If the lymph nodes appear normal, they are rarely mentioned in the context of an identifiable mass on the radiology report.

A *density* that is seen on only one projection is not confirmed three-dimensionally and may represent superimposed structures. These may appear to have scalloped edges or concave borders or both. The radiologist may request spot compression projections, rolled projections, or angled projections to confirm or rule out the presence of a real density. A suspicious density seen on only one projection within the breast is often a summation shadow of superimposed breast parenchyma and

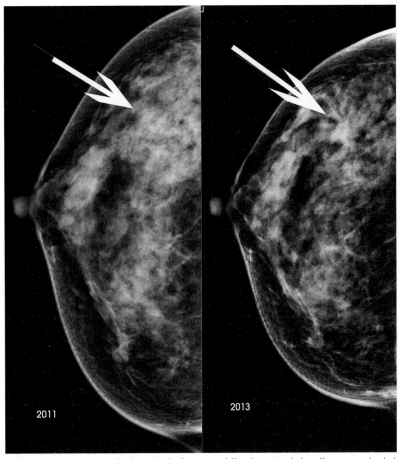

Fig. 18.15 Interval change. A change in tissue architecture and density was noted during a screening mammogram on this 51-year-old woman. Core biopsy of this area was positive for invasive ductal carcinoma.

disappears when the breast tissue is spread apart (Fig. 18.16).

Calcifications

Calcifications are often normal metabolic occurrences within the breast and are usually benign. Approximately 15% to 25% of microcalcifications found in asymptomatic women are associated with cancer, however. These calcifications can have definitive characteristics. Because of size, some microcalcifications are more difficult to interpret. The most valuable tool for defining microcalcifications is a properly performed image obtained using the magnification technique. Using this image, the radiologist can determine better whether calcifications are suspicious and warrant further work-up.

Calcifications are categorized by size, shape, and distribution. Benign calcifications are generally larger, coarser, rounder, and smoother. Typically, they are easily seen on the mammogram, whereas malignant calcifications are usually very small, often requiring magnification to be seen (Fig. 18.17).

Benign calcifications may have one or more of the following attributes: moderate size, scattered location, round shape, and, usually, bilateral occurrence. In addition, they may be eggshell (lucent center), arterial (parallel tracks), crescent, or sedimented ("teacup" milk of calcium). Calcifications may represent a fibroadenoma ("popcorn"), postsurgical scarring

Fig. 18.16 An area of increased density was noted on this MLO projection of the right breast (A). Spot compression of this area (B), also performed in the MLO position, spreads the tissue out more uniformly. The density was no longer seen, indicating that overlapped tissue was causing a summation shadow.

(sheets or large strands of calcium), skin calcifications (which can mimic suspicious microcalcifications within the breast parenchyma), and vascular calcifications. Vascular calcifications are often noted, and studies have indicated that vascular calcifications in women younger than 50 years of age may suggest potential risk for coronary artery disease.

• The projection suggested for better defined sedimented milk of calcium is the 90-degree lateral projection—lateromedial (LM) or mediolateral (ML). If possible, the mammographer should select the lateral projection that places the suspected area closest to the IR. The 90-degree lateral is also used as a triangulation projection before needle

Fig. 18.17 Examples of benign calcifications seen on mammography. (A) Coarse and round calcification. (B) Calcifications caused by dystrophic fat necrosis.

Fig. 18.17, cont'd (C) Popcorn calcification. (D) Vascular calcification. (E) Rod-like secretory calcifications.

localization and to show air-fluid-fat levels (Fig. 18.18).

Calcifications that are suspicious and arouse intermediate concern are categorized as amorphous or indistinct, or coarse heterogeneous calcifications. Amorphous or indistinct calcifications appear small and hazy. When diffusely scattered, they can usually be dismissed as benign, but when clustered, they may warrant biopsy. Coarse heterogeneous calcifications that are conspicuous and irregularly shaped, are generally larger than 0.5 mm, and can be associated with malignancy, but these calcifications may also be present in areas of fibrosis, within fibroadenomas, or in areas of trauma.

Fine pleomorphic calcifications and fine linear or branching calcifications indicate a higher probability of malignancy. The fine linear type suggests filling of the lumen of a duct involved in a breast cancer. Fine pleomorphic forms vary in shape but are generally smaller than 0.5 mm (Fig. 18.19).

The distribution of the calcifications describes the arrangement of calcifications in the breast. Diffuse or scattered calcifications are usually benign and usually bilateral. Regional distribution of calcifications indicates that a large volume of breast tissue contains calcifications. A group or cluster of calcifications indicates a minimum of five calcifications occupying a small volume of breast tissue. Linear distribution calcifications are arranged in a line, suggesting deposits within a duct. Segmental distribution suggests deposits in ducts and the possibility of extensive or multifocal breast cancer. Although benign causes of segmental calcifications are known, segmental distribution of otherwise benign-appearing calcifications elevates suspicion of carcinoma.

Architectural distortions

When the normal architecture of the breast tissue is distorted but no definitive mass is visible, this is called AD. AD is seen as a presentation of thin lines or spiculations radiating from a central point. Focal retraction or distortion of the edge of the parenchyma may also be present. AD can be associated with a mass or with asymmetry or calcifications. A history of trauma or prior surgery may present as AD, but in the absence of this history, AD is suspicious for malignancy or radial scar, and biopsy of the area is appropriate (Fig. 18.20).

Fig. 18.18 Milk of calcium occurs when residual milk remains in the alveoli following lactation. Over time, the calcium within the milk solidifies into tiny particles that become sediment. On the CC projection, it appears as rounded low-density areas (A). On the ML projection, the sediment appears crescent shaped as it settles, in a "teacup" appearance (B).

Fig. 18.19 Examples of calcifications seen on mammography that are suspicious or have a high probability of indicating cancer. (A) These amorphous, diffuse calcifications proved to be ductal carcinoma in situ (DCIS) on biopsy. (B) These linear, branching calcifications proved to be invasive ductal carcinoma on biopsy. (C) Pleomorphic linear calcifications proved to be DCIS.

Fig. 18.20 Architectural distortion is seen on this CC projection (A). Spot compression view (B) of this area confirms that this is a mass, not overlapped tissue. This proved to be invasive ductal carcinoma on biopsy.

FULL-FIELD DIGITAL MAMMOGRAPHY MANUAL TECHNIQUE CHART

Compressed thickness	Target	Fatty breast filter	kVp	mAs	Target	50% fatty–50% dense filter	kVp	mAs	Target	Dense breast filter	kVp	mAs
Amorphous selenium detector												
<3 cm	Mo	Mo	28	70	Mo	Mo	28	80	Mo	Mo	28	90
3–5 cm	Mo	Mo	28	80	Mo	Mo	28	80	Mo	Mo	28	90
5–7 cm	Mo	Rh	29	100	Rh	Rh	29	100	Rh	Rh	29	100
>7 cm	Rh	Rh	30	120	Rh	Rh	30	140	Rh	Rh	30	160
Charge-coupled device (CCD) detector												
<3 cm	Mo	Mo	25	32	Mo	Mo	26	28	Mo	Mo	26	36
3–4 cm	Mo	Mo	36	36	Mo	Rh	26	45	Mo	Rh	27	50
4–5 cm	Rh	Rh	28	50	Rh	Rh	29	56	Rh	Rh	29	63
5–6 cm	Rh	Rh	29	56	Rh	Rh	29	63	Rh	Rh	30	71
6–7 cm	Rh	Rh	29	71	Rh	Rh	29	80	Rh	Rh	30	80
7–8 cm	Rh	Rh	29	80	Rh	Rh	30	90	Rh	Rh	31	80
>8 cm	Rh	Rh	30	90	Rh	Rh	30	140	Rh	Rh	31	140

Note: Manual techniques based on use of grid and taut compression.

SUMMARY OF ANATOMY

Mammary gland (breast)	Acini	Fatty tissue
Axillary fossa	Lactiferous ductules	Superficial fascia
Nipple	Axillary lymph nodes	Pectoralis major muscle
Areola	Internal mammary lymph nodes	Serratus anterior muscle
Cooper's ligaments	Glandular tissue	Axillary prolongation (axillary tail)
Lobes	Connective tissue	

SUMMARY OF PATHOLOGY

Radiographic Findings	Definition
Masses and margins	
• Circumscribed	Smooth borders; mostly benign
• Indistinct	Ill-defined borders
• Spiculated	Mass with thin, elongated lines of tissue emerging from its center
Architectural distortion	The interruption of a regular pattern; when tissue opposes the natural breast pattern flowing from ducts to nipple
Calcifications	
Radiographic description	
• Round or punctate	Benign spherical calcium that can vary in size with well-defined margins
• Amorphous or indistinct	Small or hazy calcium with no clearly defined shape or form

Radiographic Findings	Definition
• Coarse heterogeneous	Large calcium deposits of various sizes clustered together
• Fine heterogeneous	Small calcium deposits of various sizes clustered together. Usually <0.5mm in diameter with a high probability of malignancy.

Benign calcifications
• Popcorn-type	Large, thick, dense, popcorn shaped; often result from involuting fibroadenomas
• Rim calcifications	Calcifications residing along the border of benign masses such as cysts, oil cysts, or sebaceous cysts
• Milk of calcium (teacup)	Found in microcysts, which contain radiopaque particles mixed with fluid
• Arterial calcifications	Found within vessels resulting from arterial atherosclerosis
• Skin calcifications	Found within the dermal layer of the breast, usually with smooth outlines and radiolucent centers

Benign pathologies
• Cyst	Fluid-filled sac with distinct edges and round or oval in shape
• Galactocele	Milk-filled cyst typically found in lactating women
• Fibroadenoma	Solid benign tumor of glandular and connective tissue with clearly defined margins; often easy to move
• Lipoma	Growth of fatty cells
• Hamartoma	Typically well-circumscribed lesion comprised of fibrous, glandular, and fatty tissue
• Papilloma	Growth inside the ducts; may cause discharge
• Ductal ectasia	Dilation of milk ducts with thickening of the walls; may cause discharge or fluid blockage
• Hematoma	Collection of blood within the tissue, typically resulting from trauma
• Abscess and inflammation	Accumulation of pus with swelling as a result of infection
• Fat necrosis/oil cyst	Lucent area within the breast resulting from trauma, surgery, or radiation therapy
• Gynecomastia	Benign proliferation of tissue in the male breast

High-risk conditions
• Lobular carcinoma in situ (LCIS)	Abnormal cell growth within the lobules or milk glands
• Atypical ductal hyperplasia (ADH)	Increased production or growth within breast ducts causing architectural abnormalities
• Atypical lobular hyperplasia	Increased cell growth within breast lobes
• Radial scar	Complex sclerosing lesion. Benign mass with spiculated borders not related to surgery; caused by abnormal cell growth
• Papilloma with atypia	The presence of atypical hyperplasia within a papilloma

Malignant pathologies
• Ductal carcinoma in situ (DCIS)	Abnormal, cancerous cells within the milk ducts
• Invasive/infiltrating ductal carcinoma	Cancerous cells that started in the milk ducts and have spread to surrounding breast tissue; most common type of breast cancer
• Invasive lobular carcinoma	Cancerous cells that spread from a lobule to other breast tissue
• Inflammatory carcinoma	Aggressive carcinoma that blocks the lymph vessels in the skin of the breast, causing signs of inflammation such as swelling, reddening of the skin, or an orange peel-like texture to the skin (peau d'orange)
• Paget's disease	Carcinoma in the skin of the nipple causing a sore, reddened appearance of the nipple and areola; commonly associated with other types of carcinoma within the breast tissue
• Sarcoma	Cancerous cells that begin in the connective tissue supporting the lobules and ducts of the breast

Summary of Pathology

Method of Examination

Both breasts are routinely radiographed obtaining craniocaudal (CC) and mediolateral oblique (MLO) projections. Image enhancement methods, such as spot compression and the magnification technique, are often useful as diagnostic tools. It is sometimes necessary to enhance images or vary projections to better characterize lesions and calcifications. In symptomatic patients, the examination should not be limited to the symptomatic breast. Both breasts should be examined for comparison purposes and because significant radiographic findings may be shown in a clinically normal breast.

PATIENT PREPARATION

No specific patient preparations are needed before a mammographic examination to enhance image quality. However, during the mammography procedure, the breasts will be compressed, and this may cause some discomfort to the patient. To help alleviate the discomfort and solicit patient cooperation, some practices recommend that the patient refrain from or reduce caffeine intake for 2 weeks before the examination or take ibuprofen approximately an hour before the examination.

Artifacts are common in mammography because of the sensitivity of the imaging techniques and the design of the equipment used for mammography (Fig. 18.21). To prevent artifacts caused by objects protruding into the image, you may need to ask the patient to remove eyeglasses, earrings, and necklaces. Some hairstyles may need to be pulled or clipped back to prevent the hair from falling forward into the image. It is advisable to dress patients in open-front gowns because the breast must be bared for the examination. The technologist needs to ensure before each exposure that all of the above items, as well as chins, fingers, and other body parts, are outside of the field of radiation.

Some radiology practices require that patients remove any deodorant and powder from the axillary and inframammary regions because these substances can resemble calcifications on the resultant image (Fig. 18.22). Before the breast is radiographed, a complete history is taken, and a careful physical assessment is performed, noting all biopsy scars, palpable masses, suspicious thickenings, skin abnormalities, and nipple alterations (Fig. 18.23).

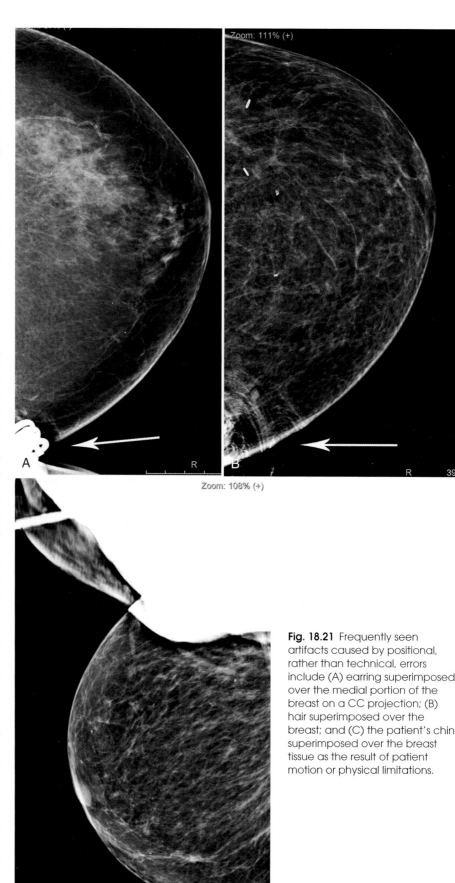

Fig. 18.21 Frequently seen artifacts caused by positional, rather than technical, errors include (A) earring superimposed over the medial portion of the breast on a CC projection; (B) hair superimposed over the breast; and (C) the patient's chin superimposed over the breast tissue as the result of patient motion or physical limitations.

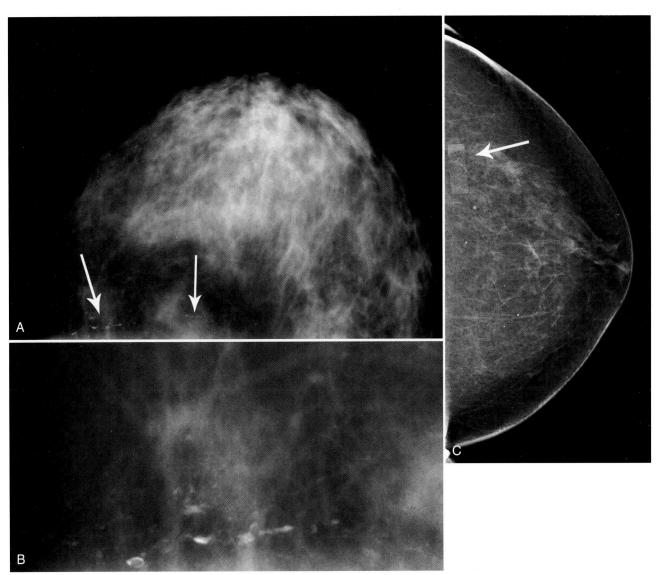

Fig. 18.22 Artifacts are often the result of poor patient preparation. (A and B) These show pseudocalcifications along the inframammary crease—the result of caked powder. (C) This shows a band-aid applied by the patient on the posterior aspect of the breast that was not noticed by the technologist until it was seen on the mammogram.

EWBC MEDICAL HISTORY FORM   M.R.#_____

*— please remember to **sign the back** of this form AND **only use ink** to fill out this form—*

1. Purpose of today's visit? _____

2. Do you use:

If discontinued

    a. Hormones?   Yes   No   Brand _____ Dosage _____ How long? _____ when? _____

    b. Oral Contraceptive?   Yes   No   Brand _____

    c. Anti-Estrogen/Breast Cancer Prevention?   Yes   No   Brand _____

3. Do you have breast implants?   Yes   No   *(type)*   Silicone Gel   Saline   Combination   Unknown

4. Are you taking aspirin or blood thinners? Yes   No

5. Are you allergic to any of the following?

    a. Medicine(s)?   Yes   No   *(type)* _____

    b. Adhesive Tape?   Yes   No

    c. Lidocaine?   Yes   No

    d. Iodine Contrast Material?   Yes   No

    e. Latex?   Yes   No

    f. Others? _____

6. Do you currently have any of the following? *– please check only those that apply to you and explain below:*

☐ Fever/Chills   ☐ Weakness   ☐ Leg Swelling   ☐ Seasonal Allergies

☐ Eye Problems   ☐ Depression   ☐ Joint Aches   ☐ Stomach Problems

☐ Kidney Problems   Explanation _____

OFFICE USE ONLY   ☐ All other systems negative

7. Questions for female patients: *(please circle your answers)*

    1. How many months since your physician examined your breasts? _____ months

    2. Your age at birth of your 1st child. _____   No biological children ☐

    3. Your age at time of 1st menstrual cycle. _____

        a. Are your periods regular?   Yes   No   *if no, date of your last period* _____

    4. Age you entered menopause. _____ (If you are no longer having periods for at least one year).

    5. Are you pregnant?   Yes   No

    6. Are you breastfeeding?   Yes   No

    7. Do you have your ovaries?   Yes   No   (RIGHT)   (LEFT)

    8. Do you have your uterus?   Yes   No

    9. Have you had breast surgery?   Yes   No

    If yes, please mark the area of surgery with the year it was done.

    10. Have you ever had radiation therapy to your breast/chest area? ☐ Yes ☐ No if yes, when? _____

    11. Have you ever had chemotherapy? ☐ Yes ☐ No   if yes, when? _____ for what? _____

8. Social History: ☐ Male ☐ Female

    Marital Status: ☐ Single ☐ Married ☐ Divorced ☐ Partner ☐ Widowed

    Occupation: _____

    Do you drink alcohol? ☐ Yes ☐ No   **if yes,** how often? _____

    Do you smoke? check one: ☐ Daily ☐ Occasional ☐ Never Smoked ☐ Former Smoker ☐ Unknown

    Race: ☐ American Indian ☐ Alaska Native ☐ Asian ☐ Black or African American

        ☐ Native Hawaiian or Pacific Islander ☐ White

    Ethnicity: ☐ Hispanic or Latino ☐ Not Hispanic or Latino

    Preferred Language: ☐ English ☐ Other _____

Please list medications *(include non-prescription medications and birth control pills, write "none" if no medications are used)*

_____ _____ _____

_____ _____ _____

_____ _____ _____

_____ _____ _____ *(over)* ➡

Mammography

Fig. 18.23 Sample mammography patient history questionnaire. Note that a good amount of emphasis is placed on patient and family history to determine risk and inclusion for *BRCA* testing and breast MRI.

(Courtesy Elizabeth Wende Breast Care, LLC, Rochester, NY.)

9. Medical/Family History: Directions-Check "None" if neither you nor anyone in your family has had this problem. Check "Self" if this is true for you. Check "Family" if a member of your family has had this problem.

	NONE	SELF	FAMILY	
Breast Cysts	☐	☐		
Breast Pain	☐	☐		
Nipple Changes				
Inversion: ☐ Left ☐ Right				
Discharge: ☐ Left ☐ Right				
Rash: ☐ Left ☐ Right				
HIV	☐	☐		
Heart Valve Replacement	☐	☐		
High Blood Pressure	☐	☐		
Pacemaker/Cardiac Stent	☐	☐		
Heart Attack	☐	☐		
Stroke	☐	☐		
Hepatitis/Liver Problems	☐	☐		type: _____
Asthma	☐	☐		
Diabetes	☐	☐	☐	
Arthritis	☐	☐	☐	type: _____
Hives	☐	☐	☐	
Pancreatic Cancer	☐	☐	☐	
Melanoma	☐	☐	☐	
Lymphoma	☐	☐	☐	type: _____
Leukemia	☐	☐	☐	type: _____
Other Cancers	☐	☐	☐	type: _____

(Please list breast and ovarian history below)

Have you ever been tested for BRCA1/BRCA2 Mutations?

☐ **NO** ☐ **YES** If yes, were the results: ☐ **Positive** ☐ **Negative** ☐ **Uncertain Variant**

Are you of Ashkenazi Jewish Ancestry? ☐ **NO** ☐ **YES**

HISTORY OF BREAST CANCER:

☐ **NO** ☐ **YES**

	Age at diagnosis	Age if diagnosed with a second NEW Breast Cancer	Mother or Father's side (PLEASE CIRCLE)
Self			
Mother			
Sister			
Daughter			
Brother			
Father			
Son			
Niece			
Nephew			
Grandmother			M F
Grandfather			M F
Aunt			M F
Uncle			M F
Cousin			M F

HISTORY OF OVARIAN CANCER:

☐ **NO** ☐ **YES**

	Age at diagnosis	Mother or Father's side (PLEASE CIRCLE)
Self		
Mother		
Sister		
Daughter		
Niece		
Grandmother		M F
Cousin		M F
Aunt		M F

If we may contact you by email, please list your email address: _____

Print Name: _____ Date of birth: _____ Date: _____

Signature: _____ Date: _____

Patient Review: _____ Date: _____ Patient Review: _____ Date: _____

OFFICE USE ONLY	MD Review: _____ Date: _____	MD Review: _____ Date: _____	MD Review: _____ Date: _____

The above information is accurate and any unanswered questions are considered not applicable or negative. May 3.12

Fig. 18.23, cont'd

Examination Procedures

This section describes procedures for conducting mammographic examinations. Only dedicated breast imaging equipment should be used to perform mammography. The following steps should be taken:

- If possible, examine previous mammographic studies of patients who are undergoing subsequent mammography screening. These images should be evaluated for positioning, compression, and exposure factors to determine whether any improvement in image quality can be obtained with the current study. Position the breast consistently so that any lesion can be accurately localized and a valid comparison with prior studies can be made.

- Determine the correct compression paddle size for the patient, and use the smallest possible size to image all of the breast tissue fully. Positioning the breast on a surface and detector that is too large causes the skin and muscles to overextend, reducing the amount of posterior tissue imaged, and may compromise the technical image quality. Occasionally, a patient may present with oversized breasts that do not fit completely on the largest detector field and compression paddle. When this happens, overlapping images are taken to visualize all of the breast tissue. This is referred to as "mosaic" imaging or tiling, as image tiles are fitted together to form a complete picture (Fig. 18.24).

- Explain the procedure simply and completely to the patient before beginning the examination. It should never be assumed that the patient is fully aware of what the mammographer is about to do, even if the patient has had prior examinations.

- In many cases, routine projections do not sufficiently show all of the breast tissue, and additional projections may be necessary. To allay patient concerns, the mammographer should explain to the patient, before beginning the procedure, why additional projections are sometimes needed and that they do not indicate a potential problem.

- Before positioning the patient's breast and applying compression, consider the natural mobility of the breast, so that patient discomfort can be minimized. The inferior and lateral portions of the breast are mobile, whereas the superior and medial portions are fixed. When possible, the mobile tissues should be moved toward the fixed tissues.

- For each of the two basic breast projections, ensure that the breast is firmly supported and adjusted, so that the nipple is directed forward.

- Profile the nipple, if possible. Obtaining an image of the posterior breast tissue should be the primary consideration, but positioning of the nipple in profile is not always possible. An additional projection can be obtained to profile the nipple, if necessary. Alternatively,

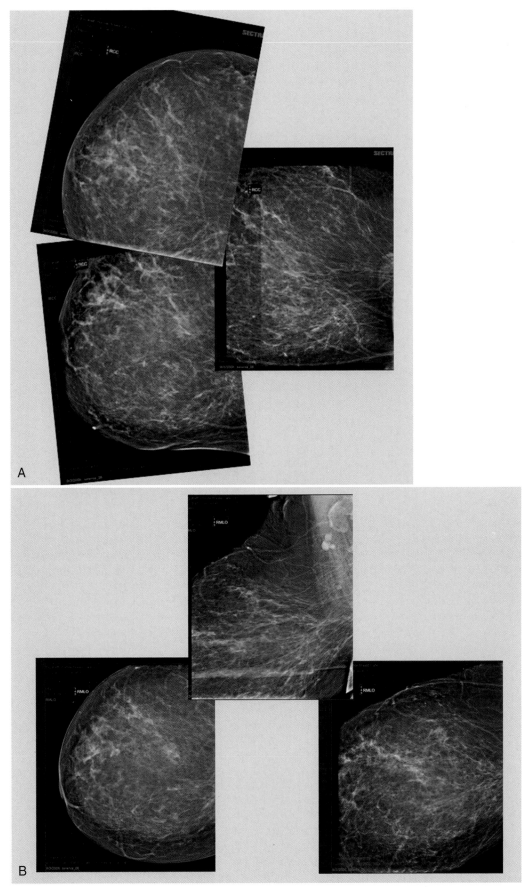

Fig. 18.24 When the breast is larger than the image receptor, several images of the breast should be taken to visualize all of the tissue. (A) Three mosaic images of the CC projection, taken to image anteromedial, anterolateral, and posterior tissue. (B) Mosaic images of the MLO view, imaging inferoposterior, anterior, and posteroaxillary tissue.

(Reprinted with permission from Andolina V, Lille S: *Mammographic imaging: a practical guide*, ed 3, Baltimore, 2011, Wolters Kluwer Health/Lippincott Williams & Wilkins.)

a marker may be used to locate clearly the nipple that is not in profile, in which case an additional image may not be needed.

- Apply adequate compression to the breast. Compression is an important factor in achieving a high-quality mammogram. The primary objective of compression is to produce uniform breast thickness from the nipple to the most posterior aspect of the breast. Properly applied compression spreads the breast so that the tissue thickness is more evenly distributed over the image and better separation of the glandular elements is achieved. A rigid, radiolucent mammography compression paddle facilitates breast compression. Generally, compression is applied initially using a hands-free control and is applied manually during the final phase of compression. The compression should be taut but not painful. The skin of a properly compressed breast should feel tight when lightly tapped with the fingertips. When evaluating images, compare the degree of compression with that of previous mammograms, and note any variations. If a patient is unable to tolerate an adequate amount of compression, document this information on the patient history form for the radiologist. Use only as much compression as the patient can tolerate.

Be sure that standard identification information is included on the image. For FFDM images, all of the pertinent information should be included in the Digital imaging and communications in medicine (DICOM) header. Often, this DICOM overlay can be turned on or off as needed by the radiologist to prevent interference during interpretation of the image. Image labeling for all mammographic images should be in accordance with ACR and FDA requirements (Table 18.1). Workstations used for interpretation have the capability to temporarily switch off the image identification information with a default setting. Image labeling for hardcopy and softcopy images must include the following information in a permanent, legible, and distinct manner, set where anatomic structures are not obscured:

1. Facility name and location, including city, state, and zip code
2. Patient's first and last names
3. Unique identification number and/or date of birth
4. Examination date
5. Technologist's initials or identification number
6. Cassette (screen) number for screen-film and computed radiography images
7. Mammographic unit identification if there is more than one unit in the facility
8. Laterality and view, placed on the image in a position near the axilla

- Facilities with more than one unit must identify the mammographic unit used (Roman numerals are suggested by the ACR).
- For patients with palpable masses, a radiopaque marker may be used to identify the location of the mass. A different type of radiopaque marker may be used to identify skin lesions, scars, or moles. This is determined by the policy of the facility, at the discretion of the reading radiologists.
- When using automatic exposure control (AEC), position the variable-position detector at the chest wall, the mid-breast, or the anterior breast, depending on breast composition and size. The appropriate location of the AEC detector must be determined for each individual patient. If possible, the detector should be placed under the most glandular portion of the breast, usually just posterior to the nipple. Most FFDM units will automatically determine these settings based on the technology used by the manufacturer.
- When reviewing images, assess contrast and density for optimal differentiation of breast tissues. Anatomic markers should be visible. The projections of one breast should be compared with the same projections of the contralateral breast so that symmetry and consistency of positioning can be evaluated. All images should be absent of motion blur, artifacts, and skin folds. Images must be evaluated for potentially suspicious lesions and calcifications that may require image enhancement methods.
- To evaluate whether sufficient breast tissue is shown, the radiographer should measure the depth of the breast from the nipple to the chest wall on the CC and MLO projections. The posterior nipple line (PNL) is an imaginary line that is "drawn" obliquely from the nipple to the pectoralis muscle or the edge of the image, whichever comes first on the MLO projection. On the CC projection, the PNL is "drawn" from the nipple to the chest wall or to the edge of the image, whichever comes first. The PNL on the CC should be within ⅓ inch (1 cm) of depth of the PNL on the MLO projection (Fig. 18.25).

- Between examinations, use a disinfectant to clean the breast tray surface, compression paddle, patient handle grips, and face guard.
- Breast cushions available through several manufacturers provide a warmer and more comfortable examination for the patient (Fig. 18.26). Check with the unit's manufacturer before implementing any patient comfort modifications.
- Mammography is a team effort involving the patient and the mammographer. Acknowledge the individual needs of each patient to facilitate the cooperation and trust necessary to complete the procedure successfully. The nature of the interaction between the radiographer and the patient is likely to determine whether the patient chooses to have subsequent mammograms.

Respiration

- To avoid patient motion and image blurring, the patient may be asked to suspend respiration during the exposure. The preferred method is to ask the patient to simply "stop breathing" rather than "hold your breath." Saying "hold your breath" often implies to the patient that she will need to take a deep breath in. This may result in an unintentional movement of the ribs and therefore the breast tissue, causing blurring or a change in the position of the breast. Alternatively, some mammographers prefer to avoid suspending respiration and simply ask the patient to remain still throughout the exposure. The verbal command to remain still is used for 3D imaging procedures, as the exposure time for these examinations lasts longer, and the patient will be unable to suspend breathing for the duration of the exam. Holding still during 3D examinations helps prevent a blurry image resulting from motion. Once the breast is vigorously compressed, the patient is not liable to take deep breaths, especially if the patient is concentrating on not moving.

Text continued on p. 396

TABLE 18.1

Labeling codes and uses for mammographic positioning

View	ACR ID	Suggested ID	Projection	C-arm angle	Image receptor placement	Tissue best visualized	Applications
Cranial-Caudal	CC		Sup-Inf	0 degrees		Subareolar, central, medial, and posteromedial tissue	Routine
Exaggerated Cranial-Caudal	XCCL	ECC	Sup-Inf	0 degrees		Posterolateral	"Wrap-around" breast
Elevated Cranial-Caudal or Pushed-Up CC	None	ECC	Sup-Inf	0 degrees		Central and medial, high on chest wall	Superior lesion not seen on CC
Caudal-Cranial	FB		Inf-Sup	0 degrees		Central and medial, high on chest wall	Non-conforming pt, superior lesion not seen on CC

Continued

TABLE 18.1

Labeling codes and uses for mammographic positioning—cont'd

View	ACR ID	Suggested ID	Projection	C-arm angle	Image receptor placement	Tissue best visualized	Applications
Mediolateral Lateral	ML		Med-Lat	90 degrees		Lateral, central, superior, and inferior	True orthogonal to CC for lesion localization, opens tissue for structural overlap
Lateromedial Lateral	LM		Lat-Med	90 degrees		Medial, central, superior, and inferior	True orthogonal to CC for lesion localization, opens tissue for structural overlap
Medial-Lateral Oblique	MLO		SM-IL	30–60 degrees		Posterior, upper outer quadrant, axillary tail, lower inner quadrant	Routine
Superolateral-Inferomedial Oblique	SIO		SL-IM	1–90 degrees		Posterior, medial, upper inner quadrant, lower outer quadrant	Additional view for encapsulated implants, non-conforming pt, orthogonal to MLO for localization

Continued

Projection				Angle	Diagram	Best Demonstrates	Notes
Inferolateral-Superomedial Oblique	LMO		IL-SM	90–180 degrees		Posterior, medial, upper outer quadrant, lower inner quadrant	Can replace MLO in pts with pacemakers, open heart surgical scars
Inferomedial-Superolateral Oblique	None	ISO	IM-SL	90–180 degrees		Lateral, upper inner quadrant, lower outer quadrant	Stereotactic positioning
Axillary Tail	AT		SM-IL	60–80 degrees		Posterior-lateral, axillary tail	

TABLE 18.1

Labeling codes and uses for mammographic positioning—cont'd

View	ACR ID	Suggested ID	Projection	C-arm angle	Image receptor placement	Tissue best visualized	Applications
Axilla	None	AX	SM-IL	70-90 degrees		Axillary content	Additional view for cancer patients on affected side, suspected inflammatory ca, lymphadenopathy, search for primary ca
Cleavage View	CV		Sup-Inf	0 degrees		Medial	Extreme medial tissue, slippery medial lesions
Rolled Lateral	RL		Sup-Inf	0 degrees		Subareolar, central, medial, and posteromedial tissue	Separation of superimposed glandular tissue
Rolled Medial	RM		Sup-Inf	0 degrees		Subareolar, central, medial, and posteromedial tissue	Separation of superimposed glandular tissue

Examination		Abbreviation		Degree of obliquity	Area demonstrated	Reason for use
Captured Lesion (Coat-Hanger View)	None	CL	All	0–90 degrees	Posterior	Palpable abnormality near chest wall or implant, often performed with magnification
Tangential View		TAN	All	0–90 degrees	All	Palpable abnormality, to visualize borders with better detail; often used in conjunction with magnification
Techniques						
Magnification		M				Improved resolution; better shows calcifications and borders of lesions
Implant Displacement		ID			Tissue anterior to subpectoral implants	Patients with implants
Nipple In Profile		NIP			Subareolar	
Spot Compression		S				Palpable abnormality, to visualize borders with better detail; often used in conjunction with magnification

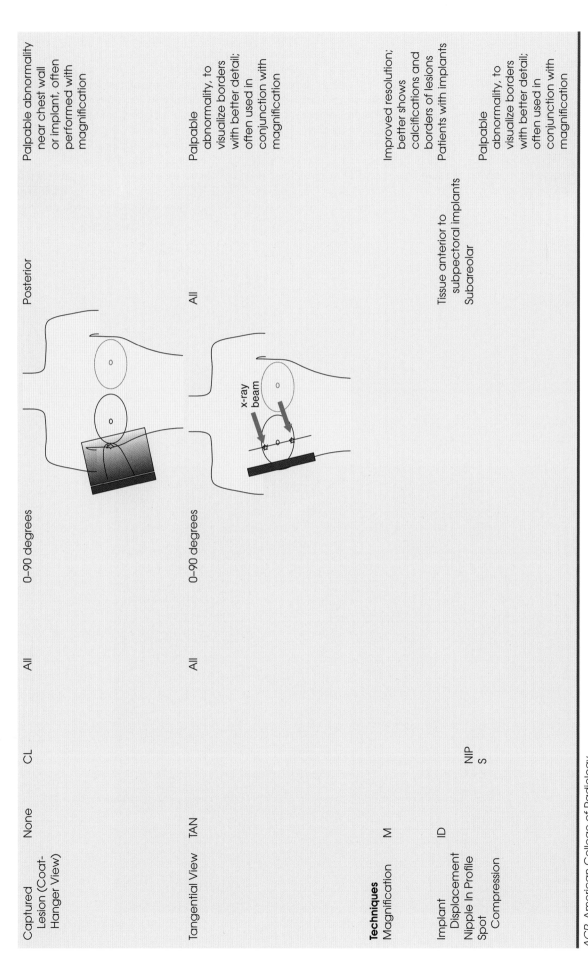

x-ray beam

ACR, American College of Radiology.
From Andolina V, Lille S: Mammographic imaging: a practical guide, ed 3, Baltimore, MD, 2011, Lippincott Williams & Wilkins.

Best Practices in Mammography

Mammography is a specialty with a goal to obtain radiographic images of breast anatomy to help aid in diagnosis. Due to the nature of the body part being examined, technologists should exhibit professionalism, sensitivity, and empathy while maintaining patient comfort. The following best practices provide some universal guidelines for the mammographer to achieve these goals.

1. *Positioning:* Careful positioning will result in high quality images to aid in accurate diagnoses. Technologists should aim to include all breast anatomy to create diagnostically useful radiographs. The images are most useful when anatomy is clearly shown and is viewable in different projections, which is a product of precise positioning. In addition to providing useful information, precise imaging also prevents repeated projections, saving patients from unnecessary radiation exposure.

2. *Empathy:* Every medical professional should be empathetic towards patients, especially in mammography, as these patients are more vulnerable because their breasts are exposed. These are very personal examinations; therefore, it is important for technologists to show compassion towards patients and empathize with them. Technologists can show empathy by demonstrating

Fig. 18.25 (A) Schematic MLO projection with PNL drawn. (B) Schematic CC projection with PNL drawn. PNL of CC projection should be within 1 cm of PNL of MLO projection, as noted on the MLO (C) and CC (D) projections of this mammogram.

caring attributes, patience, and desire to promote a positive patient experience.

3. *Professionalism:* Ethical conduct and professionalism are especially imperative with mammography. Because the relationship between the patient and technologist is intimate, it is critical for the technologist to display professional behavior since the patient is exposed. Conversing with the patient in a respectable manner demonstrates competence and professionalism.

4. *Comforting:* This is a private and personal examination, and patients are often nervous during these procedures or stressed concerning possible test results. It is the responsibility of the technologist to maximize patient comfort during an already uncomfortable exam. A relaxed conversation about any topic, ranging from the weather to complimenting the patient's shoes, helps the technologist make a connection with the patient. Prior to the exam, the technologist should explain the procedure to the patient in detail to aid in her relaxation. In addition to explaining the procedure, technologists should answer any questions the patient may have to acknowledge their concerns and alleviate their fears.

5. *Assessment:* Technologists must pay close attention to the patient's state and tolerability for compression. Some patients can be more sensitive or have a lower tolerance for pain than others. Technologists must use their best judgment to ensure that that they are obtaining optimal images without causing any pain or further harming patients. It is essential for technologists to be gentle with patients and practice safety measures.

6. *Communication:* Effective communication is of great importance when positioning patients for different projections. Communicating clear and specific instructions to the patients about what the technologist needs them to do during the exam increases patient cooperation. Speaking to the patient throughout the examination reduces anxiety. During the examination, the technologists need to tell the patients how they are going to position them before making any sudden movements.

7. *Support:* Uncertainty of results causes anxiety in patients. Patients are anxious during routine mammogram procedures; however, they are especially anxious when they are called back for a diagnostic exam or undergo a breast biopsy procedure. Technologists should be the patients' support and assure them that certain procedures are protocol and that they should not worry until there is something to worry about. When patients are emotional, technologists may support them by giving them hugs or letting them cry. Technologists can inform patients about support groups or other resources that may provide them with support during these times.

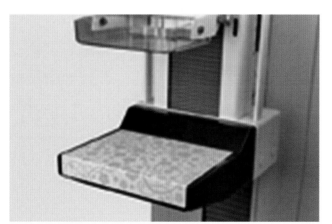

Fig. 18.26 Breast cushions are sometimes used to provide a more comfortable environment and examination for the patient.

(Courtesy Beekley Corp., Bristol, CT.)

Summary of Mammography Projections

Before beginning to learn mammography projections, the student of radiography should carefully study the illustrative summary of mammography projections shown in the box. Familiarity with the different projection names and abbreviations would enhance the student's understanding of the detailed discussions of the projections presented in this chapter.

DESCRIPTIVE TERMINOLOGY FOR LESION LOCATION

Descriptive terminology has been developed for the referring physician, the technologist, and the radiologist to communicate efficiently regarding an area of concern within a breast. When describing an area of concern, the laterality (right or left) must accompany the description (Fig. 18.27).

Each breast is divided into four quadrants: the upper outer quadrant (UOQ), the lower outer quadrant (LOQ), the upper inner quadrant (UIQ), and the lower inner quadrant (LIQ). Clock time is also used to describe the location of a specific area of concern within the breast, but it changes from the right to the left breast, that is, 2:00 in the right breast is in the UIQ, whereas 2:00 in the left breast is in the UOQ. This opposite labeling applies to all clock times; therefore, it is important to identify the correct breast, clock time, and quadrant. The distance of the abnormality from the nipple, which is the only fixed point of reference in the breast, is also noted. The terms *subareolar* and *peri-areolar* describe the area directly beneath the nipple and near (or around) the nipple area. Central describes a lesion located directly behind the nipple in both radiographic projections.

The location of a lesion seen on the mammogram is described using the clinical orientation (described above) extrapolated from the image location. The location of an imaged lesion is described by its laterality, quadrant, clock location, and depth, thus providing a consistency check for possible right-left confusion.[19] Depth of a lesion on the mammogram is described as anterior (nipple), middle, or posterior.

ILLUSTRATIVE SUMMARY OF MAMMOGRAPHY PROJECTIONS

Craniocaudal (CC)[a]

Mediolateral oblique (MLO)[a]

Mediolateral (ML)[a]

Lateromedial (LM)

Routine Projections of the Breast

Mammography is routinely performed using the CC and MLO projections. The combination of these two views best allows visualization of the greatest amount of breast tissue for screening purposes. When diagnostic examinations are performed for specific areas of concern, additional views may be indicated as desired by the radiologist.

Exaggerated craniocaudal (XCCL)[a]

Craniocaudal for cleavage (CV)

Craniocaudal with roll lateral (RL)

Craniocaudal with roll medial (RM)

Tangential (TAN)

Caudocranial (FB)

Mediolateral oblique for axillary tail (AT)

Lateromedial oblique (LMO)

Superolateral to inferomedial oblique (SIO)

[a]Essential projection.

♠ CRANIOCAUDAL (CC) PROJECTION

Paddle: 8 × 10 inches (18 × 24 cm) or 10 × 12 inches (24 × 30 cm).

Position of patient

- Have the patient stand facing the IR, with her feet pointing perpendicular to the mammography unit. If the patient is unable to stand for the duration of the exam, have the patient seated on an adjustable stool facing the unit.

Position of part

- While standing on the medial side of the breast to be imaged, elevate the inframammary fold to its maximal height.
- Adjust the height of the C-arm to the level of the inferior surface of the patient's breast.

- Have the patient lean slightly forward from the waist. Use both hands to pull the breast gently onto the IR surface, while instructing the patient to press the thorax against the IR.
- Drape the opposite breast over the corner of the IR. This maneuver improves demonstration of the medial tissue.
- Have the patient hold onto the grab bar with the contralateral hand; this helps steady the patient as you continue positioning.
- Keep the breast perpendicular to the chest wall. The technologist should use his or her fingertips to pull the inferior posterior tissue gently forward onto the IR.
- Center the breast over the AEC detector, with the nipple in profile if possible.
- Immobilize the breast with one hand, while taking care not to remove this hand until compression begins.

- While placing your arm against the patient's back with your hand on the shoulder of the affected side, make certain the patient's shoulder is relaxed and in external rotation.
- Rotate the patient's head away from the affected side, and rest the patient's head against the face guard.
- Make certain that no other objects such as jewelry or hair obstruct the path of the beam.
- With your hand on the patient's shoulder, gently slide the skin up over the clavicle.
- Using the hand that is anchoring the patient's breast, pull the lateral tissue onto the IR without sacrificing medial tissue. While holding the breast in place, use that same hand to smooth skin wrinkles anteriorly toward the nipple.
- Inform the patient that compression of the breast will begin. Using foot pedal compression controls, bring the compression paddle into contact with the breast while sliding the hand toward the nipple.
- Slowly apply compression manually until the breast feels taut.
- Check the medial and lateral aspects of the breast for adequate compression.
- Instruct the patient to indicate whether the compression becomes uncomfortable.
- After full compression is achieved and checked, instruct the patient to stop breathing (Fig. 18.28).
- Make the exposure.
- Release breast compression immediately.

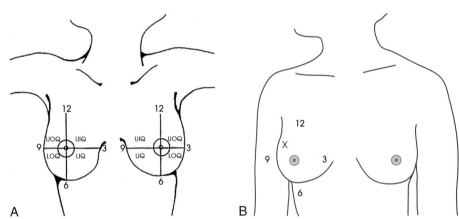

A   B

Fig. 18.27 (A) Each breast is viewed as a clock and is divided into four quadrants to describe the location of a lesion: upper outer quadrant (UOQ), upper inner quadrant (UIQ), lower outer quadrant (LOQ), and lower inner quadrant (LIQ). (B) An abnormality should always be described in a consistent manner. For example, the location of the abnormality denoted by the *x* would be described as "right breast UOQ at approximately 10:30 position."

A   B

Fig. 18.28 (A) Lift breast to adjust level of C-arm to elevated inframammary fold. (B) CC projection.

Central ray

- Perpendicular to the base of the breast

Structures shown

The CC projection shows the central, subareolar, and medial fibroglandular breast tissue. The pectoral muscle is shown in approximately 30% of all CC images.[20,21]

The following should be clearly shown:
- The PNL extending posteriorly to the edge of the image and measuring within ⅓ inch (1 cm) of the depth of the PNL on MLO projection (see Fig. 18.29)
- All medial tissue, as shown by visualization of medial retroglandular fat and the absence of fibroglandular tissue extending to the posteromedial edge of the image

- Nipple in profile (if possible) and at midline, indicating no exaggeration of positioning
- For emphasis of medial tissue, some lateral tissue may be excluded.
- Pectoral muscle seen posterior to medial retroglandular fat in about 30% of properly positioned CC images
- Slight medial skin reflection at the cleavage, ensuring adequate inclusion of posterior medial tissue
- Uniform tissue exposure if compression is adequate

Fig. 18.29 Bilateral CC projections show proper positioning and compression. The CC projection should include maximal medial breast tissue *(arrows)* with the nipple centered and in profile. As much lateral and inferior tissue as possible should be pulled onto the image receptor without compromising visualization of medial tissue. Note that pectoral muscle is seen posteriorly on these images, but this may not be possible to achieve on most CC projections.

♠ MEDIOLATERAL OBLIQUE (MLO) PROJECTION

Paddle: 8 × 10 inches (18 × 24 cm) or 10 × 12 inches (24 × 30 cm).

Position of patient
- Have the patient stand facing the IR with her feet pointed forward or seat the patient on an adjustable stool facing the unit.

Position of part
- Determine the degree of obliquity of the C-arm. The degree of obliquity should be approximately 45 degrees but will vary from 30 to 60 degrees, depending on the patient's body habitus. Draw an imaginary line from the patient's shoulder to midsternum and angle the C-arm to parallel this line.
- Adjust the height of the C-arm so that the superior border of the IR is level with the axilla.
- Instruct the patient to lean slightly forward from the waist.
- Elevate the arm of the affected side over the corner of the IR and rest the hand on the adjacent handgrip. The patient's elbow should be flexed and resting posterior to the IR.
- Place the upper corner of the IR as high as possible into the patient's axilla between the pectoral and latissimus dorsi muscles, so that the IR is behind the pectoral fold.
- Ensure that the patient's affected shoulder is relaxed and leaning slightly anterior. While placing the flat surface of the hand along the lateral aspect of the breast, gently pull the patient's breast and pectoral muscle anteriorly and medially.
- Holding the breast between the thumb and fingers, gently lift it up, out, and away from the chest wall.
- Center the breast on the IR with the nipple in profile, if possible, and hold the breast in position.
- Hold the breast up and out from the body by rotating the hand so that the base of the thumb and the heel of the hand support the breast.
- Inform the patient that compression of the breast will begin. Continue to hold the breast up and out while sliding the hand toward the nipple as the compression paddle is brought into contact with the breast. Loosen the skin at the clavicle with the opposite hand to ensure that posterior tissue is imaged while preventing injury to the shoulder. Roll the contralateral shoulder toward the unit to ensure that medial tissue is visualized.
- Slowly apply compression until the breast feels taut. The corner of the compression paddle should be inferior to the clavicle.
- Check the superior and inferior aspects of the breast for adequate compression.
- Instruct the patient to indicate whether the compression becomes uncomfortable.
- Gently pull down on the patient's abdominal tissue to open the inframammary fold.
- Instruct the patient to hold the opposite breast away from the path of the beam if necessary.
- Instruct the patient to lift her chin to clear the field of potential artifacts.
- After full compression is achieved, instruct the patient to stop breathing (Fig. 18.30).
- Make the exposure.
- Release breast compression immediately.

Central ray
- Perpendicular to the base of the breast
- The C-arm apparatus is positioned at an angle determined by the slope of the patient's pectoral muscle (30 to 60 degrees). The actual angle is determined by the patient's body habitus: Tall, thin patients require steep angulation, whereas short, stout patients require shallow angulation.

Fig. 18.30 MLO projection.

Structures shown

The MLO projection usually shows most of the breast tissue, with emphasis on the lateral aspect and AT.

EVALUATION CRITERIA

The following should be clearly shown:

- PNL measuring within ⅓ inch (1 cm) of the depth of the PNL on CC projection[5,19]
- While drawing the imaginary PNL obliquely following the orientation of breast tissue toward the pectoral muscle, use the fingers to measure its depth from nipple to pectoral muscle or to the edge of the image, whichever comes first (Fig. 18.31).
- Inferior aspect of the pectoral muscle extending to the PNL or below it if possible
- Pectoral muscle showing anterior convexity to ensure relaxed shoulder and axilla
- Nipple in profile if possible
- Open inframammary fold
- Deep and superficial breast tissues well separated when breast is adequately maneuvered up and out from the chest wall
- Retroglandular fat well visualized to ensure inclusion of deep fibroglandular breast tissue
- Uniform tissue exposure if compression is adequate

Fig. 18.31 Bilateral MLO projections show proper positioning. Images should include pectoral muscle to level of nipple *(white line)*, posterior breast tissue, and junction of inframammary fold and abdominal skin *(arrow)*.

Routine Projections of the Augmented Breast

Mammography has an 80% to 90% true-positive rate for detecting cancer in breasts that do not contain implants. For the millions of women in the United States who have undergone augmentation mammoplasty for cosmetic or reconstructive purposes, the true-positive (pathologic-mammographic) breast cancer detection rate decreases to approximately 60% because implants can obscure 85% of the breast's structures, potentially hiding a small cancer that could normally be detected with mammography at an early and curable stage.

Successful radiography of an augmented breast requires a highly skilled mammographer. During the examination, precautions must be taken to avoid rupture of the augmentation device.

Mammography of the augmented breast presents a challenge that cannot be met with the standard two-view examination of each breast. An eight-radiograph examination (four views of each breast) is preferred when possible. The tissue within the posterior and superior aspects of the augmented breast can be satisfactorily evaluated using the standard CC and MLO projections. However, these four images do not adequately show the surrounding breast parenchyma. The addition of a second set of images utilizing the implant displacement (ID) technique, also known as the Eklund method or maneuver, improves compression of the breast tissue and visualization of breast structures. For the Eklund method, the implant is pushed posteriorly against the chest wall so that it is excluded from the image, and the breast tissue surrounding the implant is pulled anteriorly and compressed. This technique is most effective when used on patients with implants that have been placed posterior to the pectoral muscle. It can be used when the implant is placed anterior to the pectoral muscle, but notably less tissue will be able to be pulled onto the IR (Fig. 18.32).

Complications frequently associated with breast augmentation include fibrosis, increased fibrous tissue surrounding the implant, shrinking, hardening, leakage, and pain. Breast augmentation does not increase the risk for developing cancer in the breast; however, the presence of the implant may make detection of cancer on a screening mammogram more difficult.[22] Because mammography alone cannot fully show all complications, ultrasonography and MRI are also used for breast examinations in symptomatic patients. Whether ultrasonography or MRI is used as the adjunct imaging after mammography for patients with suspected implant rupture varies from practice to practice.

Ultrasonography of the breast has proved useful in identifying implant leakage when implant rupture is suggested by mammographic findings and clinical examination, and occasionally when leakage is not suspected. It has also successfully identified leakage that has migrated to the axillary lymph nodes. Although ultrasonography is not yet recommended as a screening modality for implant leakage, it does enhance the mammographic examination.

MRI is also commonly used for diagnostic and screening evaluation of augmented breasts, particularly silicone-filled implants, but there is disagreement over the appropriateness of guidelines for its use.[23,24] Although MRI offers several diagnostic advantages, the cost and time-consuming nature of the procedure inhibit its use as a screening modality for patients who have undergone augmentation. It may be used as a screening tool for women who have undergone reconstruction after breast cancer surgery. MRI has proved useful as a preoperative tool in locating the position of an implant, identifying the contour of the deformity, and confirming rupture and leakage migration patterns.[25]

Fig. 18.32 (A) Eight-view mammogram of a patient with implants placed anterior to the pectoralis muscle *(arrows)*. (B) Eight-view mammogram of a patient with implants placed posterior to the pectoralis muscle *(arrows)*. Note that more pectoral muscle and breast tissue are seen when the implant is placed posterior to the muscle.

Mammography

▲ CRANIOCAUDAL PROJECTION WITH FULL IMPLANT (CC)

Paddle: 8 × 10 inches (18 × 24 cm) or 10 × 12 inches (24 × 30 cm).

Position of patient
- Have the patient stand facing the IR or seat the patient on an adjustable stool facing the unit.

Position of part
- Turn the AEC *off*, and preselect a *manual* technique. For FFDM units, be sure that Implant View processing settings are chosen if applicable.
- Follow the same positioning sequence as for the standard CC projection.
- Inform the patient that minimal compression of the breast will be used. Bring the compression paddle into contact with the breast, and slowly apply only enough compression to immobilize the breast. Compression should be *minimal*. The anterior breast tissue should still feel soft.
- Select the appropriate exposure factors and instruct the patient to stop breathing.
- Make the exposure.
- Release compression immediately.

Central ray

• Perpendicular to the base of the breast

Structures shown

The image should show the entire implant and surrounding posterior breast tissue with suboptimal compression of the anterior fibroglandular breast tissue (Fig. 18.33).

EVALUATION CRITERIA

The following should be clearly shown:
■ Implant projected over fibroglandular tissue, extending to posterior edge of image
■ Posterior breast tissue on medial and lateral aspects extending to chest wall

■ Nipple in profile, if possible, and at midline, indicating no exaggeration of positioning
■ Nonuniform compression of anterior breast tissue

Fig. 18.33 Bilateral, four-image CC and MLO examination of augmented breasts. Implants have been surgically placed behind the pectoral muscle. Additional radiographs should be obtained using the Eklund (ID) technique to complete the eight-radiograph study (see Fig. 18.35).

CRANIOCAUDAL PROJECTION WITH IMPLANT DISPLACED (CC ID)

Paddle: 8 × 10 inches (18 × 24 cm) or 10 × 12 inches (24 × 30 cm).

Position of patient

- Have the patient stand facing the IR or seat the patient on an adjustable stool facing the unit. Select an AEC technique. For FFDM units, be sure that Implant View processing settings are chosen if applicable.

Position of part

- While standing on the medial side of the breast to be imaged, elevate the inframammary fold to its maximal height.
- Adjust the height of the C-arm to the level of the inferior surface of the breast.

- Standing behind the patient, place both arms around the patient and locate the anterior border of the implant by walking the fingers back from the nipple toward the chest wall, or
- Stand beside the patient lateral to the breast being imaged. Have the patient hold the grip with the opposite hand to retain her balance. Locate the anterior border of the implant by walking the fingers back from the nipple toward the chest wall.
- When the anterior border of the implant has been located, gently pull the anterior breast tissue forward onto the IR (Fig. 18.34). Use the hands and the edge of the IR to keep the implant displaced posteriorly.
- Center the breast over the AEC detector with the nipple in profile if possible.
- Hold the implant back against the chest wall. Slowly apply compression to the

anterior skin surface, being careful not to allow the implant to slip under the compression paddle. As compression continues, the implant should be seen bulging behind the compression paddle.
- Apply compression until the anterior breast tissue is taut. Compared with the full-implant projection, an additional ¾ to 2 inches (2 to 5 cm) of compression should be achieved with the implant displaced.
- Instruct the patient to indicate if the compression becomes too uncomfortable or intolerable.
- When full compression is achieved, move the AEC detector to the appropriate position and instruct the patient to stop breathing.
- Make the exposure.
- Release breast compression immediately.

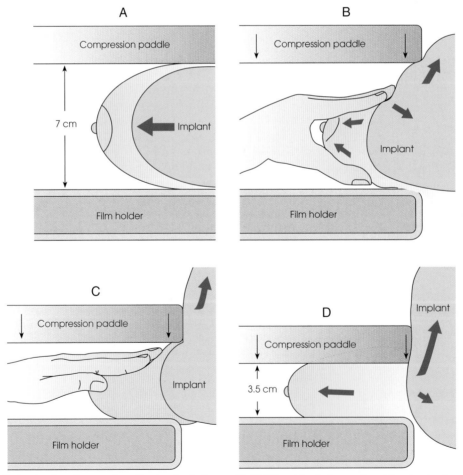

Fig. 18.34 (A) Breast with implant and normal positioning techniques. (B–D) Eklund technique of pushing implant posteriorly against chest wall, pulling breast anteriorly, and compressing tissue.

(From Eklund GW, Busby RC, Miller SH, Job JS: Improved imaging of the augmented breast. *AJR Am J Roentgenol* 151:469, 1988.)

Central ray
- Perpendicular to the base of the breast

Structures shown
This projection shows the anterior and central breast tissue projected free of superimposition with uniform compression and improved tissue differentiation. The implant is displaced posteriorly and should not be visualized on the image (Fig. 18.35).

The following should be clearly shown:
- Breast tissue superior and inferior to the implant pulled forward with the anterior breast tissue projected free of the implant
- PNL extending posteriorly to edge of implant, measuring within ⅓ inch (1 cm) of depth of PNL on MLO projection with implant displaced
- Implant along posterior edge of image, flattened against chest wall, should not be visualized on the image, but often remnants of the implant may be seen.
- Image sharpness is enhanced by increased compression of the breast tissue and reduced scatter due to removal of the implant from the path of the beam.

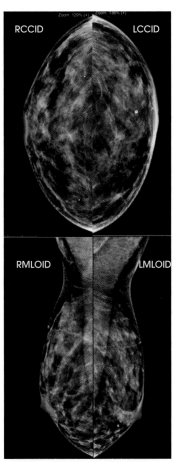

Fig. 18.35 Bilateral, four-image CC and MLO projections with ID of the same patient as in Fig. 18.33, using Eklund (ID) technique. Implants are pushed back for better visualization of surrounding breast tissue.

♠ MEDIOLATERAL OBLIQUE (MLO) PROJECTION WITH FULL IMPLANT

Paddle: 8 × 10 inches (18 × 24 cm) or 10 × 12 inches (24 × 30 cm).

Position of patient

- Have the patient stand facing the IR or seat the patient on an adjustable stool facing the unit.

Position of part

- Turn the AEC *off*, and preselect a *manual* technique. For FFDM units, be sure that Implant View processing settings are chosen if applicable.
- Follow the same positioning sequence as for the standard MLO projection.
- Inform the patient that minimal compression of the breast will be used. Continue to hold the breast up and out while sliding the hand toward the nipple as the compression paddle is brought into contact with the breast.

- Slowly apply only enough compression to immobilize the breast. Compression should be minimal, and the anterior breast tissue should still feel soft.
- Pull down on the patient's abdominal tissue to open the inframammary fold.
- Select the appropriate exposure factors and instruct the patient to stop breathing.
- Make the exposure.
- Release breast compression immediately.

Central ray

- Perpendicular to the IR
- The C-arm apparatus is positioned at an angle determined by the slope of the patient's pectoral muscle (30 to 60 degrees). The actual angle is determined by the patient's body habitus: Tall, thin patients require steep angulation, whereas short, stout patients require shallow angulation.

Structures shown

The image shows the entire implant and surrounding posterior breast tissue as well as axillary tissue and pectoral muscle, with suboptimal compression of the anterior fibroglandular breast tissue (see Fig. 18.33).

EVALUATION CRITERIA

The following should be clearly shown:
- Implant projected over fibroglandular tissue, extending to posterior edge of image
- Posterior breast tissue on the inferior aspect, extending to chest wall
- Nipple in profile if possible
- Open inframammary fold
- Breast adequately maneuvered up and out from chest wall
- Nonuniform compression of anterior breast tissue

MEDIOLATERAL OBLIQUE PROJECTION WITH IMPLANT DISPLACED (MLO ID)

Paddle: 8 × 10 inches (18 × 24 cm) or 10 × 12 inches (24 × 30 cm).

Position of patient
- Have the patient stand facing the IR or seat the patient on an adjustable stool facing the unit.
- Select an AEC technique. For FFDM units, be sure that Implant View processing settings are chosen if applicable.

Position of part
- Determine the degree of obliquity of the C-arm apparatus by rotating the tube until the long edge of the IR is parallel to the upper third of the pectoral muscle of the affected side. The degree of obliquity should be between 30 and 60 degrees, depending on the patient's body habitus.
- Adjust the height of the C-arm so that the superior border is level with the axilla.
- Instruct the patient to elevate the arm of the affected side over the corner of the IR and to rest the hand on the adjacent handgrip. The patient's elbow should be flexed.
- Standing in front of the patient, locate the anterior border of the implant by walking the fingers back from the patient's nipple toward the chest wall.
- After locating the anterior border of the implant, gently pull the anterior breast tissue forward onto the IR. Use the edge of the IR and the hands to keep the implant displaced posteriorly.

- Center the breast tissue over the AEC detector with the nipple in profile if possible.
- Hold the anterior breast tissue up and out so that the base of the thumb and the heel of the hand support the breast.
- Hold the implant back against the chest wall while using fingers to bring the anterior breast tissue forward onto the IR. Slowly apply compression to the anterior skin surface, taking care not to allow the implant to slip under the compression paddle. As compression continues, the implant should be seen bulging behind the compression paddle.
- Apply compression until the anterior breast tissue is taut. Compared with the full-implant projection, an additional ¾ to 2 inches (2 to 5 cm) of tissue should be adequately visualized with the implant displaced.
- Instruct the patient to indicate if the compression becomes uncomfortable or intolerable.
- Pull down on the patient's abdominal tissue to open the inframammary fold.
- Instruct the patient to hold the opposite breast away from the path of the beam, as necessary.
- When full compression is achieved, move the AEC detector to the appropriate position if necessary and instruct the patient to stop breathing.
- Make the exposure.
- Release breast compression immediately.

Central ray
- Perpendicular to the IR
- The C-arm apparatus is positioned at an angle determined by the slope of the patient's pectoral muscle (30 to 60 degrees). The actual angle is determined by the patient's body habitus: Tall, thin patients require steep angulation, whereas short, stout patients require shallow angulation.

Structures shown
This image shows the anterior and central breast tissue projected free of superimposition of the implant, with uniform compression and improved tissue differentiation (see Fig. 18.35).

EVALUATION CRITERIA
The following should be clearly shown:
- Breast tissue superomedial and inferolateral to the implant with anterior breast tissue projected free of the implant
- Pectoral muscle showing anterior convexity to ensure relaxed shoulder and axilla
- PNL extending obliquely to edge of implant, measuring within ⅓ inch (1 cm) of depth of PNL on CC projection with implant displaced
- Implant should not be visualized on the image, but often some remnants of the implant may be seen posteriorly.
- Posterior breast tissue on inferior aspect of breast, extending to chest wall
- Nipple in profile if possible
- Open inframammary fold
- Breast adequately maneuvered up and out from chest wall
- Image sharpness is enhanced by increased compression of the breast tissue and reduced scatter due to removal of the implant from the path of the beam.

Male Mammography
EPIDEMIOLOGY OF MALE BREAST DISEASE

In the United States, more than 2400 men develop invasive breast cancer every year, and nearly 20% of these men die of the disease.[1] Although most men who develop breast cancer are 60 years of age and older, juvenile cases have been reported. Nearly all male breast cancers are primary tumors. An estimated 4% to 40% of male breast cancers are due to inherited mutations. Men typically have significantly less breast tissue and screening mammograms typically are not performed for male patients; therefore, most male breast cancers are diagnosed as palpable lumps and are more likely to be diagnosed at advanced stages. The overall 5-year survival rate for male breast cancer is 84%, compared to 90% in women, which reflects this fact.[26] Other symptoms of breast cancer in men include nipple retraction, crusting, discharge, and ulceration.

Gynecomastia, a benign excessive development of the male mammary gland, can make malignant breast lesions more elusive to palpation. Gynecomastia occurs in 40% of male breast cancer patients; however, a histologic relationship between gynecomastia and male breast cancer has not been definitively established. Because gynecomastia is caused by a hormonal imbalance, it is believed that abnormal hormonal function may increase the risk of male breast cancer in these patients.[27] Other associated risk factors for male breast cancer include increasing age, positive family history, *BRCA1* and *BRCA2* gene mutations, and Klinefelter syndrome.[28]

Breast cancer treatment options are limited among male patients. Because men have less breast tissue, lumpectomy is not considered practical. Most of the male glandular tissue is located directly posterior to the nipple. Therefore, a modified radical mastectomy, including dissection of the nipple, is usually the preferred surgical procedure.[29–31] Radiation and systemic therapy are considered when the tumor is located near the chest wall or when indicated by lymph node analysis. Similar to female breast cancer, the prognosis for male breast cancer is directly related to the stage of the disease at diagnosis. An early diagnosis indicates a better chance of survival. Survival rates among male patients with localized breast carcinomas are positive: 98% survive for 5 years.[26]

Routine Projections of the Male Breast

Male breast anatomy varies significantly from female breast anatomy. The pectoral muscle is more highly developed in men, and most of the glandular breast tissue is located directly posterior to the nipple. The radiographer must take this variance into consideration. The standard CC and MLO projections may be applied with success in most male patients (Figs. 18.36–18.38). For men (or women) with large pectoral muscles, the radiographer may perform the caudocranial (FB) projection instead of the standard CC because it may be easier to compress the inferior portion of the breast. In addition, the lateromedial oblique (LMO) projection may replace the standard MLO.

Keep in mind that these unconventional views are rarely necessary but are viable alternatives in extreme cases. These projections may allow the radiographer to accommodate more successfully a patient with prominent pectoral muscles. Some facilities also use narrower quadrant compression paddles (3 inches [8 cm] wide) to compress the male breast or the extremely small female breast.[32] The smaller paddle permits the radiographer to hold the breast in position while applying final compression. A wooden spoon or a plastic spatula

Fig. 18.36 Positioning for CC projection of male breast.

Fig. 18.37 Positioning for MLO projections of male breast.

can be used to hold the breast in place, then can be slowly removed as the compression paddle replaces it.

Because most men who undergo mammography present with outward symptoms, mammography of the male breast is usually considered a diagnostic examination. It can be considered a screening examination for men who know they carry the *BRCA1* or *BRCA2* gene, or who have a history of breast cancer. The radiographer should work closely with the radiologist to achieve a thorough demonstration of the potential abnormality. In the male breast, most tumors are located in the subareolar region. Careful attention should be given to positioning the nipple in profile and to providing adequate compression of this area to allow the best visualization of this tissue.

Calcifications are rare in male breast cancer cases. When present, they are usually larger, rounder, and more scattered than the calcifications associated with female breast cancer. Spot compression and the magnification technique are common image enhancement methods for showing the morphology of calcifications.

Procedures other than mammography are used to diagnose male breast cancer. FNAB and excisional biopsy of palpable lesions are standard methods of diagnosis. Histologically, most breast cancers in men are ductal, and most are infiltrating ductal carcinomas. Very few in situ cancers are found in male patients.

Because breast cancer is traditionally considered a "woman's disease," the radiographer should remain sensitive to the feelings of the male patient by offering not only physical comfort but also psychological and emotional support during the procedure.

Image Enhancement Methods

The spot compression technique and the magnification technique are designed to enhance the image of the area under investigation.

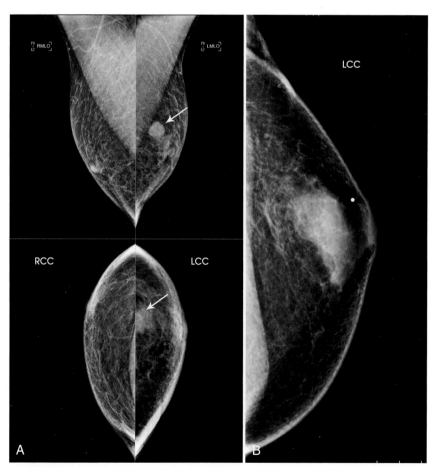

Fig. 18.38 (A) Four-view mammogram of a 55-year-old man with a new palpable lump *(arrow)*. This proved to be cancer on biopsy. (B) Left CC view of a 49-year-old male with a new lump. This proved to be gynecomastia, a benign process, on biopsy.

MAGNIFICATION TECHNIQUE (M USED AS PREFIX)

Paddle: 8 × 10 inches (18 × 24 cm).

Position of patient

- Have the patient stand facing the IR or seat the patient on an adjustable stool facing the unit.
- Use only equipment designed to be used for magnification mammography to perform this maneuver and use the equipment according to the manufacturer's directions.

Position of part

- Attach the firm, radiolucent magnification platform to the unit. The patient's breast is positioned on the platform between the compression device and a nongrid IR.

- Select the smallest focal spot target size (≤0.1 mm is preferred). Most units allow magnification images to be exposed only when the correct focal spot size is used.
- Select the appropriate compression paddle (regular, quadrant, or spot compression). Collimate according to the size of the compression paddle.
- Position the patient's breast to obtain the projection that best shows the area of interest. The angle of the C-arm can be adjusted to accommodate any projection normally performed using a traditional grid technique.
- When full compression is achieved, move the AEC detector to the chest wall position (if necessary) and instruct the patient to stop breathing (Fig. 18.39).
- Make the exposure.
- Release breast compression immediately.

Central ray

- Perpendicular to the area of interest

Structures shown

This technique optically magnifies the compressed area of interest with improved detail, facilitating determination of the characteristics of microcalcifications (Fig. 18.40)[33,34] and the margins (or lack of definitive margins) of suspected lesions (Fig. 18.41).

EVALUATION CRITERIA

The following should be clearly shown:

- Area of interest within collimated and compressed margins
- Improved delineation of number, distribution, and morphology of microcalcifications
- Enhanced architectural characteristics of focal density or mass
- Uniform tissue exposure if compression is adequate

Fig. 18.39 Radiolucent platform placed between breast and film holder causes breast image to be enlarged.

(Courtesy Lorad Corp.)

Fig. 18.40 MLO projection using the magnification technique and a quad paddle to better visualize microcalcifications.

✹ SPOT COMPRESSION TECHNIQUE

Image receptor: 8 × 10 inches (18 × 24 cm).

Position of patient

- Have the patient stand facing the IR or seat the patient on an adjustable stool facing the unit.
- This technique is often performed in conjunction with the magnification technique, especially for determination of number, distribution, and morphology of microcalcifications.

Position of part

In conjunction with magnification technique

- Place a firm, radiolucent magnification platform, designed for use with the dedicated mammography equipment on the unit, between the patient's breast and a nongrid IR.
- Select the smallest focal spot target size (≤0.1 mm is preferred).

For palpable masses

A tangential (TAN) projection combined with spot compression and the magnification technique is most often used to image a palpable mass; however, the spot compression technique in a previously imaged projection is also requested by many radiologists.

- Select the appropriate spot compression device.
- Mark the location of the palpable mass with a felt-tip pen or with a radiopaque beebee (BB) marker placed on the lump, according to the policy of the facility.
- Center the area of interest under the compression device in the position indicated by the radiologist.
- Inform the patient that compression of the breast will be used and may be

051Y
JAG
C: 2047.0, W: 4096.0
C=2047.0, W=4096.0 1/2
RML ⌐RMML⌐

A

8/22/2013
Dimensions 3
48 mm, 0.029 dGy, 30 kV, 81 mAs   F

Fig. 18.41 Right MLO projection using the magnification technique and a spot paddle to perform a tangential view of a palpable mass. This proved that the mass was smoothly outlined with uniform edges and was shown to be a cyst on ultrasound.

uncomfortable. Bring the compression paddle into contact with the breast, and slowly apply compression until the breast feels taut.

- Instruct the patient to indicate if the compression becomes too uncomfortable.
- When full compression is achieved, move the AEC detector to the chest wall position if necessary, and instruct the patient to stop breathing (Fig. 18.42).
- Make the exposure.
- Release breast compression immediately.

For nonpalpable masses

- While viewing the routine mammogram, measure the location of the area of interest from a reference point (the nipple), using a tape measure or the fingertips (Fig. 18.43).
- Select the appropriate spot compression device.
- Reposition the patient's breast to obtain the projection from which the measurements were taken.
- Using the same reference point, transfer onto the patient the measurements taken from the mammogram.
- Mark the area of interest with a felt-tip pen, or mentally note the location on the breast.
- Center the area of interest under the compression device in the requested view, which may be different from the original projection.
- Inform the patient that compression of the breast will be used. Bring the compression paddle into contact with the breast, and slowly apply compression until the breast feels taut. Adequate compression is especially important for spot views of nonpalpable masses, as the objective is to use targeted compression to separate tissue islands that may be overlapped, causing an area of suspicious density.
- Instruct the patient to indicate if the compression becomes too uncomfortable.
- When full compression is achieved, move the AEC detector to the appropriate position if necessary, and instruct the patient to stop breathing.
- Make the exposure.
- Release breast compression immediately.

Fig. 18.42 Spot compression used with CC projection.

Fig. 18.43 To find the area of interest in the breast for a spot view, measure how far posterior the area is by using the nipple as a reference point. This image illustrates how measurement of the lesion from the nipple on the CC view approximates measurement of the lesion from the nipple on the magnified spot view.

Central ray

- Perpendicular to the area of interest

Structures shown

The spot compression technique resolves superimposed structures seen on only one projection, better visualizes small lesions located in the extreme posterior breast, separates superimposed ductal structures in the subareolar region, and improves visualization in areas of dense tissue through localized compression (Fig. 18.44).

The following should be clearly shown:

- Area of interest clearly seen within compressed margins
- Close collimation to the area of interest unless contraindicated by radiologist
- Improved recorded detail through the use of close collimation and the magnification technique employing a spot compression device
- Uniform tissue exposure if compression is adequate

NOTE: Densities caused by the superimposition of normal breast parenchyma disappear on spot compression images.

Fig. 18.44 (A) This 45-year-old woman with extremely dense tissue was recalled for a questionable mass *(arrow)* in the left breast on screening mammography. (B) A spot view was performed to spread the tissue and more clearly delineate the borders of the mass. This proved to be a fibroadenoma on biopsy.

Supplemental Projections

The routine projections are not always adequate in completely showing a patient's breast tissue, or a specific area may require clearer delineation. Supplemental projections complement the routine projections and have distinct applications (Table 18.2). The mammographer should fully understand the value of each projection and its potential to show significant findings in the breast. This section provides a brief overview of significant mammographic findings in their most common radiographic presentation and provides suggested correlative supplemental projections. The language related to mammographic findings must be appreciated for the mammographer and the radiologist to work collaboratively toward a successful diagnostic examination.

The mass is the most common presentation of a potential abnormality in the breast. It is identified on two projections of the affected breast. A mass has a convex shape or an outward contour to its margins. If a suspected mass is identified on only one projection, the mammographer must strive to position the breast so that the area in question is shown on at least two projections. If the suspected mass is seen only on the MLO projection in the deep medial aspect of the breast, a CC projection for cleavage may complement the standard CC projection. Conversely, if the mass is seen in the extreme lateral aspect, an exaggerated craniocaudal (XCCL) projection laterally would be the projection of choice. In a sense, the radiographer is collecting evidence to prove whether the mass is real or is merely a summation shadow of superimposed breast parenchyma.

Other supplemental projections are intended to offer alternative methods for tailoring the mammographic procedure to the specific abilities of the patient and the requirements of the interpreting physician.

Often the need for additional projections is determined only after careful examination of the standard projections. Throughout mammographic procedures, the radiographer should consistently evaluate the images, keeping foremost in mind the optimal demonstration of possible findings. For example, when performing lateral projections, the mammographer should place the area of interest closest to the IR. The mammographer may develop the expertise to predict and perform supplemental projections that confirm or rule out suspected breast abnormalities. As with all radiographic procedures, image evaluation is a crucial component of high-quality imaging. In evaluating images, the mammographer becomes an integral member of the breast imaging team, actively participating in the work-up of an asymptomatic patient.

TABLE 18.2

Supplemental projections or methods and their suggested applications

Projection or method	Application
Spot compression	Defines lesion or area through focal compression; separates overlying parenchyma
Magnification (M)	Combines with spot compression to show margins of lesion; delineates microcalcifications
Mediolateral (ML)	Localization; shows air-fluid-fat levels; defines lesion located in lateral aspect of breast; complements mediolateral oblique (MLO) projection
Lateromedial (LM)	Localization; shows air-fluid-fat levels; defines lesion located in medial aspect of breast
Exaggerated craniocaudal (XCCL)	Visualizes lesions in deep outer aspect of breast that are not seen on standard CC
CC for cleavage (CV)	Visualizes deep medial breast tissue; shows medial lesion in true transverse or axial plane
CC with roll (RL, RM)	Triangulates lesion seen only on CC projection; defines location of lesion as in superior or inferior aspect of breast
Tangential (TAN)	Confirms dermal vs. breast calcifications; shows obscure palpable lump over subcutaneous fat
Captured lesion	Shows palpable lump in posterior tissue that is difficult to immobilize with conventional techniques
Caudocranial (FB)	Visualizes superior breast tissue; defines lesion located in superior aspect of breast; replaces standard CC for patients with kyphosis or prominent pectoral muscles
MLO for axillary tail (AT)	Focal compression projection of AT
Lateromedial oblique (LMO)	Shows medial breast tissue; replaces standard MLO for patients with pectus excavatum, prominent pacemakers, prominent pectoral muscles, Hickman catheters, and postoperative open heart surgery
Superolateral to inferomedial oblique (SIO)	Visualizes upper-inner quadrant and lower-outer quadrant, which normally are superimposed on MLO and LMO projections

⚕ 90-DEGREE MEDIOLATERAL (ML) PROJECTION

Paddle: 8 × 10 inches (18 × 24 cm) or 10 × 12 inches (24 × 30 cm).

Position of patient

- Have the patient stand facing the IR or seat the patient on an adjustable stool facing the unit.

Position of part

- Rotate the C-arm assembly 90 degrees, with the x-ray tube placed on the medial side of the patient's breast.
- Have the patient bend slightly forward from the waist. Position the superior corner of the IR high into the axilla, with the patient's elbow flexed and the affected arm resting behind the IR.
- Ask the patient to relax the affected shoulder.
- Pull the breast tissue and the pectoral muscle superiorly and anteriorly, ensuring that the lateral rib margin is pressed firmly against the edge of the IR.
- Rotate the patient slightly laterally to help bring the medial tissue forward.
- Gently pull the medial breast tissue forward from the sternum and position the nipple in profile.
- Hold the patient's breast up and out by rotating the hand so that the base of the thumb and the heel of the hand support the breast.
- Inform the patient that compression of the breast will be used. Continue to hold the patient's breast up and out while sliding the hand toward the nipple as the compression paddle is brought into contact with the breast. Do not allow the breast to droop (Fig. 18.45).
- Slowly apply compression until the breast feels taut.
- Instruct the patient to indicate if compression becomes too uncomfortable.
- Ask the patient to hold the opposite breast away from the path of the beam.
- Instruct the patient to lift her chin to clear the field of potential artifacts.
- When full compression is achieved, move the AEC detector to the appropriate position if necessary, and instruct the patient to stop breathing (Fig. 18.46).
- Make the exposure.
- Release breast compression immediately.

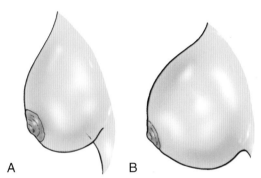

Fig. 18.45 (A) Lateral profile of breast showing inadequate compression and drooping breast. (B) Lateral profile of properly compressed breast. Note how compression has overcome the effect of gravity and how the breast is spread out over a greater area.

Fig. 18.46 ML projection.

Central ray

• Perpendicular to the base of the breast

Structures shown

This projection shows lesions on the lateral aspect of the breast in the superior and inferior aspects. It resolves superimposed structures seen on the MLO projection, localizes a lesion seen on one (or both) of the initial projections, and shows air-fluid and fat-fluid levels in breast structures (e.g., milk of calcium, galactoceles) and in pneumocystography (a rarely performed procedure involving injection of air into an aspirated cyst to image the cyst lining for intracystic lesions). The ML view is an orthogonal view to the CC and is often used to localize the depth of breast lesions.

EVALUATION CRITERIA

The following should be clearly shown:
- Nipple in profile
- Open inframammary fold
- Deep and superficial breast tissues well separated when breast is adequately maneuvered up and out from chest wall (Fig. 18.47)
- Retroglandular fat well visualized to ensure inclusion of deep fibroglandular breast tissue
- Uniform tissue exposure if compression is adequate

Fig. 18.47 ML projection.

90-DEGREE LATEROMEDIAL (LM) PROJECTION

Paddle: 8 × 10 inches (18 × 24 cm) or 10 × 12 inches (24 × 30 cm).

Position of patient
- Have the patient stand facing the IR or seat the patient on an adjustable stool facing the unit.

Position of part
- Rotate the C-arm assembly 90 degrees, with the x-ray tube placed on the lateral side of the patient's breast.
- Position the superior corner of the IR at the level of the jugular notch.
- Have the patient flex the neck slightly forward.
- Have the patient relax the affected shoulder, raise her arm on the affected side and flex the elbow, then rest the affected arm over the top of the IR.
- Pull the breast tissue and pectoral muscle superiorly and anteriorly, ensuring that the patient's sternum is pressed firmly against the edge of the IR.
- Rotate the patient slightly medially to help bring the lateral tissue forward.

- Have the patient rest the chin on the top edge of the IR to help loosen the skin in the medial aspect of the breast.
- Position the nipple in profile.
- Hold the patient's breast up and out. Do not let it droop.
- Inform the patient that compression of the breast will be used. Bring the compression paddle past the latissimus dorsi muscle and into contact with the breast. Slowly apply compression while sliding the hand out toward the nipple until the patient's breast feels taut.
- Instruct the patient to indicate whether the compression becomes uncomfortable.
- When full compression is achieved, move the AEC detector to the appropriate position if necessary, and instruct the patient to stop breathing (Fig. 18.48).
- Make the exposure.
- Release breast compression immediately.

Fig. 18.48 Lateromedial projection.

Central ray

• Perpendicular to the base of the breast

Structures shown

This projection shows lesions on the medial aspect of the breast in the superior or inferior aspects (Fig. 18.49). It resolves superimposed structures seen on the MLO projection, localizes a lesion seen on one (or both) of the initial projections, and shows air-fluid and fat-fluid levels in breast structures (e.g., milk of calcium, galactoceles) and in pneumocystography (a rarely performed procedure involving injection of air into an aspirated cyst to image the cyst lining for intracystic lesions). The LM view is an orthogonal view to the CC and is often used to localize the depth of breast lesions.

EVALUATION CRITERIA

The following should be clearly shown:
■ Nipple in profile
■ Open inframammary fold
■ Deep and superficial breast tissues well separated when breast is adequately maneuvered up and out from chest wall
■ Retroglandular fat well visualized to ensure inclusion of deep fibroglandular breast tissue
■ Uniform tissue exposure if compression is adequate

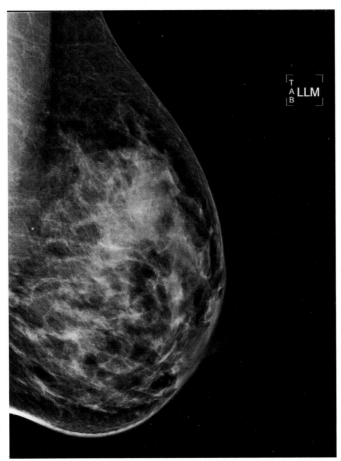

Fig. 18.49 LM projection.

⚞ EXAGGERATED CRANIOCAUDAL (XCCL) PROJECTION

Paddle: 8 × 10 inches (18 × 24 cm) or 10 × 12 inches (24 × 30 cm).

Position of patient

- Have the patient stand facing the IR or seat the patient on an adjustable stool facing the unit.

Position of part

- The contralateral side should be turned away from the image receptor.
- The lateral aspect of the ipsilateral breast should be closest to the image receptor.
- Elevate the inframammary fold to its maximal height.
- Adjust the height of the C-arm accordingly.
- Use one hand to scoop the inferior and posterior breast tissue up from the inframammary fold and place the breast onto the IR.
- This should be done with the technologist's right hand when the left breast is positioned, and with the left hand when the right breast is positioned.
- Use both hands to pull the breast gently onto the IR while instructing the patient to press the thorax against the breast tray.

- Slightly rotate the patient medially to place the lateral aspect of the breast on the IR.
- Place an arm against the patient's back with the hand on the shoulder of the affected side, ensuring that the shoulder is relaxed in external rotation.
- Slightly rotate the patient's head away from the affected side.
- Have the patient lean toward the machine and rest the head against the face guard.
- Rotate the C-arm assembly mediolaterally approximately 5 degrees, if necessary, to eliminate overlapping of the humeral head.
- Inform the patient that compression of the breast will be used. Smooth and flatten the breast tissue toward the nipple while bringing the compression paddle into contact with the breast.
- Slowly apply compression until the breast feels taut.
- Instruct the patient to indicate if the compression becomes uncomfortable.
- When full compression is achieved, move the AEC detector to the appropriate position if necessary, and instruct the patient to stop breathing (Figs. 18.50 and 18.51).
- Make the exposure.
- Release breast compression immediately.

Fig. 18.50 XCCL projection.

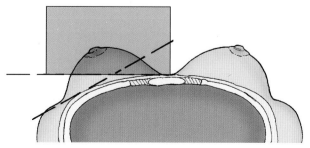

Fig. 18.51 Superior profile illustrates how placement of flat edge of IR against curved chest wall excludes a portion of breast tissue *(shaded area). Dashed line* indicates placement of IR for exaggerated position.

Central ray

- Angled 5 degrees mediolaterally to the base of the breast, if necessary

Structures shown

This projection shows a superoinferior projection of the lateral fibroglandular breast tissue and posterior aspect of the pectoral muscle. It also shows a sagittal orientation of a lateral lesion located in the AT of the breast.

The following should be clearly shown:

- Retroglandular fat well visualized to ensure inclusion of deep fibroglandular breast tissue on lateral aspect of breast and lower axillary region
- Pectoral muscle visualized over lateral chest wall (Fig. 18.52)
- Humeral head projected clear of image with use of a 5-degree ML angle
- Uniform tissue exposure if compression is adequate

Fig. 18.52 (A) CC projection of right breast. (B) XCCL projection of right breast. This projection is exaggerated laterally to show AT (*arrow*). Note also some visualization of pectoral muscle.

CRANIOCAUDAL PROJECTION FOR CLEAVAGE (CV)

Paddle: 8 × 10 inches (18 × 24 cm) or 10 × 12 inches (24 × 30 cm).

Position of patient

- Have the patient stand facing the IR or seat the patient on an adjustable stool facing the unit

Position of part

- Turn the AEC *off*, and preselect a *manual* technique. The radiographer may use AEC only if enough breast tissue is positioned over the AEC detector. The cleavage may be intentionally offset for this purpose.
- Determine the proper height of the breast tray by elevating the inframammary fold to its maximal height.
- Adjust the height of the C-arm accordingly.

- Lift and pull both breasts gently forward onto the IR while instructing the patient to press the thorax against the IR.
- Pull as much medial breast tissue as possible onto the IR.
- Slightly rotate the patient's head away from the affected side.
- Have the patient lean toward the machine and rest the head against the face guard.
- Ask the patient to hold the grip bars with both hands to keep in position on the IR.
- Raise the height of the IR slightly to loosen the superior tissue.
- Place one hand at the level of the patient's jugular notch, and then slide the hand down the patient's chest while pulling forward as much deep medial tissue as possible.
- Inform the patient that compression of the breast will be used. Bring the compression paddle into contact with the breasts, and slowly apply compression until the medial tissue feels taut. Using a quadrant compression paddle allows better compression of the cleavage area and allows more of the area of interest to be pulled into the imaging area. If a quadrant paddle is used, collimate to the area of compression to better visualize the detail of the tissue.
- Instruct the patient to indicate if the compression becomes uncomfortable.
- When full compression is achieved, move the AEC detector to the appropriate position if AEC is used, and instruct the patient to stop breathing (Fig. 18.53).
- Make the exposure.
- Release breast compression immediately.

Fig. 18.53 (A) Craniocaudal projection for cleavage. Cleavage is slightly off-center, so that AEC is under breast tissue. (B) Craniocaudal projection for cleavage using a smaller-quadrant paddle for maximum posterior visualization.

Central ray

• Perpendicular to the area of interest or the centered cleavage

Structures shown

This projection shows lesions located in the deep posteromedial aspect of the breast.

The following should be clearly shown:

■ Area of interest over the central portion of the IR (over the AEC detector if possible) with cleavage slightly off-centered or with cleavage centered to the IR and manual technique selected (Fig. 18.54)

■ Deep medial tissue of affected breast

■ All medial tissue included, as shown by visualization of medial retroglandular fat and the absence of any fibroglandular tissue extending to the posteromedial edge of imaged breasts

■ Uniform tissue exposure. It is not necessary to image all of the breast tissue on this projection.

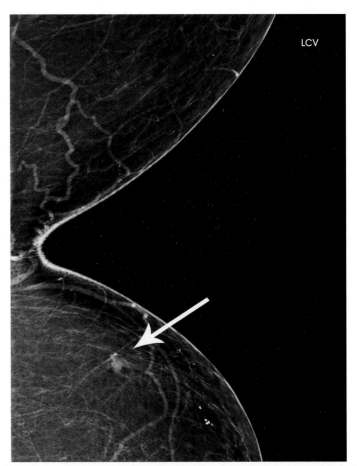

Fig. 18.54 This cleavage view was off-center to the left (LCV) but was performed to view the medial aspect of the right breast. A mass was seen on the right MLO but was not visualized on the standard RCC view. This extremely medial mass *(arrow)* proved to be invasive carcinoma on biopsy.

CRANIOCAUDAL PROJECTION WITH ROLL LATERAL OR ROLL MEDIAL (RL OR RM USED AS SUFFIX)

Paddle: 8 × 10 inches (18 × 24 cm) or 10 × 12 inches (24 × 30 cm).

Position of patient

- Have the patient stand facing the IR or seat the patient on an adjustable stool facing the unit.

Position of part

- Reposition the patient's breast in the CC projection.
- Place the hands on opposite surfaces of the patient's breast (superior/inferior), and roll the surfaces in opposite directions. The direction of the roll is not important as long as the mammographer rolls the superior surface in one direction and the inferior surface in the other direction. In a sense, the mammographer is very gently rotating the breast approximately 10 to 15 degrees (Fig. 18.55).

- Place the patient's breast onto the IR surface with the lower hand while holding the rolled position with the upper hand.
- Note the direction of the superior surface roll (lateral [RL] or medial [RM]) and label the image accordingly. If the superior aspect of the breast is rolled medially, the image should be labeled RM.
- Inform the patient that compression of the breast will be used. Bring the compression paddle into contact with the breast, and slide the hand out while rolling the breast tissue.
- Slowly apply compression until the breast feels taut.
- Instruct the patient to indicate if the compression becomes uncomfortable.
- When full compression is achieved, move the AEC detector to the appropriate position if necessary and instruct the patient to stop breathing (Fig. 18.56).
- Make the exposure.
- Release breast compression immediately.

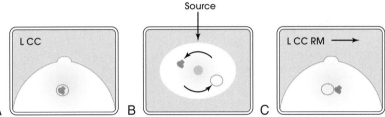

Fig. 18.55 (A) CC projection showing lesion that may represent superimposition of two structures. If spot compression fails to resolve these structures, CC projection with the roll position may be performed. (B) Anterior view of CC projection, with *arrows* indicating rolling of superior and inferior breast surfaces in opposite directions to separate superimposed structures. (C) CC projection with RM, showing resolution of two lesions. *Arrow* indicates direction of roll of superior surface of breast.

Fig. 18.56 CC projection with lateral and medial roll.

427

Central ray

- Perpendicular to the base of the breast

Structures shown

This position shows separation of superimposed breast tissues (also known as *summation shadow*), particularly those seen only on the CC projection. The position also helps determine whether a lesion is located in the superior or inferior aspect of the breast (Fig. 18.57). Alternatively, the standard CC projection may be performed using the spot compression technique, or with the C-arm assembly rotated 10 to 15 degrees mediolaterally or lateromedially to eliminate superimposition of breast tissue. These methods are often preferred because they allow for easier duplication of the projection during subsequent examinations.

The following should be clearly shown:
- Suspected superimposition adequately resolved
- Suspected lesion in superior or inferior aspect of breast
- All medial tissue included, as shown by visualization of medial retroglandular fat and the absence of fibroglandular tissue extending to posteromedial edge of image
- Nipple in profile and at midline, indicating no exaggeration of positioning. The nipple is used as a point of reference to distinguish the location of the suspected lesion, if it exists.
- Some lateral tissue possibly excluded to emphasize medial tissue visualized
- Slight medial skin reflection at cleavage, ensuring that posterior medial tissue is adequately included
- Uniform tissue exposure if compression is adequate

Fig. 18.57 CC projection with RL.

TANGENTIAL (TAN) PROJECTION

Paddle: 8 × 10 inches (18 × 24 cm).

Position of patient
- Have the patient stand facing the IR or seat the patient on an adjustable stool facing the unit.

Position of part
For a palpable mass. The TAN projection is most often performed with use of the magnification technique.
- Select a standard, quadrant, or spot compression paddle, as appropriate.
- Place the AEC detector at the chest wall.
- Locate the area of interest by palpating the patient's breast.
- Place a radiopaque marker or BB on the mass, or have the patient place the BB on the area of concern.
- Using the imaginary line between the nipple and the BB as the angle reference

(Fig. 18.58), rotate the C-arm apparatus parallel to this line. The central ray is directed tangential to the breast at the point identified by the BB marker.
- Place the breast on the IR or magnification stand with the area of interest marked by the BB on the edge of the skin.
- The "shadow" of the BB will be projected onto the IR surface.
- Using the appropriate compression paddle, compress the breast while ensuring that enough breast tissue covers the AEC detector area.
- Slowly apply compression until the breast feels taut.
- Instruct the patient to indicate if the compression becomes uncomfortable.
- When full compression is achieved, instruct the patient to stop breathing (Figs. 18.59 and 18.60).
- Make the exposure.
- Release breast compression immediately.

Central ray
- Perpendicular to the area of interest

Structures shown
This projection shows superficial lesions close to the skin surface with minimal parenchymal overlapping. It also shows skin calcifications or palpable lesions projected over subcutaneous fat (Fig. 18.61).

EVALUATION CRITERIA
The following should be clearly shown:
- Palpable lesion visualized over subcutaneous fat
- TAN radiopaque marker or BB marker accurately correlated with palpable lesion
- Minimal overlapping of adjacent parenchyma
- Calcification in parenchyma or skin
- Uniform tissue exposure if compression is adequate

Fig. 18.58 Degree of angle for TAN projection. Correlation of location of abnormality with degree of rotation of C-arm; an angle of the C-arm shows upper quadrant and lower quadrant abnormality tangentially.

Fig. 18.59 TAN projection.

Fig. 18.60 TAN projection of palpable mass in LOQ. (A) IR is angled parallel to nipple-to-mass line. (B) The mass, marked by *BB*, is positioned on edge of skin line. (C) Radiograph of mass imaged in tangent using the magnification technique. Spiculated borders indicate cancer.

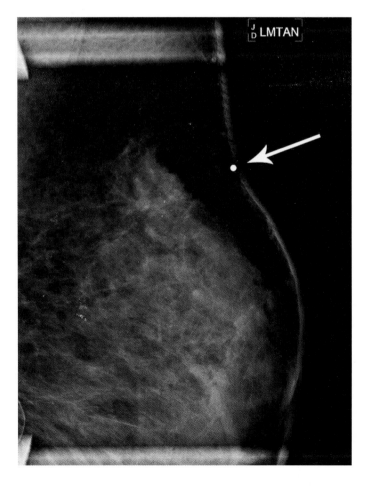

Fig. 18.61 Left magnified tangential view of a palpable mass with a BB placed on it shows the area of interest in the subdermal fatty tissue. The magnified view showed an area of architectural distortion with scattered clusters of coarse calcifications. This proved to be a cancer on biopsy.

CAPTURED LESION OR COAT-HANGER PROJECTION (CL)

This specialized positioning is seldom used but is very useful when a palpable lesion located in the extreme posterior or lateral breast tissue is imaged. Sometimes lesions in these areas tether themselves to the chest wall and resist being pulled forward to be visualized on a routine projection. This procedure is a variation of the TAN projection and should be labeled as such. It is generally performed using magnification and tight collimation. The captured lesion (CL) or coat-hanger projection captures and isolates the palpable lump for imaging (Figs. 18.62 and 18.63).

Paddle: 8 × 10 inches (18 × 24 cm).

Position of patient
- Have the patient stand facing the IR or seat the patient on an adjustable stool facing the unit.

Position of part
- Place the magnification platform designed for use with the dedicated mammography unit on the equipment.
- Place a lead BB over the palpable mass.
- Using your hands, determine the projection most likely to image the lump with no superimposition of other tissue. Place the area of clinical concern at the edge of the breast in a tangent plane to the imaging plate.
- The palpable area of clinical concern is captured with a corner of a wire coat-hanger or an inverted spot compression device. No additional compression is needed.
- It may be necessary to use a manual technique if the amount of tissue captured within the coat-hanger or inverted compression device does not cover the AEC detector.

Central ray
- Perpendicular to the imaging plate.

Structures shown
The area of clinical concern is positively identified and visualized with the advantages of magnification mammography.

EVALUATION CRITERIA

The following should be clearly shown:
- Area of interest within collimated and self-compressed margins

Supplemental Projections

Fig. 18.62 Coat-hanger projection. (A and B) A slippery lesion is captured for imaging by the angle of a wire coat-hanger. (C) Inverted spot compression device can sometimes achieve the same results. (D) Radiograph of lesion imaged using coat-hanger projection. This lesion could not be viewed on routine projections because of its position within the breast and the elastic nature of the lesion, which was determined to be a cancer on biopsy.

Fig. 18.63 This 40-year-old patient presented with a palpable lump on the left breast extremely posterior at 1:00. A BB was placed on the lump before imaging. The area was not visualized on the standard MLO view (A). Subsequent tangential imaging was unsuccessful because of the proximity of the pectoral muscle (B and C). A CL view was performed (D) to stabilize the lump within the imaged area. This proved to be a lipoma.

CAUDOCRANIAL PROJECTION (FB, OR FROM BELOW)

Paddle: 8 × 10 inches (18 × 24 cm) or 10 × 12 inches (24 × 30 cm).

Position of patient
- Have the patient stand facing the IR.

Position of part
- Rotate the C-arm apparatus 180 degrees from the rotation used for a routine CC projection. The tube head will be near the floor and the IR will be above the patient's breast.
- Standing on the medial side of the breast to be imaged, elevate the inframammary fold to its maximal height.
- Adjust the height of the C-arm so that the IR is in contact with the superior breast tissue.
- Lean the patient slightly forward while gently pulling the elevated breast out and perpendicular to the chest wall. Hold the breast in position.
- Have the patient rest the affected arm over the top of the IR.
- Inform the patient that compression of the breast will be used. Bring the compression paddle from below into contact with the patient's breast while sliding the hand toward the nipple.
- Slowly apply compression until the breast feels taut.
- Instruct the patient to indicate if the compression becomes uncomfortable.
- To ensure that the patient's abdomen is not superimposed over the path of the beam, have the patient pull in the abdomen or move the hips back slightly.
- When full compression is achieved, move the AEC detector to the appropriate position, and instruct the patient to stop breathing (Fig. 18.64).
- Make the exposure.
- Release breast compression immediately.

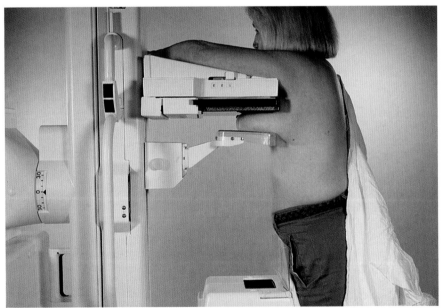

Fig. 18.64 FB projection.

Central ray

- Perpendicular to the base of the breast

Structures shown

This projection shows an inferosuperior projection of the breast for improved visualization of lesions located in the superior aspect as a result of reduced object–to–IR distance. The FB projection may facilitate a shorter route for needle-wire insertion to localize an inferior lesion (Fig. 18.65) or during prone stereotactic core biopsy. The projection may also be used as a replacement for the standard CC projection in patients with prominent pectoral muscles or kyphosis.

EVALUATION CRITERIA

The following should be clearly shown:

- Superior breast tissue and lesions clearly visualized
- For needle localization images, inferior lesion visualized within specialized fenestrated compression plate
- Patient's abdomen projected clear of image
- Inclusion of fixed posterior tissue of superior aspect of breast
- PNL extending posteriorly to edge of image, measuring within ⅓ inch (1 cm) of depth of PNL on MLO projection
- All medial tissue included as shown by visualization of medial retroglandular fat and absence of fibroglandular tissue extending to posteromedial edge of image
- Nipple in profile, if possible, and at midline, indicating no exaggeration of positioning
- Some lateral tissue possibly excluded to emphasize medial tissue
- Slight medial skin reflection at cleavage, ensuring that posterior medial tissue is adequately included
- Uniform tissue exposure if compression is adequate

Fig. 18.65 (A) FB projection performed in a 57-year-old woman to access the shortest route for localizing lesions identified in the inferior aspect of the breast *(arrow)*. (B) Orthogonal 90-degree ML projection of the same patient, showing successful placement of needle-wire system within lesion *(arrow)*. The lesion was found to be a 9-mm infiltrating ductal carcinoma.

MEDIOLATERAL OBLIQUE PROJECTION FOR AXILLARY TAIL (AT)

Paddle: 8 × 10 inches (18 × 24 cm) or 10 × 12 inches (24 × 30 cm).

Position of patient
- Have the patient stand facing the IR or seat the patient on an adjustable stool facing the unit.

Position of part
- Determine the degree of obliquity of the C-arm apparatus by rotating the tube until the long edge of the IR is parallel with the AT of the affected side. The degree of obliquity varies between 10 and 35 degrees.
- Adjust the height of the C-arm so that the superior border of the IR is just under the axilla.

- Instruct the patient to elevate the arm of the affected side over the corner of the IR and to rest the hand on the adjacent handgrip. The patient's elbow should be flexed.
- Have the patient relax the affected shoulder and lean it slightly anterior. Using the flat surface of the hand, gently pull the tail of the breast anteriorly and medially onto the IR, keeping the skin and tissue smooth and free of wrinkles.
- Ask the patient to turn the head away from the side being examined and to rest the head against the face guard.
- Inform the patient that compression of the breast will be used. Continue to hold the breast in position while sliding the hand toward the nipple as the compression paddle is brought into contact with the AT (Fig. 18.66).

- Slowly apply compression until the breast feels taut. The corner of the compression paddle should be inferior to the clavicle. To avoid patient discomfort caused by the corner of the paddle and to facilitate even compression, remind the patient to keep the shoulder relaxed.
- Instruct the patient to indicate if the compression becomes uncomfortable.
- When full compression is achieved, move the AEC detector to the appropriate position, and instruct the patient to stop breathing. It may be necessary to increase exposure factors if compression is not as taut as in the routine projections.
- Make the exposure.
- Release breast compression immediately.

Fig. 18.66 MLO projection for AT.

Central ray

- Perpendicular to the IR
- The angle of the C-arm apparatus is determined by the slope of the patient's AT.

Structures shown

This projection shows the AT of the breast, with emphasis on its lateral aspect.

The following should be clearly shown:

- AT with inclusion of axillary lymph nodes under focal compression (Fig. 18.67)
- Uniform tissue exposure if compression is adequate
- Slight skin reflection of affected arm on superior border of image

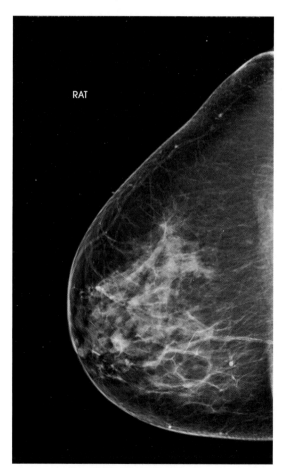

RAT

Fig. 18.67 Right AT projection.

Supplemental Projections

AXILLA PROJECTION FOR AXILLARY TAIL (AT)

Paddle: 8 × 10 inches (18 × 24 cm).

Position of patient
- Have the patient stand facing the IR or seat the patient on an adjustable stool facing the unit.

Position of part
- Rotate the C-arm to approximately 70 degrees.
- Adjust the height of the C-arm so that the superior edge of the IR is even with the top of the patient's shoulder.
- Select the appropriate compression device. A quadrant paddle will capture more deep axillary tissue; a standard 18 × 24 cm compression paddle will capture additional lateral tissue and AT.

- Instruct the patient to elevate the arm of the affected side so that it is perpendicular to the body.
- Place the arm against the IR so that the posterior aspect of the shoulder is resting against the IR. The patient's arm is draped across the IR with the forearm resting on the grip bar.
- Have the patient relax the affected shoulder and lean slightly anterior. Using the flat surface of the hand placed under the axillary region, gently pull the tail of the breast anteriorly and medially onto the IR, keeping the skin and tissue smooth and free of wrinkles.
- Inform the patient that compression of the breast will be used. Slowly bring compression down along the patient's ribs, with the top edge of the compression paddle skimming the lower edge of the patient's upper arm.

- Slowly apply compression until the axillary tissue feels taut. The corner of the compression paddle should be inferior to the clavicle. To avoid patient discomfort caused by the corner of the paddle and to facilitate even compression, remind the patient to keep the shoulder relaxed.
- Instruct the patient to indicate if the compression becomes uncomfortable. Vigorous compression is not necessary for this view (Fig. 18.68).
- When full compression is achieved, move the AEC detector to the appropriate position, and instruct the patient to stop breathing. It may be necessary to increase exposure factors if compression is not as taut as in the routine projections.
- Make the exposure.
- Release breast compression immediately.

Fig. 18.68 Axilla projection for AT.

Structures shown

This projection shows the axilla and the AT of the breast, with emphasis on its lateral aspect.

The following should be clearly shown:

■ AT with inclusion of axillary lymph nodes under focal compression (Fig. 18.69)

■ Uniform tissue exposure if compression is adequate

■ Slight skin reflection of affected arm on superior border of image

Fig. 18.69 Left AT projection demonstrating the axilla and its contents. Note ductal carcinoma and metastasized lymph nodes *(arrows)*.

LATEROMEDIAL OBLIQUE (LMO) PROJECTION

Paddle: 8 × 10 inches (18 × 24 cm) or 10 × 12 inches (24 × 30 cm).

Position of patient

- Have the patient stand facing the IR or seat the patient on an adjustable stool facing the unit.

Position of part

- Determine the degree of obliquity of the C-arm apparatus by rotating the assembly until the long edge of the IR is parallel with the upper third of the pectoral muscle of the affected side. The central ray enters the inferior aspect of the breast from the lateral side. The degree of obliquity should be between 30 and 60 degrees, depending on the body habitus of the patient.

- Adjust the height of the C-arm so that the superior border of the IR is level with the jugular notch.
- Ask the patient to place the opposite hand on the C-arm. The patient's elbow should be flexed.
- Lean the patient toward the C-arm apparatus and press the sternum against the edge of the IR, which is slightly off-center toward the opposite breast.
- Have the patient relax the affected shoulder and lean it slightly anterior. Gently pull the patient's breast and pectoral muscle anteriorly and medially, with the flat surface of the hand positioned along the lateral aspect of the breast.
- Scoop breast tissue up with the hand, gently grasping the breast between fingers and thumb.
- Center the breast with the nipple in profile, if possible, and hold the breast in position.

- Inform the patient that compression of the breast will be used. Continue to hold the patient's breast up and out while sliding the hand toward the nipple as the compression paddle is brought into contact with the LOQ of the breast.
- Slowly apply compression until the breast feels taut.
- Instruct the patient to indicate if the compression becomes uncomfortable.
- Pull down on the patient's abdominal tissue to open the inframammary fold.
- Ask the patient to rest the affected elbow on the top edge of the IR.
- When full compression is achieved, move the AEC detector to the appropriate position, and instruct the patient to stop breathing (Fig. 18.70).
- Make the exposure.
- Release breast compression immediately.

Fig. 18.70 LMO projection.

Central ray

- Perpendicular to the IR
- The C-arm apparatus is positioned at an angle determined by the slope of the patient's pectoral muscle (30 to 60 degrees). The actual angle is determined by the patient's body habitus: Tall, thin patients require steep angulation, whereas short, stout patients require shallow angulation.

Structures shown

This projection shows a true reverse projection of the routine MLO projection and is typically performed to better show the medial breast tissue. It is also performed if the routine MLO cannot be completed because of one or more of the following conditions: pectus excavatum, extreme kyphosis, post open-heart surgery, prominent pacemaker, men or women with prominent pectoralis muscles, or Port-A-Cath/MediPort (Hickman catheters).

EVALUATION CRITERIA

The following should be clearly shown:

- Medial breast tissue clearly visualized (Fig. 18.71)
- PNL measuring within ⅓ inch (1 cm) of the depth of the PNL on the CC projection. (While drawing the PNL obliquely, following the orientation of the breast tissue toward the pectoral muscle, measure its depth from nipple to pectoral muscle or to the edge of the image, whichever comes first.)
- Inferior aspect of the pectoral muscle extending to nipple line or below it if possible

- Pectoral muscle with anterior convexity to ensure a relaxed shoulder and axilla
- Nipple in profile if possible
- Open inframammary fold
- Deep and superficial breast tissues well separated when breast is adequately maneuvered up and out from chest wall
- Retroglandular fat well visualized to ensure inclusion of deep fibroglandular breast tissue
- Uniform tissue exposure if compression is adequate

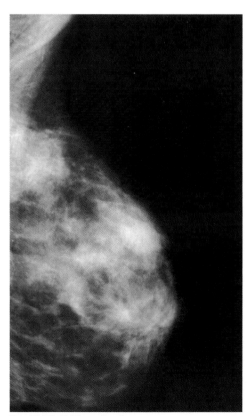

Fig. 18.71 LMO projection.

(From Svane G: Screening mammography, St Louis, 1993, Mosby.)

Supplemental Projections

SUPEROLATERAL TO INFEROMEDIAL OBLIQUE (SIO) PROJECTION

Paddle: 8 × 10 inches (18 × 24 cm) or 10 × 12 inches (24 × 30 cm).

Position of patient

- Have the patient stand facing the IR or seat the patient on an adjustable stool facing the unit.

Position of part

- Rotate the C-arm apparatus so that the central ray is directed at an angle to enter the superior and lateral aspect of the affected breast. The LIQ is adjacent to the IR.
- Adjust the degree of C-arm obliquity according to the body habitus of the patient, or, when the superolateral to inferomedial oblique (SIO) projection is being used as an additional projection to image an area of the tissue more clearly without superimposition of surrounding tissue, adjust the C-arm to the degree of angulation required by the radiologist, generally a 20- to 30-degree angle.

- Adjust the height of the C-arm to position the patient's breast over the center of the IR.
- Instruct the patient to rest the hand of the affected side on the handgrip adjacent to the IR holder. The patient's elbow should be flexed. For shallow-angled SIO projections, the arm on the affected side should lie straight against the patient's side. The handgrip is held by the hand on the contralateral side.
- Place the upper corner of the IR along the sternal edge adjacent to the upper inner aspect of the patient's breast.
- With the patient leaning slightly forward, gently pull as much medial tissue as possible away from the sternal edge while holding the breast up and out. The breast should not droop. Ensure that the patient's back remains straight during positioning, and that the patient does not lean to the side or toward the IR.
- Inform the patient that compression of the breast will be used. Continue to hold the breast up and out.
- Bring the compression paddle under the affected arm and into contact with the patient's breast while sliding the hand toward the patient's nipple. For shallow-angled SIO, the affected arm at the patient's side should be bent at the elbow to avoid superimposition of the humeral head over the breast tissue.
- Slowly apply compression until the breast feels taut. The upper corner of the compression paddle should be in the axilla for the standard SIO projection.
- Instruct the patient to indicate if the compression becomes uncomfortable.
- When full compression is achieved on the standard SIO, help the patient bring the arm up and over with the flexed elbow resting on top of the IR.
- Gently pull down on the patient's abdominal tissue to smooth out any skin folds.
- Move the AEC detector to the appropriate position and instruct the patient to stop breathing (Fig. 18.72).
- Make the exposure.
- Release breast compression immediately.

Fig. 18.72 (A) SIO projection. (B) Shallow-angled SIO with arm down.

Central ray

- Perpendicular to the IR
- The C-arm apparatus is positioned at an angle determined by the patient's body habitus or tissue composition.

Structures shown

This projection shows the UIQ and LOQ of the breast free of superimposition. In addition, lesions located in the lower inner aspect of the breast are shown with better recorded detail. This projection may also be used to replace the MLO ID projection in patients with encapsulated implants (Fig. 18.73).

The following should be clearly shown:

- UIQ and LOQ free of superimposition (these quadrants are superimposed on MLO and LMO projections)
- Lower inner aspect of breast visualized with greater detail
- Nipple in profile if possible
- Deep and superficial breast tissues well separated when breast is adequately maneuvered up and out from chest wall
- Retroglandular fat well visualized to ensure inclusion of deep fibroglandular breast tissue
- Uniform tissue exposure if compression is adequate.

Supplemental Projections

Fig. 18.73 Patient presented with a palpable mass at 1:00 in the right breast. A BB was placed on the skin over the lump, and standard MLO and CC projections were taken (A and B). A tangential view taken in an SIO projection (C) places the palpable lump within the dermis for best visualization. This proved to be invasive ductal carcinoma on biopsy.

Ductography (Examination of Milk Ducts)

Ductography is indicated in a patient who presents with a unilateral spontaneous discharge from the nipple that is either bloody or clear and watery. This type of discharge can be associated with a ductal carcinoma that is mammographically occult. More often, nipple discharge is the product of a papilloma within the duct. The ductogram can help the radiologist determine the cause and location of the origin of the discharge by injecting an opaque contrast medium into the duct. These patients can often be biopsied immediately using stereotactic methods with contrast-enhanced ducts (Fig. 18.74).

Equipment and supplies for the examination include a sterile hypodermic syringe (usually 1 to 3 mL); a 30-gauge ductography cannula with a smooth, round tip; a skin cleansing agent; sterile gauze sponges or cotton balls; paper tape; a waste basin; and an organic, water-soluble, iodinated contrast medium.

Fig. 18.74 This 55-year-old patient presented with a spontaneous brown discharge from the left nipple. Ductography was performed for visualization of the ducts. A probable papilloma was noted as an area of lucency *(arrows)* on CC (A) and ML (B) views. This patient was sent for stereotactic core biopsy (C, pre-fire images) where the area was excised. It proved to be a papilloma.

Continued

Fig. 18.74, cont'd

After the nipple is cleaned, a small amount of discharge is expressed to identify the correct ductal opening. The cannula is inserted into the orifice of the duct, and undiluted iothalamate meglumine or iopamidol is gently injected. So that the patient does not experience unnecessary discomfort and extravasation does not occur, the injection is terminated as soon as the patient experiences a sense of fullness, pressure, or pain. The cannula is taped in place before the patient is positioned for the radiographs. If cannulation is unsuccessful, a sterile local anesthetic gel or warm compress may be applied to the nipple and areola, and the procedure is reattempted. If ductography is unsuccessful after several attempts, the procedure may be rescheduled in 7 to 14 days. On successful injection, the following guidelines are observed:

- Immediately obtain radiographs with the patient positioned for the CC and lateral projections of the subareolar region using the magnification technique (see Fig. 18.74A and B). If needed, MLO or rolled CC and rolled MLO magnification projections may be obtained to resolve superimposed ducts.
- Employ the exposure techniques used in general mammography.
- Leave the cannula in the duct to minimize leakage of contrast material during compression and to facilitate reinjection of the contrast medium without the need for recannulation.
- If the cannula is removed for the images, do not apply vigorous compression because this would cause the contrast medium to be expelled.

Localization and Biopsy of Suspicious Lesions

Approximately 80% of nonpalpable lesions identified by mammography are not malignant. Nonetheless, a breast lesion cannot be definitively judged benign until it has been microscopically evaluated. When mammography identifies a nonpalpable lesion that warrants biopsy, the abnormality must be accurately located so that the smallest amount of breast tissue is removed for microscopic evaluation, minimizing trauma to the breast. This technique conserves the maximal amount of normal breast tissue unless extensive surgery is indicated by pathologic findings.

Suspicious breast lesions can be biopsied using three techniques: (1) FNAB, (2) large-core needle biopsy (LCNB), and (3) open surgical biopsy. FNAB uses a hollow small-gauge needle to extract tissue cells from a suspicious lesion. The location of the lesion is identified by the doctor using palpation, ultrasonography, or mammographic or stereotactic guidance. FNAB can potentially decrease the need for surgical excisional biopsy by identifying benign lesions and by diagnosing malignant lesions that require extensive surgery rather than excisional biopsy.

LCNB obtains small samples of breast tissue by means of a larger-gauge (generally sized between 9-gauge and 14-gauge) hollow needle with a trough adjacent to the tip of the needle, using the same localizing techniques. A vacuum suction system is frequently employed during this procedure to pull the target tissue through the trough into a collecting chamber. Once the tissue sample has been obtained, a titanium clip is often placed in the breast through the needle to mark the exact location of the biopsy. This clip can be used by the surgeon to locate the area of concern during an open surgical excision, or to indicate the area of a prior LCNB during subsequent mammography. Because larger tissue samples are obtained with LCNB, and because results are very accurate, clinical support is available for use of this technique instead of surgical excisional biopsy to diagnose pathology of a lesion. LCNB may be used with clinical, ultrasound, stereotactic, and MRI guidance. The method used depends on the preference of the radiologist and the surgeon and is typically determined by the modality with which the lesion is most visible.

When a patient is a candidate for an open surgical biopsy, preoperative localization is used to locate and guide the surgeon to a nonpalpable lesion. Several types of preoperative localization methods are in use today, but all require imaging assistance to tag the nonpalpable area of concern.

The most common method of preoperative localization is needle-wire localization. A long needle containing a hooked guidewire is inserted into the breast to lead the surgeon directly to the lesion. The four most common needle-wire localization systems are the Kopans, Homer (18-gauge), Frank (21-gauge), and Hawkins (20-gauge) biopsy guides. A small incision (1 to 2 mm) at the entry site may be necessary to facilitate insertion of a larger-gauge needle. With each system, a long needle containing a hooked wire is inserted into the breast until the needle's tip is adjacent to the lesion. When the needle and wire are in place, the needle is withdrawn over the wire. The hook on the end of the wire anchors the wire within the breast tissue. Some radiologists also inject a small amount of methylene blue dye to label the proper biopsy site visually. After needle-wire localization, the patient is bandaged and taken to the surgical area for excisional biopsy (Fig. 18.75). The surgeon then cuts along the guidewire and removes the breast tissue around the wire's hooked end. Alternatively, the

surgeon may choose an incision site that intercepts the anchored wire distant from the point of wire entry. Ideally, the radiologist and the surgeon should review the localization images together before the excisional biopsy is performed.

Newer methods of preoperative localization that utilize breast imaging include radioguided occult lesion localization (ROLL), radioactive iodine seed localization (RSL), and SAVI Scout (Cianna Medical) radar localization. The ROLL method involves the injection of a radioisotope into the tissue in the area to be excised. With RSL, a radioactive seed is placed in the tissue through a localizing needle. Both of these methods require the surgeon to locate the tissue to be excised using a gamma probe. Surgical outcomes with this method have been found to be similar to those of wire-guided localizations.[35,36] The SAVI Scout method utilizes radar technology. A reflector is placed into the target tissue by the radiologist up to 30 days prior to surgery using mammographic or ultrasound guidance. The surgeon uses the SCOUT guide, which emits the radar signal, to detect the location of the reflector and target tissue. Real-time audible and visual indicators from the radar console assist the surgeon in accurately locating the reflector and target tissue.[37] This is a newer and nonradioactive method of localization.[38]

Fig. 18.75 Material for breast localization using specialized compression plate: alphanumeric localization compression plate, sterile gloves, topical antiseptic, alcohol wipe, local anesthetic, 5-mL syringe, 25-gauge needle, scalpel blade, sterile gauze, tape, and needle-wire localization system.

BREAST LESION LOCALIZATION WITH A SPECIALIZED COMPRESSION PLATE

Most breast cancers that are surgically removed are nonpalpable lesions that have been found during mammography. Preoperative localization of these lesions is often performed to aid the surgeon in locating the area of concern to ensure excision of the lesion. Most mammography units are adaptable with specialized compression plates with openings that can be positioned over a breast lesion. Through the opening, a specialized localizing needle-wire set can be introduced into the breast. The initial mammogram and a 90-degree lateral projection are usually reviewed together to determine the shortest distance from the skin to the breast lesion. A lesion in the inferior aspect of the breast may be best approached from the medial, lateral, or inferior surface of the breast but not from the superior surface.

Two styles of fenestrated localization compression paddles are currently in use: a rectangular cutout with radiopaque alphanumeric grid markings along at least two adjacent sides, and a device in which the plate may be fenestrated with several rows of holes, each large enough to accommodate insertion of a localization needle (Fig. 18.76). There are proponents for each of the paddles, and the radiologist performing the localization procedure usually decides which one to use. The device with fenestrated holes allows the breast tissue to be more firmly fixed and compressed; this in turn allows the area to be localized, making it more discernible from the surrounding tissue.

Needle-localization procedures vary from radiologist to radiologist. As a result, no standardized procedure is known. The following steps are typically taken:

• Perform preliminary routine full-breast projections to confirm the existence of the lesion (Figs. 18.77 and 18.78). Orthogonal views will be more helpful in visualizing the exact location of the lesion; therefore, the MLO projection may be replaced by a 90-degree lateral projection.

• Obtain informed consent after discussing the following topics with the patient:
  1. Full explanation of the procedure
  2. Full description of potential problems per facility policy: These may include vasovagal reaction, excessive bleeding, allergic reaction to lidocaine, and possible failure of the procedure (failure rate of 0% to 20%).[39–41]
  3. Answers to patient's preliminary questions

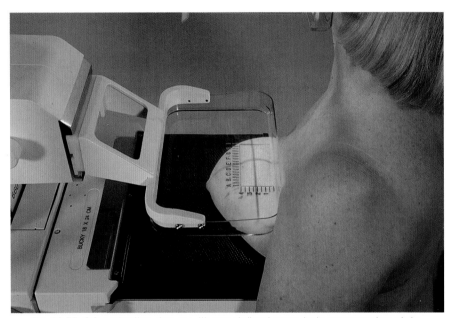

Fig. 18.77 CC projection shown with specialized open-hole compression plate.

Fig. 18.76 Compression plates specifically designed for breast localization procedure.

Fig. 18.78 ML projection shown with specialized open-hole compression plate.

- Position the patient so that the compression plate is against the skin surface closest to the lesion as determined from preliminary images.
- Tell the patient that compression will not be released until the needle has been successfully placed and that the patient is to hold as still as possible.
- Disable the automatic release of the compression paddle.
- Make a preliminary exposure using compression. Ink marks may be placed at the corners of the paddle window or in several of the concentric holes away from the area to be localized to determine whether the patient moves during the procedure.

- Process the image without removing compression. The resultant image shows where the lesion lies in relation to the compression plate openings (Fig. 18.79). If using the circularly fenestrated paddle, count the holes visible on the image to determine the correct entry point of the needle. If using rectangular hole, use the alphanumeric marker system supplied with the paddle to determine the location of the lesion and the needle entry point.
- Clean the skin of the breast over the entry site with a topical antiseptic. Some radiologists may prefer to do this before compression.
- Apply a topical anesthetic if necessary.

- Insert the localizing needle and guidewire into the breast perpendicular to the compression plate and parallel to the chest wall, moving the needle directly toward the underlying lesion. Advance the needle to the estimated depth of the lesion. Because the breast is compressed in the direction of the needle's insertion, it is better to pass beyond the lesion than to be short of the lesion. Do not advance the guidewire into the tissue until the depth of the lesion has been determined by the orthogonal view.
- With the needle in position, make an exposure. Be sure that the shadow of the hub of the needle projects directly over the insertion point of the needle during the exposure to precisely indicate the location of the tip. Slowly release the compression plate, leaving the needle-wire system in place. Obtain an additional projection after the C-arm apparatus has been shifted 90 degrees. (These two orthogonal radiographs are used to determine the position of the end of the needle-wire relative to the depth of the lesion.)
- If the needle is not located adjacent to or within the area of interest, reposition the needle-wire, and repeat the exposures.
- When the needle is accurately placed within the lesion, withdraw the needle, but leave the hooked guidewire in place.
- Place a gauze bandage over the breast.
- Transport the patient to surgery along with the final localization images.

Fig. 18.79 CC and ML projections (A and B) taken to verify area to be excised. Clips from prior core biopsy *(arrows)* indicate correct area for wire localization. These images show that inserting the localization needle from the lateral aspect of the breast uses the closest route, thereby minimizing trauma and scarring from surgery. The breast is positioned in the LM projection using the alphanumeric fenestrated paddle. The needle is inserted, and an image is taken to verify that it has been inserted over the lesion (C). The arrow indicates the hub of the needle. A final image (D) is taken in the CC projection to affirm that the needle passes through the area to be biopsied.

Localization of dermal calcifications

For localization of nonpalpable dermal calcifications, two projections are necessary: (1) a localization projection (which depends on the area of interest) and (2) a TAN projection.

- From the routine CC and MLO projections, determine the quadrant in which the area of interest is located.
- Determine which projection would best localize the area of interest—the CC or 90-degree lateral projection.
- Turn off the automatic compression release, and inform the patient that compression will be continued while the first image is processed.
- Using a localization compression paddle, position the C-arm and breast so that the paddle opening is positioned over the quadrant of interest.
- Slowly apply compression until the breast feels taut.
- Instruct the patient to indicate if the compression becomes uncomfortable.
- When full compression is achieved, move the AEC detector to the appropriate position, and instruct the patient to stop breathing.
- Make the exposure.
- *Do not release compression.* Keep the breast compressed while the initial image is processed.

Tangential projection

- Check the initial image, and locate the area of interest using the alphanumeric identifiers.
- With the patient's breast still under compression, locate the corresponding area on the breast and place a radiopaque marker or BB over the area.
- Release breast compression, and replace the localization compression paddle with a regular or spot compression paddle.
- Rotate the C-arm apparatus until the central ray is directed TAN to the breast at the point identified by the BB marker (the "shadow" of the BB is projected onto the IR surface).
- Compress the area while ensuring that enough breast tissue covers the AEC detector area.
- Slowly apply compression until the breast feels taut.
- Instruct the patient to indicate whether the compression becomes uncomfortable.
- When full compression is achieved, move the AEC detector to the appropriate position, and instruct the patient to stop breathing.
- Make the exposure.
- Release breast compression immediately.

Central ray

- Perpendicular to the area of interest

Structures shown

This projection shows superficial lesions close to the skin surface with minimal parenchymal overlapping. It also shows skin calcifications or palpable lesions projected over subcutaneous fat (see Fig. 18.61).

EVALUATION CRITERIA

The following should be clearly shown:

- Palpable lesion visualized over subcutaneous fat
- TAN radiopaque marker or BB marker accurately correlated with palpable lesion
- Minimal overlapping of adjacent parenchyma
- Calcification in parenchyma or skin
- Uniform tissue exposure if compression is adequate

STEREOTACTIC IMAGING AND BIOPSY PROCEDURES

Stereotactic imaging, or *stereotaxis*, is a method of calculating the exact location of a specific lesion in the breast using mammographic imaging. Stereotaxis uses three-dimensional triangulation to identify the exact location of a breast lesion by taking two *stereo images* 30 degrees apart (Fig. 18.80). Once the lesion has been identified in a perpendicular *scout image*, the x-ray tube is rotated +15 degrees for the first stereo exposure, then −15 for the second. At a computer workstation, the lesion is marked in each stereo image, and a digitizer calculates X, Y, and Z coordinates (Fig. 18.81).

The X, Y, and Z coordinates allow the physician to calculate the exact location of the breast lesion in three dimensions. The X coordinate identifies the transverse location, right to left, or the inferior breast versus the lateral breast. The Y coordinate designates depth, front to back, or anterior versus posterior breast. The Z coordinate identifies the height of the lesion, top to bottom, or superficial to the skin versus the center of the breast (Fig. 18.82). Different stereotactic systems have different methods for calculating a Z value depending on the location of the center reference point. The operator should be familiar with the system in use so that accurate adjustments of the localization device can be made.

Imaging with stereotactic units is available as digital imaging, or DBT. DBT units have the capacity to image two-dimensionally, tomographically, or with a combination of images if needed. The operator can select the type of views within each case that best suits each biopsy. With DBT biopsies, one scout image is taken with tomosynthesis. The multiple tomographic images at varying angles eliminate the need for two additional stereotactic images. The operator finds the slice where the area of interest is best visualized, and that allows the computer to calculate the Z coordinate. DBT biopsies reduce the overall images and the time spent on the biopsy table. This is important as the breast is held in compression throughout the procedure. Any slight movement changes the X, Y, and Z values.

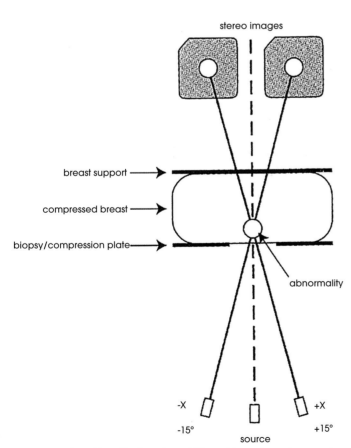

Fig. 18.80 Three-dimensional localization. Acquisition of two planar images from different source positions provides the means for 3D localization.

(Reprinted with permission from Willison KM: Fundamentals of stereotactic breast biopsy. In Fajardo LL, Willison KM, Pizzutello RJ, editors: *A comprehensive approach to stereotactic breast biopsy*, Cambridge, 1996, Blackwell Science, p 14.)

Fig. 18.81 Digitizer calculates and transmits X, Y, and Z coordinates to stage, or "brain," of biopsy system, where biopsy gun is attached. This information is used to determine placement of biopsy needle.

(Courtesy Hologic, Bedford, MA.)

Once the lesion is localized using stereotaxis, three general methods can be used to biopsy a breast lesion. The physician's preference generally determines the procedure that is performed. The lesion can be mapped with hooked guidewire in needle-wire localization for subsequent surgery, or it can be biopsied through FNAB or LCNB. In FNAB, cells are extracted from a suspicious lesion with a thin needle. For LCNBs, core samples of tissue are obtained by means of a larger needle with a trough adjacent to its tip. Samples are then evaluated to determine the benign or malignant nature of the suspicious breast lesion. Given that LCNB using stereotactic imaging is a minor outpatient procedure and the preferred biopsy method, it is discussed in depth in this chapter.

The benefits of *stereotactic core needle biopsy* over open surgical biopsy include less pain, less scarring, shorter recovery time, less patient anxiety, and lower cost. Most women with a mammographic or clinical breast abnormality are candidates for stereotactic core needle biopsy. The only exceptions are patients who cannot cooperate for the procedure, patients with physical limitations prohibiting use of the equipment, patients who have mammographic findings at the limits of perception, and patients with lesions of potentially ambiguous histology.

Stereotactic biopsies are generally quicker and easier to schedule than conventional surgery. This can expedite pathology results, so potential surgical decisions regarding lumpectomy or mastectomy can be made with minimal delay. When operating on the basis of a core biopsy diagnosis of cancer, surgeons are more likely to obtain clean (negative) lumpectomy margins with the first excision. Axillary lymph nodes, which are evaluated to ascertain metastases, are also sampled at the time of the initial surgery. A woman with a known diagnosis of breast cancer may avoid a second operation.

Two types of mammographic equipment are commercially available for stereotactic biopsy procedures: prone biopsy tables and upright add-on devices.

Disadvantages of the upright add-on system include a limited working space, increased potential for patient motion, and greater potential for vasovagal reactions as the patient can watch the biopsy procedure (Fig. 18.83). The dedicated prone system allows the patient to lie face down with the breast hanging pendulous through a hole in the table (Figs. 18.84 and 18.85). This gives the technologists and doctors more work space underneath the raised table, and the procedure is out of sight of the patient. The prone table is more expensive than the add-on system, requires a larger space, and should not be used for conventional mammography. It can be more difficult to locate suspicious lesions close to the chest wall with the prone table versus the upright add-on system. But the success or failure of core needle breast biopsy ultimately depends more on the experience and interest of the diagnostic team, including a radiologist, a mammographer, a pathologist, and a specially trained nurse or technologist, than on the particulars of the system that is used.

Frontal View

Fig. 18.82 Cartesian coordinates. A Cartesian system identifies the location of a unique point by three axes intersecting at right angles.

(Reprinted with permission from Willison KM: Fundamentals of stereotactic breast biopsy. In Fajardo LL, Willison KM, Pizzutello RJ, editors: A comprehensive approach to stereotactic breast biopsy, Cambridge, 1996, Blackwell Science, p 16.)

Fig. 18.83 Upright stereotactic system attached to dedicated mammography unit.

(Courtesy Hologic, Bedford, MA.)

Fig. 18.84 Prone stereotactic biopsy system with digital imaging.

(Courtesy Hologic, Bedford, MA.)

Before beginning the procedure, the physician reviews the initial mammographic images to determine the best approach and projection of the breast to allow for the shortest distance from the surface of the skin to the breast lesion. The biopsy needle should be inserted through the least amount of tissue, limiting the amount of trauma to the breast. A lesion located in the lateral aspect of the UOQ is approached from the lateral aspect, whereas a lesion located in the medial and superior portion of the breast is approached from above. After the best approach to the lesion has been determined, the affected breast is positioned and compressed with an open compression paddle for a scout image to localize the breast lesion. Once the breast lesion has been localized, stereo images are taken to triangulate the lesion and measure its X, Y, and Z coordinates (Fig. 18.86).

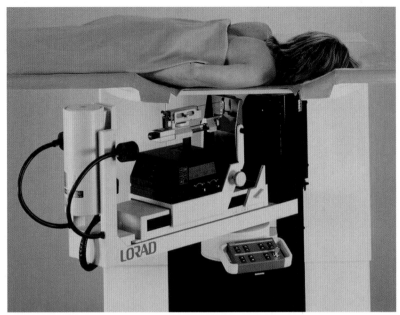

Fig. 18.85 Open aperture in table for prone biopsy system allows breast to be positioned beneath table.

(Courtesy Trex Medical Corp., LORAD Division, Danbury, CT.)

Fig. 18.86 Stereo images showing three-dimensional view of breast lesion before intervention.

At the computer workstation, the physician reads the two side-by-side stereotactic images and identifies the center of the lesion on each image. Or with a DBT biopsy, the physician uses the one scout image to locate and mark the lesion. The computer is then used to calculate the exact X, Y, and Z coordinates. At this point the physician must determine whether the Z value, or depth of the lesion, is within range for the biopsy. If the lesion is very deep within the breast with a high Z value, it may be appropriate to change the approach and positioning of the breast to minimize trauma. If the Z value is too low, the lesion is very shallow and close to the surface of the skin; there may not be enough breast tissue to cover the trough and tip of the biopsy needle. In this case, another approach would be justified. Once an appropriate Z value is found, the physician transmits the coordinates from the computer workstation to the biopsy table stage (Fig. 18.87).

At the biopsy table, the breast is aseptically cleansed to minimize infection, and the skin is anesthetized at the area where the biopsy needle enters. The physician can effectively manage the pain associated with the procedure by anesthetizing the tissue within the breast at the biopsy site. The biopsy needle is then placed on the *stage*, which holds it in place and interprets the coordinates sent by the computer. Next, the tip of the needle must be *zeroed* by aligning it with the center reference point. The needle is then moved into position within the opening of the compression plate based on the appropriate X and Y values sent from the workstation. A small incision is made with a scalpel to facilitate entry of the needle into the breast and proper positioning of the Z axis. Before the needle enters the lesion at the exact Z axis, the needle is "dialed back," and "pre-fire" images are obtained with stereotaxis to ensure proper positioning (Fig. 18.88).

After the pre-fire images verify the needle's tip adjacent to the lesion, the needle is fired into the lesion quickly to penetrate the tissue without pushing it deeper within the breast. With vacuum-assisted core biopsies, the probe is fired with the use of air pressure. Or the physician may use a spring-loaded biopsy device to power the needle back and forth through the target. Once the first pass is made, stereotactic "post-fire" images confirm correct needle placement. These images determine the course of subsequent passes. Redigitization (use of a digitizer to repeat the steps needed to calculate the new triangulation coordinates) can be performed to obtain additional samples. Alternatively, the physician can estimate where to move the biopsy needle based on the initial needle location within the breast.

After post-fire images are acquired, vacuum-assisted biopsies gently aspirate the tissue through a trough in a rotating cutter into the probe's aperture and collected in a basket. With the probe in the center of the lesion, the cutter can be spun in a circle to move the trough and collect samples from every direction without multiple insertions. When the biopsy is complete, the cutter is removed, and a radiopaque clip can be deployed through the probe and into the biopsy site to mark the area for future reference.

Fig. 18.87 Stage of biopsy system supports biopsy gun. X, Y, and Z coordinates are displayed.

Fig. 18.88 Pre-fire stereo images showing placement of the biopsy needle adjacent to calcium to be biopsied.

If a multi-fire, spring-loaded biopsy device is used, the sheath, or needle cover, slides over the trough of the needle. The sheath cuts the tissue sample within the trough and holds the sample in place while the needle is removed from the breast. The sheath is then pulled back exposing the tissue for collection. Subsequent passes can then be made for additional sampling. This method requires the clip marker to be placed within the breast separately.

Radiopaque clips are placed following most LCNBs. The titanium clip serves as a marker, allowing radiologists to know the location of past biopsies for subsequent mammograms or for surgical guidance. Immediately after the clip is seeded, "post-clip" images are obtained to ensure proper deployment and placement (Fig. 18.89). After this is done, the patient is released from compression and is given follow-up care.

With each technique, a minimum of 5 to a maximum of 20 tissue samples are obtained to ensure proper sampling of the abnormality. For vacuum-assisted biopsies, a larger amount of tissue sample is obtained; this has been reported to improve accuracy in diagnosing atypical ductal hyperplasia (ADH) and DCIS lesions.[42] If the abnormality contains radiopaque calcium, the radiologist may choose to x-ray the sample to guarantee the presence of calcium for accurate diagnosis. Following this image, the tissue samples are transferred into a formalin specimen container for transportation to the pathology laboratory.

After the LCNB procedure is completed, the breast is cleaned and bandaged using sterile technique. Compression to the biopsy site is necessary to prevent excessive bleeding, and a cold compress is applied to minimize discomfort and swelling of related tissues. The patient should limit strenuous activity and keep the affected breast immobilized for at least 8 hours to prevent future bleeding or excessive bruising. The patient may be asked to return within 24 to 48 hours, so the breast can be examined to ensure that no bleeding or infection has occurred. The physician who performed the biopsy discusses the biopsy results and subsequent treatment options, if applicable, with the patient.

Fig. 18.89 Post-biopsy images in standard CC and lateral projections to document accuracy of biopsy site and marker clip placement.

Breast Specimen Radiography

When open surgical biopsy is performed, the suspected lesion must be contained in its entirety in the tissue removed during the biopsy. Very small lesions that are characterized by tissue irregularity or microcalcifications on a mammographic image and that are nonpalpable in the excised specimen may be undetectable on visual inspection; a radiographic image of the biopsied tissue may be necessary to determine that the entire lesion has been removed. Compression of the specimen is necessary to identify lesions, especially lesions that do not contain calcifications. Magnification imaging is used to better visualize microcalcifications. Specimen radiography is often performed as an immediate postexcision procedure while the patient is still under anesthesia. Speed is essential.

The procedure for handling the specimen must be established before the procedure is started. Cooperation among radiologist, mammographer, surgeon, and pathologist is imperative. Together, a system of identifying the orientation of the tissue sample to the patient's breast (anterior, posterior, medial, or lateral aspect of the sample) can be applied to help the clinician confirm that the lesion has been completely removed.[43]

The specimen may be imaged using the magnification technique, with or without compression, as ordained by the policy of the facility. As patient radiation exposure and patient motion are no longer factors, imaging for high resolution, regardless of dose, is appropriate. Exposure factors depend on the thickness of the specimen and the imaging modality that is used (Fig. 18.90). Alternatively, radiographic equipment is manufactured specifically for imaging tissue specimens. These units are self-contained, are often portable, and allow specimens to be imaged directly in the operating suite. Digital technology allows the image to be seen by the surgeon and the radiologist and the pathologist in remote locations, almost immediately and simultaneously.[44,45]

The pathologist often uses the specimen radiograph to precisely locate the area of concern, so a copy of the image should be sent with the specimen. The next step is to match the actual specimen to the specimen radiograph before the specimen is dissected. Marking the area of concern within the specimen by placing a radiopaque object, such as a 1- or 2-inch (2.5- or 5-cm) needle, directly at the area of concern helps the pathologist locate the abnormality more accurately.

Specimens of tissue from LCNBs are frequently radiographed, particularly when the biopsy is performed for calcifications. Radiographing tissue specimens can confirm that the area of interest has been sampled and is included within the tissue sent for examination by the pathologist (Fig. 18.91).

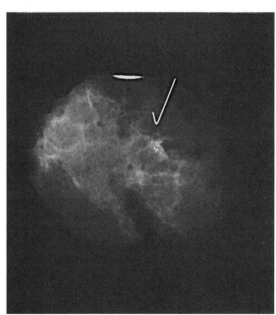

Fig. 18.90 Radiograph of surgical specimen containing suspicious microcalcifications.

Fig. 18.91 Magnified radiograph of specimen obtained from core biopsy shown in Figs. 18.86–18.89. Note calcium indicating successful biopsy.

Breast Magnetic Resonance Imaging

Breast MRI has proved most useful in patients with proven breast cancer or at high risk for breast cancer, to assess for multifocal or multicentric disease, chest wall involvement, chemotherapy response, or tumor recurrence, or to identify the primary site in patients with occult breast disease.[46]

INDICATIONS

Assessment of extent of disease and residual disease

MRI can be helpful for patients who have had a lumpectomy and have positive margins and no evidence of residual disease on conventional imaging (mammography, ultrasound). Postoperative mammography can help detect residual calcifications but is limited for residual mass. MRI is very sensitive for detection of residual mass and identifies other potentially suspicious sites seen only on MRI.

Assessment of tumor recurrence

Assessment of tumor recurrence on MRI can be very complicated because scars can become enhanced for 1 to 2 years after surgery. Suggestion of recurrence can be made by MRI, yet the cost of the procedure should be weighed against a less expensive needle biopsy of the area.

Occult primary breast cancer

Patients with axillary metastases suspicious for primary breast cancer with a negative physical examination, mammogram, and ultrasound are good candidates for MRI because of its high sensitivity for invasive cancers. MRI has been shown to detect 90% to 100% of cancers if tumor is present in the breast. If the primary site is detected, the patient may be spared a mastectomy, and MRI can influence patient surgical management.

Neoadjuvant chemotherapy response

In patients with advanced breast cancer, MRI may be used to predict earlier which patients are responding to chemotherapy. Mammography and physical examination can sometimes be limited by fibrosis. Studies suggest that MRI may be better for assessing patients' response to treatment.[47–49]

High-risk screening

Breast MRI is recommended as an annual screening examination for patients at high risk for developing breast cancer.[18] These include women

1. Who have a first-degree relative (parent, sibling, child) with a *BRCA1* or *BRCA2* mutation, even if they have yet to be tested themselves.
2. Whose lifetime risk of breast cancer has been scored at 20% to 25% or greater, based on one of several accepted risk assessment tools that look at family history and other factors.
3. Who have received radiation to the chest between 10 and 30 years of age.
4. Who have Li-Fraumeni syndrome, Cowden syndrome, or Bannayan-Riley-Ruvalcaba syndrome, or who may have one of these syndromes based on history in a first-degree relative.

A study published in the *New England Journal of Medicine* concluded that MRI is "more sensitive than mammography in detecting tumors in women with an inherited susceptibility of breast cancer."[50]

Breast MRI is recommended for women at high risk to be used as an adjunct to mammography. The most beneficial method for screening is to schedule 6-month intervals alternating MRI with mammography. Women who are found to have MRI-detected foci suspicious of cancer need to have these verified by biopsy. Often these areas are reexamined with mammography and directed ultrasound for potential biopsy. If these lesions are not found by conventional imaging, confirmation with MRI-guided biopsy would be necessary before the patient is committed to potential lumpectomy or mastectomy or both.

Thermography and Diaphanography

Beginning in the 1950s, thermography and diaphanography were actively investigated in the hope that breast cancer and other abnormalities could be diagnosed using nonionizing forms of radiation. These two diagnostic tools are seldom used today.

Thermography is the photographic recording of the infrared radiation emanating from a patient's body surface. The resulting thermogram shows areas of increased temperature, with a temperature increase often suggesting increased metabolism. (More complete information on this technique is provided in the fourth through eighth editions of this atlas.)

Diaphanography is an examination in which a body part is transilluminated using selected light wavelengths and special imaging equipment. With this technique, the interior of the breast is inspected using light directed through its exterior wall. The light exiting the patient's body is recorded and interpreted. Rapid advances in mammography have essentially eliminated the use of this technique for evaluating breast disease. (More complete information on diaphanography is given in this chapter in the fourth through eighth editions of this atlas.)

Conclusion

Radiographic examination of the breast is a technically demanding procedure. Success depends in large part on the skills of the mammographer—more so than in most other areas of radiology. In addition to skill, the mammographer must have a strong desire to perform high-quality mammography and must be willing to work with the patient to allay qualms and to obtain cooperation. In the course of taking the patient's history and physically assessing and radiographing the breasts, the mammographer may be asked questions about breast disease, BSE, screening guidelines, and breast radiography that the patient has been reluctant to ask other health care professionals. The knowledge, skill, and attitude of the mammographer may be lifesaving for the patient. Although most patients do not have significant breast disease when first examined, statistics show that approximately 12% of patients develop breast cancer at some time during their lifetime. An early positive mammography encounter may make the patient more willing to undergo mammography in the future. When properly performed, breast radiography is safe, and presently, it offers the best hope for significantly reducing the mortality of breast cancer.

References

1. American Cancer Society. *Cancer facts and figures*. Atlanta; 2017, 10.
2. American Cancer Society. *Cancer facts and figures*. Atlanta; 2013, 9.
3. Thomas AMK, Banerjee AK, Busch U. *Classic papers in modern diagnostic radiology*. Berlin: Springer; 2005:540.
4. U.S. Food and Drug Administration. *MQSA Scorecard Statistics*. FDA MQSA National Statistics; 2017. www.fda.gov. (Accessed June 20, 2017).
5. Bassett L. Clinical image evaluation. *Radiol Clin North Am*. 1995;33:1027.
6. Barkhausen J, Achim R, Schaefer F. *Digital Breast Tomosynthesis*. Stuttgart, Germany: Thieme; 2016.
7. Peppard HR, Nicholoson BE, Rochman CM, et al. Digital breast tomosynthesis in the diagnostic setting. indications and clinical applications. *Radiographics*. 2015;35(4):975–990. https://doi.org/10.1148/rg.2015140204.
8. Zuley ML, Guo B, Catullo VJ, et al. Comparison of two-dimensional synthesized mammograms versus original digital mammograms alone and in combination with tomosynthesis images. *Radiology*. 2015;276(1):65–72. https://doi.org/10.1148/radiol.15142009.
9. Friedewald SM, Rafferty EA, Rosa SL, et al. Breast cancer screening using tomosynthesis in combination with digital mammography. *JAMA*. 2014;311(24):2499–2507. https://doi.org/10.1001/jama.2014.6095.
10. Kopans DB. Double-reading. *Radiol Clin North Am*. 2000;38:719.
11. Destounis SV, et al. Can computer-aided detection with double reading of screening mammograms help decrease the false-negative rate? Initial experience. *Radiology*. 2004;232:578.
12. Fenton JJ, Xing G, Elmore JG, et al. Short-term outcomes of screening mammography using computer-aided detection: a population-based study of medicare enrollees. *Ann Intern Med*. 2013;158:580–587.
13. American Cancer Society. *Cancer facts and figures*. Atlanta; 2017, 12.
14. American Cancer Society. *Cancer facts and figures*. Atlanta; 2017, 11.
15. Feig SA. Adverse effects of screening mammography. *Radiol Clin North Am*. 2004;42:807–819.
16. Campeau P, Foulkes WD, Tischkowitz MD. Hereditary breast cancer: new genetic developments, new therapeutic avenues. *Hum Genet*. 2008;124(1):31–42.
17. Amir E, Freedman OC, Seruga B, et al. Assessing women at high risk of breast cancer: a review of risk assessment models. *J Natl Cancer Inst*. 2010;102(10):680–691.
18. American Cancer Society. *Cancer facts and figures*. Atlanta; 2017.
19. American College of Radiology (ACR). ACR BI-RADS-mammography 2013. In: *ACR breast imaging reporting and data system, breast imaging atlas*. ed 5. Reston, VA: American College of Radiology; 2013.
20. Bassett L, Heinlein R. Good positioning key to imaging of breast. *Diagn Imaging*. 1993;9:69.
21. Shaw de Paredes E. *Atlas of mammography*. ed 3. Lippincott Williams & Wilkins; 2007:6.
22. McIntosh SA, Horgan K. Augmentation mammoplasty: effect on diagnosis of breast cancer. *J Plastic Reconstr Aesthet Surg*. 2008;61:124.
23. Stoblen F, et al. Imaging in patients with breast implants: results of the first international breast (implant) conference 2009. *Insights Imaging*. 2010;1:93.
24. Kleimeyer AE, Mahoney MC. MRI for breast implant evaluation. In: Molleran VM, Mahoney MC, eds. *Breast MRI*. Philadelphia: Elsevier; 2014:140–151.
25. Orel SG. MR imaging of the breast. *Radiol Clin North Am*. 2000;38:899.
26. American Cancer Society. *Cancer facts and figures*. Atlanta; 2017:37.
27. Weiss JR, et al. Epidemiology of male breast cancer. *Cancer Epidemiol Biomarkers Prev*. 2005;14:20.
28. Ruddy KJ, Winer EP. Male breast cancer: risk factors, biology, diagnosis, treatment and survivorship. *Ann Oncol*. 2013;24:1434–1443.
29. Fields EC, DeWitt P, Fisher CM, et al. Management of male breast cancer in the United States: a surveillance, epidemiology and end results analysis. *Int J Radiat Oncol Biol Phys*. 2013;87(4):747. https://doi.org/10.1016/j.ijrobp.2013.07.016.
30. Camus C, et al. Ductal carcinoma in situ of the male breast. *Cancer*. 1994;74:1289.
31. Hill T, et al. Comparison of male and female breast cancer incidence trend, tumor characteristics, and survival. *Ann Epidemiol*. 2005;15:773.
32. Eklund GW, Cardenosa G. The art of mammographic positioning. *Radiol Clin North Am*. 1992;30:21.
33. Kim HH, et al. Comparison of calcification specificity in digital mammography using soft-copy display versus screen-film mammography. *AJR Am J Roentgenol*. 2006;187:47.
34. Andolina V. *Lille S: Mammographic imaging, a practical guide*. ed 3. Philadelphia: Wolters Kluwer/Lippincott Williams & Wilkins; 2011:236–237.
35. Nadeem R, Chagla LS, Harris O, et al. Occult breast lesions: A comparison between radioguided occult lesion localisation (ROLL) vs. wire-guided lumpectomy (WGL). *Breast*. 2005;14(4):283–289.
36. Duarte C, Bastidas F, de los Reyes A, et al. Randomized controlled clinical trial comparing radioguided occult lesion localization with wire-guided lesion localization to evaluate their efficacy and accuracy in the localization of nonpalpable breast lesions. *Surgery*. 2016;159(4):1140–1145.
37. Kalambo M, Parikh JR. Implementing the SAVI SCOUT system in community radiology practice. *J Am Coll Radiol*. 2017;14(9):1234–1238.
38. Mango V, Ha R, Gomberwalla A, et al. Evaluation of the SAVI SCOUT surgical guidance system for localization and excision of nonpalpable breast lesions: a feasibility study. *AJR Am J Roentgenol*. 2016;207(4):W69–W72.
39. Jackman RJ, Marzoni Jr FA. Needle-localized breast biopsy: why do we fail? *Radiology*. 1997;204(3):677.
40. Abrahamson PE, et al. Factors predicting successful needle-localized breast biopsy. *Acad Radiol*. 2003;10(6):601.
41. Kouskos E, et al. Wire localisation biopsy of non-palpable breast lesions: reasons for unsuccessful excision. *Eur J Gynaecol Oncol*. 2006;27(3):262.
42. Dershaw DD. Equipment, technique, quality assurance, and accreditation for image-guided breast biopsy procedures. *Radiol Clin North Am*. 2000;38:773.
43. Britton SE, et al. Breast surgical specimen radiographs: how reliable are they? *Eur J Radiol*. 2011;79:245.
44. Kim SH, et al. An evaluation of intraoperative digital specimen mammography versus conventional specimen radiography for the excision of nonpalpable breast lesions. *Am J Surg*. 2013;S0002-9610(13).00081-0.
45. Layfield DM, et al. The effect of introducing an in-theatre intra-operative specimen radiography (IOSR) system on the management of palpable breast cancer within a single unit. *The Breast*. 2012;21:459.
46. American College of Radiology. *ACR practice parameter for the performance of contrast enhanced magnetic resonance imaging (MRI) of the breast*. Revised 2013.
47. Yeh E, Slanetz P, Kopans DB, et al. Prospective comparison of mammography, sonography, and MRI in patients undergoing neoadjuvant chemotherapy for palpable breast cancer. *AJR Am J Roentgenol*. 2005;184(3):868–877.
48. Chen JH, Bahri S, Mehta R, et al. Breast cancer: evaluation of response to neoadjuvant chemotherapy with 3.0-t MR imaging. *Radiology*. 2011;261(3):735–743.
49. Loo CE, Rigter LS, Pengel KE, et al. Survival is associated with complete response

on MRI after neoadjuvant chemotherapy in ER-positive HER2-negative breast cancer. *Breast Cancer Res.* 2016;18(1):82.

50. Kriege M, Brekelmans CT, Boetes C, et al. Efficacy of MRI and mammography for breast-cancer screening in women with a familial or genetic predisposition. *N Engl J Med.* 2004;351(5):427–437.

Suggested readings

American Cancer Society. *Cancer facts and figures.* Atlanta; 2017.

Andolina V. *Lille S: Mammographic imaging: a practical guide.* ed 3. Philadelphia: Lippincott, Williams & Wilkins; 2011.

Appelbaum AH, Evans GF, Levy KR, et al. Mammographic appearance of male breast disease. *Radiographics.* 2001;19:559–568.

Bassett L. Imaging of breast masses. *Radiol Clin North Am.* 2000;38:669–691.

Bassett L, et al., ed. *Quality determinants of mammography.* AHCPR pub No 95-0632. Rockville, MD: U.S. Department of Health and Human Services; 1994.

Burbank F. Stereotactic breast biopsy of atypical hyperplasia and ductal carcinoma in situ lesions: improved accuracy with directional, vacuum-assisted biopsy. *Radiology.* 1997;202:843–847.

Carr JJ, Hemler PF, Halford PW, et al. Stereotactic localization of breast lesions: how it works and methods to improve accuracy. *Radiographics.* 2001;21:463–473.

Dershaw DD. Equipment, technique, quality assurance, and accreditation for image-guided breast biopsy procedures. *Radiol Clin North Am.* 2000;38:773–789.

Digital mammography quality control manual. rev ed. Chicago: American College of Radiology; 2016.

Eklund GW, Busby RC, Miller SH, et al. Improved imaging of the augmented breast. *AJR Am J Roentgenol.* 1988;151:469–473.

Eklund GW, Cardenosa G. The art of mammographic positioning. *Radiol Clin North Am.* 1992;30:21–53.

F-D-C Reports, Inc: ImageChecker unanimously endorsed by radiology panel. Medical devices, diagnostics, and instrumentation: "the gray sheet," 24:20.

Feig SA. Breast masses: mammographic and sonographic evaluation. *Radiol Clin North Am.* 1992;30:67–92.

Fields EC, DeWitt P, Fisher CM, et al. Management of male breast cancer in the United States: a surveillance, epidemiology and end results analysis. *Int J Radiat Oncol Biol Phys.* 2013;87(4):747–752.

Healy B. BRCA genes: bookmarking, fortunetelling, and medical care. *N Engl J Med.* 1997;336:1448–1449. editorial.

Henderson IC. Breast cancer. In: Murphy GP, Lawrence WL, Lenhard RE, eds. *Clinical oncology.* Atlanta: American Cancer Society; 1997.

Jackson VP. The status of mammographically guided fine needle aspiration biopsy of nonpalpable breast lesions. *Radiol Clin North Am.* 1992;30:155–166.

Kopans DB. Double reading. *Radiol Clin North Am.* 2000;38:719–724.

Krainer M, Silva-Arrieta S, FitzGerald MG, et al. Differential contributions of BRCA1 and BRCA2 to early-onset breast cancer. *N Engl J Med.* 1997;336:1416–1421.

Liberman L. Clinical management issues in percutaneous core breast biopsy. *Radiol Clin North Am.* 2000;38:791–807.

Logan-Young W, Dawson AE, Wilbur DC, et al. The cost effectiveness of fine-needle aspiration cytology and 14-gauge core needle biopsy compared with open surgical biopsy in the diagnosis of breast cancer. *Cancer.* 1998;82:1867–1873.

National Cancer Institute. Available at: https://www.cancer.gov/ (Accessed September 2018).

Nishikawa RM, Doi K, Giger ML, et al. Computerized detection of clustered microcalcifications: evaluation of performance on mammograms from multiple centers. *Radiographics.* 1995;15:443–452.

Orel SG. MR imaging of the breast. *Radiol Clin North Am.* 2000;38:899–913.

Parker SH, Burbank F. A practical approach to minimally invasive breast biopsy. *Radiology.* 1996;200:11–20.

Parker SH, Burbank F, Jackman RJ, et al. Percutaneous large-core breast biopsy: a multi-institutional study. *Radiology.* 1994;193:359–364.

Prechtel K, Pretchel V. Breast carcinoma in the man: current results from the viewpoint of clinic and pathology. *Pathologe.* 1997;18:45–52.

Rozenberg S, Liebens F, Kroll M, et al. Principal cancers among women: breast, lung, and colorectal. *Int J Fertil Menopausal Stud.* 1996;41:166–171.

Ruddy KJ, Winer EP. Male breast cancer: risk factors, biology, diagnosis, treatment and survivorship. *Ann Oncol.* 2013;24:1434–1443.

Schmidt R, et al. Computer-aided diagnosis in mammography. In: *RSNA categorical course in breast imaging* [syllabus]. Oak Park, IL: RSNA; 1995.

Skolnick AA. Ultrasound may help detect breast implant leaks. *JAMA.* 1992;267:786.

Slawson SH, Johnson BA. Ductography: how to and what if? *Radiographics.* 2001;21:133–150.

Vyborny CJ, Giger ML, Nishikawa RM. Computer-aided detection and computer-aided diagnosis of breast cancer. *Radiol Clin North Am.* 2000;38:725–740.

19

BONE DENSITOMETRY

SHARON R. WARTENBEE

Principles of Bone Densitometry

Bone densitometry[a] is a general term that encompasses the art and science of measuring the *bone mineral content* (BMC) and *bone mineral density* (BMD) of specific skeletal sites or the whole body. The bone measurement values are used to assess bone strength, diagnose diseases associated with low bone density (especially *osteoporosis*), monitor the effects of therapy for such diseases, and predict risk of future fractures.

Several techniques are available to perform bone densitometry using ionizing radiation or ultrasound. The most versatile and widely used is *dual energy x-ray absorptiometry* (DXA) (Fig. 19.1).[1] This procedure has the advantages of low radiation dose, wide availability, ease of use, short scan time, high-resolution images, good *precision,* and stable calibration. DXA is the focus of this chapter, but summaries of other procedures are also presented.

---

[a] Almost all italicized words on the succeeding pages are defined at the end of this chapter.

A

B

C

Fig. 19.1 (A) Hologic model, Horizon. (B) GE Lunar model, Prodigy. (C) Norland model, XR-46.

(A, Courtesy Hologic, Inc, Bedford, MA; B, courtesy GE Lunar Corp, Madison, WI; C, courtesy Norland/Swissray Inc, Ft. Atkinson, WI.)

DUAL ENERGY X-RAY ABSORPTIOMETRY AND CONVENTIONAL RADIOGRAPHY

The differences between DXA and conventional radiography are as follows:

1. DXA can be conceptualized as a *subtraction technique.* To quantitate BMD, it is necessary to eliminate the contributions of soft tissue and measure the x-ray attenuation of bone alone. This is achieved by scanning two x-rays at different photon energies (hence the term *dual energy x-ray*) and mathematically manipulating the recorded signal to take advantage of the differing attenuation properties of soft tissue and bone at the two energies. The density of the isolated bone is calculated on the basis of the principle that dense, more mineralized bone attenuates (absorbs) more x-ray. Adequate amounts of artifact-free soft tissue are essential to help ensure the reliability of the bone density results.

2. The bone density results are computed by proprietary software from the x-ray attenuation pattern striking the detector, not from the scan image. Scanned images are only for the purpose of confirming correct positioning of the patient and correct placement of the *regions of interest* (ROI). The images may not be used for diagnosis, and any apparent medical conditions must be followed up by appropriate diagnostic tests.

3. In conventional radiography, x-ray machines from different manufacturers are operated in essentially the same manner and produce identical images. This is not the case with DXA. Three DXA manufacturers are in the United States (see Fig. 19.1), and technologists must be educated about the specific scanner model in their facility. The numeric bone density results cannot be compared among manufacturers. This chapter presents general scan positioning and analysis information, but the manufacturers' specific procedures must be used when actual scans are performed and analyzed.

4. The effective radiation dose for DXA is considerably lower than the effective radiation dose for conventional radiography. The specific personnel requirements vary among states and countries. All bone density technologists should be instructed in core competencies, including radiation protection, patient care, history taking, basic computer operations, knowledge of scanner quality control, patient positioning, scan acquisition and analysis, and proper record keeping and documentation.

History of Bone Densitometry

Osteoporosis was an undetected and overlooked disease until the 1920s, when the advent of x-ray film methods allowed the detection of markedly decreased bone densities. The first publications indicating an interest in *bone mass* quantification methods appeared in the 1930s, and much of the pioneering work was performed in the field of dentistry. *Radiographic absorptiometry* involved taking a radiograph of bone with a known standard, placing it in the ROI, and optically comparing the densities.

Radiogrammetry was introduced in the 1960s, partly in response to the measurements of bone loss performed in astronauts. As bone loss progresses, the thickness of the outer shell of phalanges and metacarpals decreases while the inner cavity enlarges. Indices of bone loss are established by measuring and comparing the inner and outer diameters.

In the late 1970s the emerging technique of computed tomography (CT) (see Chapter 25) was adapted, through the use of specialized software and reference phantoms, enabling quantitative measurement of the central area of the vertebral body, where early bone loss occurs. This technique, called *quantitative computed tomography* (QCT), is still used.

The first scanners dedicated to bone densitometry appeared in the 1970s and early 1980s. *Single photon absorptiometry* (SPA) (Fig. 19.2) and *dual photon absorptiometry* (DPA) are based on physical principles similar to those for DXA. The SPA approach was not a subtraction technique but relied on a water bath or other medium to eliminate the effects of soft tissue. SPA found application only in the peripheral skeleton. DPA used photons of two energies and was used to assess sites in the central skeleton (lumbar spine and proximal femur). The radiation source was a highly collimated beam from a radioisotope (iodine-125 [^{125}I] for SPA and gadolinium-153 [^{153}Gd] for DPA). The intensity of the attenuated beam was measured by a collimated *scintillation counter,* and the bone mineral was quantified.

The first commercial DXA scanner was introduced in 1987. In this scanner, the expensive, rare, and short-lived radioisotope source was replaced with an x-ray tube. Improvements over time have included the choice of *pencil-beam* or *array-beam collimation*; a rotating C-arm to allow supine lateral spine imaging; shorter scan time; improved detection of low bone density; improved image quality; and enhanced computer power, multimedia, and networking capabilities.

Since the late 1990s, renewed attention has been given to smaller, more portable, less complex techniques for measuring the peripheral skeleton. This trend has been driven by the introduction of new therapies for osteoporosis and the resultant need for simple, inexpensive screening tests to identify persons with osteoporosis who are at increased risk for fracture. However, DXA of the hip and spine is still the most widely accepted method for measuring bone density, and it remains a superior procedure for monitoring the effects of therapy.

Fig. 19.2 SPA wrist scan being performed on a Lunar model, SP2. This form of bone densitometry is obsolete.

(Courtesy GE Lunar Corp, Madison, WI.)

Bone Biology and Remodeling

The skeleton serves the following purposes:

- Supports the body and protects vital organs
- Manufactures red blood cells
- Stores minerals that are necessary for life, including calcium and phosphate

The two basic types of bone are *cortical* (or compact) and *trabecular* (or cancellous). Cortical bone forms the dense, compact outer shell of all bones, and the shafts of the long bones. It supports weight, resists bending and twisting, and accounts for approximately 80% of the skeletal mass. Trabecular bone is the delicate, latticework structure within bones that adds strength without excessive weight. It supports compressive loading in the spine, hip, and calcaneus, and it is also found at the ends of long bones, such as the distal radius. The relative amounts of trabecular and cortical bone differ by bone densitometric technique used and anatomic site measured (Table 19.1).

Bone is constantly going through a remodeling process in which old bone is replaced with new bone. With this *bone remodeling* process (Fig. 19.3), the equivalent of a new skeleton is formed approximately every 7 years. Bone-destroying cells called *osteoclasts* break down and remove old bone, leaving pits. This part of the process is called *resorption,* whereas bone-building cells called *osteoblasts* fill the pits with new bone. This process is called *formation.* The comparative rates of resorption and formation determine whether bone mass increases (more formation than resorption), remains stable (equal resorption and formation), or decreases (more resorption than formation).

Osteoclasts and osteoblasts operate as a bone-remodeling unit. A properly functioning bone remodeling cycle is a tightly coupled physiologic process in which resorption equals formation, and the net bone mass is maintained. The length of the resorption process is approximately 1 week compared with a longer formation process of approximately 3 months. At any point in time, millions of remodeling sites within the body are in different phases of the remodeling cycle or at rest.

TABLE 19.1

Bone densitometry regions of interest: estimated percentage of trabecular and cortical bone and preferred measurement sites

Region of interest	Trabecular bone (%)	Cortical bone (%)	Preferred measurement site
PA spine (by DXA)	66	34	Cushing disease, corticosteroid use
PA spine (by QCT)	100		
Femoral neck	25	75	Type II osteoporosis Second choice for hyperparathyroidism
Trochanteric region	50	50	
Calcaneus	95	5	
33% radius	1	99	First choice for hyperparathyroidism
Ultradistal radius	66	34	
Phalanges	40	60	
Whole body	20	80	Pediatrics

Data from Bonnick SL. *Bone Densitometry in Clinical Practice: Application and Interpretation.* Totowa, NJ: Humana Press; 1998.

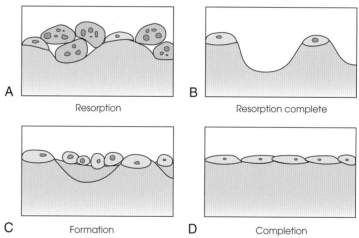

Fig. 19.3 Bone remodeling process. (A) Osteoclasts break down bone in the process of resorption. (B) Pits in the bone. (C) Osteoblasts form new bone. (D) With equal amounts of resorption and formation, the bone mass is stable.

(From National Osteoporosis Foundation. *Boning up on osteoporosis.* Washington, DC: National Osteoporosis Foundation; 1997.)

Fig. 19.4 Osteoporotic vertebral body *(right)* shortened by compression fractures, compared with a normal vertebral body. The osteoporotic vertebra exhibits a characteristic loss of horizontal trabeculae and thickened vertical trabeculae.

(From Kumar V, Abbas AK, Aster JC, Cotran RS, Robbins SL. *Robbins and Cotran pathologic basis of disease.* 8th ed. Philadelphia: Saunders/Elsevier; 2010.)

When the cycle becomes uncoupled, the result is a net loss of bone mass. Some reasons for uncoupling include enhanced osteoclastic recruitment, impaired osteoblastic activity, and increased number of cycles which results in a shorter time for each cycle. The increased number of cycles favors the shorter resorption phase over the longer formation phase.

Bone mass increases in youths until *peak bone mass* is reached at approximately 20 to 30 years of age. This is followed by a stable period in middle age. A period of decreasing bone mass starts at approximately age 50 in women and approximately age 65 in men. The decrease in bone mass becomes pronounced in women at menopause because of the loss of bone-preserving estrogen. If the peak bone mass is low or the resorption rate is excessive, or both, at menopause, osteoporosis may result (Fig. 19.4).

Osteoporosis

Osteoporosis is a disease characterized by low bone mass and structural deterioration of bone tissue. This decrease in bone mass and degradation of bone architecture may not support the mechanical stress and loading of normal activity. As a result, the bones are at increased risk for *fragility fractures.* In 2014, the National Osteoporosis Foundation (NOF) released an estimate that stated 54 million adults over the age of 50 were affected by osteoporosis or low bone mass. With current trends, the NOF expects this number to grow to 71.2 million by the year 2030. Persons with osteoporosis may experience decreased life quality due to the pain, deformity, and disability of fragility fractures. An increased risk of morbidity and mortality exists, especially from hip fractures.

Many risk factors for osteoporosis have been identified and studied. The following are considered primary risk factors:
- Female gender
- Increased age
- Estrogen deficiency
- Caucasian race
- Low body weight (<127 lb [<58 kg]), low body mass index (BMI) (weight in kilograms divided by height in meters squared), or both
- Family history of osteoporosis or fracture
- History of prior fracture as an adult
- Smoking tobacco

Osteoporosis is often overlooked in older men because it is considered a woman's disease. However, the NOF found that 2 million American men have osteoporosis, and another 12 million are at risk. Of Americans diagnosed with osteoporosis, 20% are men.

The exact cause of osteoporosis is unknown, but it is clearly a multifactorial disorder. Major contributors are genetics, metabolic factors regulating internal calcium equilibrium, lifestyle, aging, and menopause. Peak bone mass attained in young adulthood, coupled with the rate of bone loss in older age, will determine whether an individual's bone mass becomes low enough to be diagnosed as osteoporosis. Genetic factors are estimated to account for 70% of the peak bone mass attained, which is why family history is an important risk factor for osteoporosis and fracture. Calcium equilibrium is maintained by a complex mechanism involving hormones (parathyroid, calcitonin, and vitamin D) controlling key ions (calcium, magnesium, and phosphate) within target tissues (blood, intestine, and bone). Calcium and phosphate enter the blood from the intestine and are stored in bone. The process also occurs in reverse, moving calcium out of the bones for other uses within the body. Nutritional and lifestyle factors can upset the balance and cause too much calcium to move out of bone. In the course of normal aging, the loss of estrogen at menopause tends to increase the rate of bone turnover, which increases the number of remodeling cycles and shortens the length of each cycle. Enough time is allowed for the shorter resorption process, but the longer formation process is cut short. Various combinations of these factors can result in a net loss of bone mass and increase the risk of osteoporosis and fracture.

Two points are important to note about osteoporosis. First, an older person with a normal bone loss rate may still develop osteoporosis if their peak bone mass is low. Second, a common misconception is that proper exercise and diet at menopause prevents bone loss associated with a decrease in estrogen. Persons concerned about their risk of osteoporosis should consult their physician.

Osteoporosis can be classified as primary or secondary. A DXA scan result does not automatically lead to a diagnosis of primary osteoporosis. Secondary causes of systemic or localized disturbances in bone mass must be ruled out before a final diagnosis can be made. Proper choice of treatment should be based on the type of osteoporosis and the underlying cause, if secondary osteoporosis is present (see Table 19.1).

Primary osteoporosis can be *type I* (postmenopausal), *type II* (senile or age related), or both. Type I osteoporosis is caused by bone resorption exceeding bone formation owing to estrogen deprivation in women. Type II osteoporosis occurs in aging men and women and results from a decreased ability to build bone.

Secondary osteoporosis is osteoporosis caused by a heterogeneous group of skeletal disorders resulting in an imbalance of bone turnover. Disorder categories include genetic, endocrine and metabolic, hypogonadal, connective tissue, nutritional and gastrointestinal, hematologic, malignancy, and use of certain prescription drugs. Common causes of secondary osteoporosis include the following:

- Hyperparathyroidism
- Gonadal insufficiency (including estrogen deficiency in women and hypogonadism in men)
- Osteomalacia (rickets in children)
- Rheumatoid arthritis
- Anorexia nervosa
- Gastrectomy
- Celiac disease (hypersensitivity to gluten [wheat protein])
- Multiple myeloma
- Use of corticosteroids, heparin, anticonvulsants, or excessive thyroid hormone treatment

Several prescription medications arrest bone loss and may increase bone mass, including traditional estrogen or hormone replacement therapies, bisphosphonates, selective estrogen receptor modulators, parathyroid hormone, receptor activator of nuclear factor kappa-B ligand (RANKL) inhibitors, and calcitonin (Table 19.2). The availability of therapies beyond the traditional estrogens has led to the widespread use of DXA to diagnose osteoporosis.

Laboratory tests for *biochemical markers* of bone turnover may be used in conjunction with DXA to determine the need for or the effectiveness of the therapy. Problems of poor precision and individual variability have limited their use. Some markers of bone formation found in blood are alkaline phosphatase, osteocalcin, and C- and N-propeptides of type I collagen. Some markers of bone resorption excreted in urine are pyridinium cross-links of collagen, C- and N-telopeptides of collagen, galactosyl hydroxylysine, and hydroxyproline.

TABLE 19.2
Osteoporosis medicines: National Osteoporosis Foundation 2020

FDA approved for:	Postmenopausal women	Men	Prevents osteoporosis	Treats osteoporosis	Prevents osteoporosis caused by steroid medicines	Treats osteoporosis caused by steroid medicines
Bisphosphonates						
Alendronate (Fosamax, Fosamax Plus D)	■	■a	■	■		■
Ibandronate (Boniva)	■		■	■b		
Risedronate (Actonel, Actonel with Calcium)	■	■a	■	■	■	■
Zoledronic Acid (Reclast)	■	■		■	■	■
Calcitonins						
Calcitonin (Fortical)	■			■		
Calcitonin (Miacalcin)	■			■		
Estrogen agonists/antagonists						
Raloxifene (Evista)	■		■	■		
Estrogen therapy (ET) and hormone therapy (HT)						
Many brands	■		■			
Parathyroid hormone						
Tomosozumab (Evenity)	■			■		
Teriparatide (Forteo)	■	■		■		
Abaloparatide (Tymlos)	■			■		
RANK ligand (RANKL)						
Denosumab (Prolia)	■			■		

aFor men, alendronate and risedronate are approved for treatment only.
bIbandronate as an intravenous (IV) injection is approved for treatment only.

FRACTURES AND FALLS

Fractures occur when bones encounter an outside force that exceeds their strength. Fragility fractures occur with minimal trauma from a standing height or less. A small percentage of fragility fractures are spontaneous, meaning that they occur with no apparent force being applied. The most common sites for fractures associated with osteoporosis are the hip, spinal vertebrae, wrist (Colles fracture), ribs, and proximal humerus, but other bones can be affected. Current estimates of fracture in the United States are that approximately 1.5 million osteoporotic fractures occur each year; these include 700,000 vertebral (only one-third are clinically diagnosed), 300,000 hip, 250,000 wrist, and 300,000 other fractures.

One in two women and one in four men above 50 years of age, have an osteoporotic fracture in their remaining lifetime. Risk factors for fracture include being female, low bone mass, personal history of fracture as an adult, history of fracture in a first-degree relative, current cigarette smoking, and low body weight (<127 lb [<58 kg]).

Hip fractures account for 20% of osteoporotic fractures and are the most devastating for the patient in terms of health costs. Important points about hip fracture include the following:

- The overall 1-year mortality rate after hip fracture is one in five.[2]
- Two to three times as many women as men sustain hip fractures, but the 1-year mortality rate for men is twice as high.
- Two-thirds of patients with hip fracture never regain their preoperative activity status. One-fourth requires long-term care.
- A woman's risk of hip fracture is equal to her combined risk of breast, uterine, and ovarian cancer.
- Protective undergarments with side padding, called *hip pads,* have proven effective in preventing hip fractures from falling in elderly adults. Resistance to wearing the garment is the only limitation.

Vertebral fractures are the most common osteoporotic fracture, but only approximately one-third are clinically diagnosed. The effects of vertebral fractures have traditionally been underestimated but are beginning to be recognized and quantified. These fractures cause pain, disfigurement, and dysfunction and decrease the quality of life. More recent studies link them to an increased risk of mortality. Vertebroplasty is a minimally invasive procedure for managing acute painful vertebral fractures. This procedure involves injecting bone cement into the fractured vertebra under fluoroscopic guidance (see Fig. 14.16). Balloon kyphoplasty is a minimally invasive procedure that can reduce back pain and restore vertebral body height and spinal alignment. This procedure involves reducing the vertebral compression and injecting the cement into this space created within the vertebral body (Fig. 19.5). Fluoroscopic guidance is used for this procedure.

The presence of one osteoporotic vertebral fracture significantly increases the risk of future vertebral fractures and progressive curvature of the spine. Most osteoporotic fractures are caused by falls. Identifying elderly persons at increased risk for falls and instituting fall prevention strategies are important goals. Some risk factors for falling are the use of some medications including sedatives, sleep aids, and antidepressants; impaired muscle strength, range of motion, balance, and gait; impaired psychological functioning, including dementia and depression; and environmental hazards, including lighting, rugs, furniture, bathroom, and stairs. Fall prevention strategies through a physical therapy program include balance, gait, and strengthening exercises. Addressing psychological issues, reviewing medication regimens, and counseling patients on correct dosing are other prevention methods. Homes and living areas should be inspected for hazards, and safety measures should be implemented.

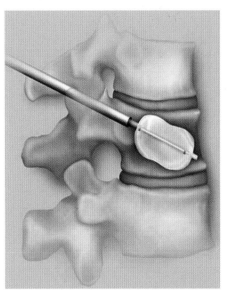

Fig. 19.5 Diagram of balloon kyphoplasty.

BONE HEALTH RECOMMENDATIONS

The NOF's Bone Health and Prevention Recommendations are as follows:
- Obtain daily recommended amounts of calcium and vitamin D.
- Engage in regular weight-bearing and resistance exercise.
- Avoid smoking and excessive alcohol.
- Talk to a health care provider about bone health.
- Have a bone density test and take medication when appropriate.

Surgeon General's Report on Bone Health and Osteoporosis

The Surgeon General's Report on Bone Health and Osteoporosis includes an extensive review of the factors affecting bone health, including the health consequences associated with poor bone health. The report provides the following list of recommendations to promote better bone health and health status in general:
- Getting adequate levels of calcium and vitamin D
- Engaging in physical activity
- Reducing hazards in the home that can lead to fractures and falls
- Talking with a physician about preventive strategies to promote bone health
- Maintaining a healthy weight
- Not smoking
- Limiting alcohol use

Many Americans fail to meet currently recommended guidelines for optimal calcium intake. The Surgeon General's Report on Bone Health and Osteoporosis recommends the following calcium intake: 1000 mg/daily for women 19 to 50 years of age and 1200 mg/daily for females over the age of 50; 1000 mg/daily is recommended for males 51 to 70 years of age. Dietary calcium is the best source, including yogurt, milk, and some cheeses. Dietary shortfall should be met with calcium supplements with the United States Pharmacopeia (USP) designation that supply the appropriate amount of elemental calcium. The individual needs to check the number of pills to meet the serving size and whether or not to take with food (Table 19.3).

Adequate intake of vitamin D is essential for calcium absorption and bone health. Some calcium supplements and most multivitamins contain vitamin D. The Surgeon General's Report on Bone Health and Osteoporosis recommends at least 800 IU/day for adults older than 50 years. Dietary sources are vitamin D–fortified milk and cereals, egg yolks, saltwater fish, and liver.

Weight-bearing exercise occurs when bones and muscles work against gravity as the feet and legs bear the body's weight. Some examples are weightlifting to improve muscle mass and bone strength, low-impact aerobics, walking or jogging, tennis, dancing, stair climbing, gardening, and household chores.

TABLE 19.3

Daily recommended needs for calcium intake

Your body needs calcium	
If this is your age	then you need this much calcium each day (mg)
0–6 months	200
6–12 months	260
1–3 years	700
4–8 years	1000
9–18 years	1300
19–50 years	1000
51–70-year-old males	1000
51–70-year-old females	1200
>70 years old	1200

A cup of milk or fortified orange juice has approximately 300 mg of calcium.
From the Office of the Surgeon General's Report.

Physical and Mathematic Principles of Dual Energy X-Ray Absorptiometry

The measurement of bone density requires separation of the x-ray attenuating effects of soft tissue and bone. The mass attenuation coefficients of soft tissue and bone differ and depend on the energy of the x-ray photons. The use of two different photon energies (dual energy x-ray) optimizes the differentiation of soft tissue and bone. GE Lunar model Advance (GE Lunar Corp, Madison, WI) and Norland model XR-46 (Norland/Swissray, Inc, Ft. Atkinson, WI) use a different method of producing the two energies than Hologic model Horizon (Hologic, Inc, Bedford, MA).

GE Lunar and Norland Swissray use a rare-earth, filtered x-ray source. The primary x-ray beam is passed through selected rare-earth filters to produce a spectrum with peaks near 40 kiloelectron volts (keV) and 70 keV compared with the usual continuous spectrum with one peak near 50 keV (Fig. 19.6A and B). Sophisticated pulse-counting detectors are used to separate and measure the low-energy and high-energy photons (Fig. 19.7). Calibration must be performed externally by scanning a calibration phantom on a regular basis.

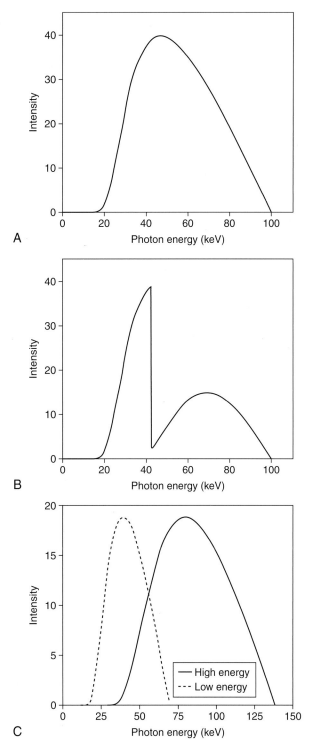

Fig. 19.6 Energy spectra (keV) for x-ray sources used in bone densitometry instruments. (A) Continuous spectrum from x-ray tube. (B) Continuous x-ray spectrum modified by K-edge filter. (C) High-energy and low-energy spectra from kV-switching system.

(From Blake G et al. *The evaluation of osteoporosis: DXA and ultrasound in clinical practice.* London: Martin Dunitz; 1998.)

Hologic scanners use an energy-switching system that synchronously switches the x-ray potential between 100 and 140 kVp. This system produces a primary beam with two photon energies with peaks near 40 and 80 keV (see Fig. 19.6C). The energy-switching system continuously calibrates the beam by passing it through a calibration wheel or drum (Fig. 19.8) containing three sectors for an open-air gap, a soft tissue equivalent, and a bone equivalent. Each sector is divided so that it can differentiate and measure the low-energy and high-energy photons. This permits the use of a relatively simple current-integrating detector that does not have to separate the photons.

Common physics problems of DXA are as follows:

- *Beam hardening in energy-switching systems.* With increasing body thickness, a higher proportion of low-energy photons are absorbed within the body, shifting the spectral distribution toward high-energy photons.
- *Scintillating detector pileup in K-edge filtration systems.* A detector can process only one photon at a time and assign it to the high-energy or low-energy channel. An incoming photon may be missed if the preceding photon has not yet been processed. Digital detectors do not have this problem.
- *Crossover in K-edge filtration systems.* Some high-energy photons lose energy passing through the body and are counted as low-energy photons by the detector. This problem is solved by subtracting a fraction of the high-energy counts from the low-energy channel, depending on body thickness.

The low-energy and high-energy x-rays are attenuated differently within each patient, producing a unique attenuation pattern at the detector, which is transmitted electronically to the computer. Mathematic computations are then performed to subtract the soft tissue signals, producing a profile of the bone (Fig. 19.9). Proprietary bone edge detection algorithms are next applied, and a two-dimensional area is calculated. The average BMD is calculated for all areas, and finally the *BMD* is calculated as BMD = BMC/Area. The three bone densitometry parameters reported on the DXA printouts are area in centimeters squared (cm^2), BMC in grams (g), and BMD in g/cm^2. BMD is the most widely used parameter because it reduces the effect of body size.

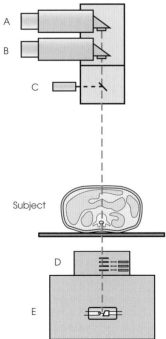

Fig. 19.7 Schematic drawing of a Norland model XR-35 illustrating the principle of operation of a rare-earth filtered system. (A) High-energy detector. (B) Low-energy detector. (C) Laser indicator. (D) Samarium filter module (one fixed, three selectable). (E) Ultrastable 100-kV x-ray source.

Fig. 19.8 Calibration drum used as internal reference standard in Hologic energy-switching instruments. Different segments represent bone standard, soft tissue standard, and empty segment for air value.

BMD can be calculated if BMC and the area is known by the equation BMD = BMC/Area. This equation can be used to determine if a change in BMD is due to a change in BMC, area, or both. A decrease in BMC results in a decrease in BMD; conversely, a decrease in area results in an increase in BMD. If BMC and area move proportionally in the same direction, BMD remains unchanged. In general, a change in a patient's BMD over time should be from a change in BMC, not area. A change in area could be from the technologist not reproducing the baseline positioning or from a change in the software's bone edge detection. Changes in area over time should be investigated and corrected, if possible.

BMD is based on a two-dimensional area, not a three-dimensional volume, making DXA a *projectional,* or *areal, technique.* Techniques to estimate *volumetric density* from DXA scans have been developed but have not been shown to have any improved diagnostic sensitivity over traditional areal density. Fig. 19.10 shows the lateral spine areal and estimated volumetric BMDs.

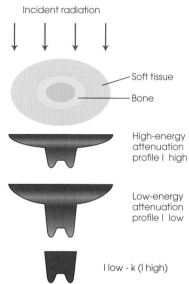

Fig. 19.9 Soft tissue compensation using DXA. By obtaining data at two energies, the soft tissue attenuation can be mathematically eliminated. The remaining attenuation is due to the amount of bone present.

(From Faulkner KG. *DXA Basic science, radiation use and safety, quality assurance, unpublished certification report.* Madison, WI: Personal Communication; 1996.)

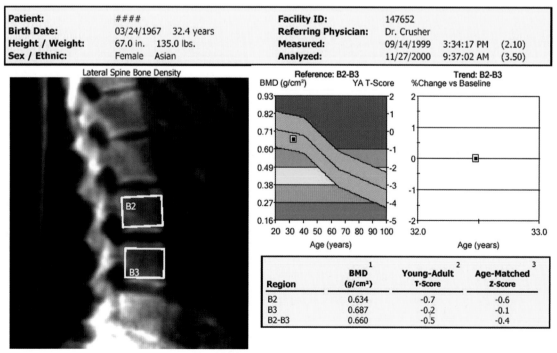

Patient:	####		Facility ID:	147652		
Birth Date:	03/24/1967	32.4 years	Referring Physician:	Dr. Crusher		
Height / Weight:	67.0 in.	135.0 lbs.	Measured:	09/14/1999	3:34:17 PM	(2.10)
Sex / Ethnic:	Female	Asian	Analyzed:	11/27/2000	9:37:02 AM	(3.50)

Region	BMD [1] (g/cm²)	Young-Adult [2] T-Score	Age-Matched [3] Z-Score
B2	0.634	-0.7	-0.6
B3	0.687	-0.2	-0.1
B2-B3	0.660	-0.5	-0.4

Fig. 19.10 Lateral spine BMD scan.

Pencil-Beam and Array-Beam Techniques

The original DXA scanners used a pencil-beam system. With this system, a circular pinhole x-ray collimator produces a narrow (or pencil-beam) stream of x-ray photons that are received by a single detector. The pencil-beam of x-ray moves in a serpentine (also called *rectilinear* or *raster*) fashion across or along the length of the body (Fig. 19.11). This system has a good resolution and it is reproducible, but the early scanners had relatively long scanning periods of 5 to 7 minutes.

The array-beam (also called fan-beam) system has a wide "slit" x-ray collimator and a multielement detector (Fig. 19.12). The scanning motion is reduced to only one direction, which greatly reduces scan time and permits supine lateral lumbar spine scans to be performed. The array-beam system introduces geometric magnification and a slight geometric distortion at the outer edges. Consequently, careful centering of the object of interest is necessary to avoid parallax (Fig. 19.13). The software takes into account the known degree of magnification and produces an *estimated* BMC and an estimated area.

Fig. 19.11 DXA system using pencil-beam single detector.

Fig. 19.12 DXA system using an array-beam multiple detector.

Fig. 19.13 Potential array-beam errors including magnification *(top)* and parallax *(bottom)*. Area and BMC are influenced by magnification to the same degree, such that BMD is not significantly affected. Parallax errors can cause changes in BMD by altering the beam path through the object being measured.

(From Faulkner KG. *DXA Basic science, radiation use and safety, quality assurance, unpublished certification report.* Madison, WI: Personal Communication; 1996.)

ACCURACY AND PRECISION

Three statistics are particularly important in bone densitometry: mean, standard deviation (SD), and percent coefficient of variation (%CV).

1. The mean is commonly called the average. It is the sum of the data values divided by the number of values.
2. The SD is a measure of variability that measures the spread of the data values around their mean. It takes into account the average distance of the data values from the mean. The smaller the average distance or the spread, the smaller the SD. This is the goal in bone densitometry—a smaller SD is better. Fig. 19.14 plots two sets of phantom BMD data measured over 6 months. The means are the same (1.005 g/cm^2), but the red data set has an SD that is twice as large as that of the green data set (0.008 g/cm^2 versus 0.004 g/cm^2). It is better to have phantom BMD data that looks like the green data set.
3. The %CV is a statistic that allows the comparison of variability between different data sets, whether or not they have the same mean. A smaller %CV means less variability and is preferred

in bone densitometry. The %CV is calculated using the following equation:

$$\% \, CV = \left(\frac{SD}{Mean} \right) \times 100$$

In Fig. 19.14, the green data set has a %CV of 0.35 and the red data set has a %CV of 0.81. This is the %CV that must be checked on a Hologic spine phantom plot (Fig. 19.15). The red data set would not pass the criteria that the %CV should be less than or equal to 0.6. The %CV is also used to express precision.

Bone densitometry differs from diagnostic radiology in that, it has a good image quality, which can tolerate variability in technique though it is not the ultimate goal, but it is very important. With bone densitometry, the goal is accurate and precise quantitative measurement by the scanner software, which requires stable equipment and careful, consistent work from the technologist. Two important performance measures in bone densitometry are *accuracy* and *precision*. Accuracy relates to the ability of the system to measure the true value of an object. Precision relates to the ability of the system to reproduce the same (but

not necessarily accurate) results in repeat measurements of the same object. A target may be used to illustrate this point. In Fig. 19.16A, the archer is precise but not accurate. In Fig. 19.16B, the archer is accurate but not precise. Finally, in Fig. 19.16C, the archer is precise and accurate.

In bone densitometry practice, accuracy is most important at baseline when the original diagnosis of osteoporosis is made. Accuracy is determined primarily by the calibration of the scanner, which is set and maintained by the manufacturer. Preventive maintenance once or twice a year is recommended. Precision is followed closely because it is easy to determine and is the most important performance measure in following a patient's BMD over time. Precision can be measured in vitro (in an inanimate object, e.g., phantom) or in vivo (in a live body). Precision is commonly expressed as %CV, and a smaller value indicates better precision.

In vitro precision is the cornerstone of the quality control systems built into the scanners to detect drifts or shifts (variations) in calibration. Each manufacturer provides a unique phantom for this purpose.

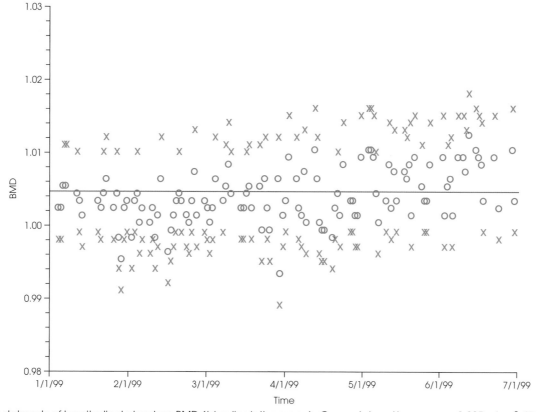

Fig. 19.14 Two data sets of longitudinal phantom BMD (*blue line* is the mean). *Green data set* has mean = 1.005 g/cm^2, SD = 0.004 g/cm^2, and %CV = 0.35. *Red data set* has mean = 1.005 g/cm^2, SD = 0.008 g/cm^2, and %CV = 0.81.

In vivo precision has two main aspects in bone densitometry:

1. The variability within a patient makes it easy or difficult to obtain similar BMD results from several scans on the same patient, on the same day, with repositioning between scans. (Patients with abnormal anatomy, very low bone mass, or thick or thin bodies are known to reflect a larger precision error.)

2. The variability is related to the technologist's skill and how attentive he or she is to obtaining the best possible baseline scan and then reproducing the positioning, scanning parameters, and placement of ROI on all *follow-up scans.*

The primary factors affecting precision are as follows:

• Reproduction of positioning, acquisition parameters (e.g., mode, speed, current), and ROI placement. It is important to note that with a faster scan mode, there is less precision.

• Anatomic variations and pathology and their degeneration over time.

• Body habitus (e.g., excessive thickness or thinness).

• Large weight changes over time.

• Geometric factors on array scanners.

• Stability of scanner calibration and bone edge detection.

Performing precision assessment

Each DXA laboratory should determine its precision error and calculate the *least significant change* (LSC). This precision is used to determine the magnitude of change in BMD that must occur over time to ensure the change is due to a change in the patient's BMD and not to the precision error of the technologist and scanner. The precision error supplied by the manufacturer should not be used because it is the error rate for the machine and not the technologist. If a DXA laboratory has more than one technologist, an average precision error that combines the data from all technologists should be used to establish the precision error and LSC for the facility. Every technologist should perform an in vivo precision assessment using patients who are representative of

the patient population of the facility. Each technologist should do one complete precision assessment after basic scanning skills have been learned, and after having performed at least 100 patient scans. If a new DXA system is installed, a repeat precision assessment should be done. A repeat assessment should also be done if a technologist's skill level has changed (International Society for Clinical Densitometry [ISCD] 2019 Position Statements).

Procedure to determine precision error for each technologist

Measure 15 patients three times or 30 patients two times, repositioning the patient after each scan. Use the ISCD Precision Assessment tool (http://www.iscd.org) to calculate precision. Calculate LSC for the group at 95% confidence interval. The clinician uses this information to interpret all serial scans. The minimum acceptable precision values for an individual technologist are as follows:

• Lumbar spine: 1.9% (LSC = 5.3%)
• Total hip: 1.8% (LSC = 5.0%)
• Femoral neck: 2.5% (LSC = 6.9%)

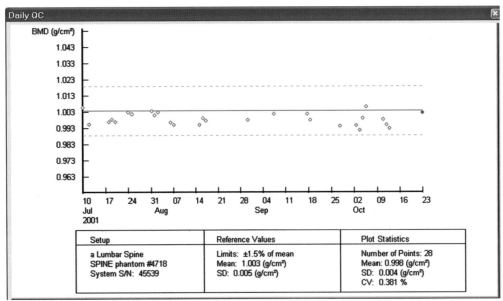

Fig. 19.15 Hologic spine phantom quality control plot. All plotted BMD points are within the control limits *(dotted lines),* which indicate 1.5% of the mean. The coefficient of variation (CV) (under *Plot Statistics*) is within acceptable limits at 0.43%.

Fig. 19.16 Illustration of accuracy versus precision, assuming an archer is shooting for the center of the target. (A) Precise but not accurate. (B) Accurate but not precise. (C) Accurate and precise.

Retraining is required if a technologist's precision is worse than these values.

Precision assessment should be standard clinical practice. This research should not require approval from an institutional review board and may potentially benefit patients. Adherence to local or state radiologic safety regulations is necessary. A precision assessment requires the consent of participating patients (ISCD 2019 Position Statements).

CROSS-CALIBRATION OF DUAL ENERGY X-RAY ABSORPTIOMETRY MACHINES

- It is impossible to quantitatively compare BMD or to calculate LSC between facilities/scanners without cross-calibration of the machines.
- DXA facilities should always cross-calibrate machines when changing hardware, replacing a system with the same technology, changing the entire system, or changing to a system by a different manufacturer.
- Scan patients as suggested in ISCD position statements. Calculate the average BMD relationship and LSC between the initial machine and new machine using the ISCD Machine Cross-Calibration tool (http://www.iscd.org).
- If a cross-calibration assessment is not performed, no quantitative comparison to the prior machine can be made. Consequently, a new baseline BMD and intrasystem LSC should be established (ISCD 2019 Position Statements).

Z-SCORES AND T-SCORES

A BMD measurement from a patient is most useful when it is compared statistically with an appropriate sex-matched *reference population*. The three DXA manufacturers have separately collected reference population databases, which vary because different populations, entrance criteria, and statistical methods were used. To correct this problem, the Third National Health and Nutrition Examination Survey (NHANES III) DXA total hip database was adapted to provide a *standardized hip* reference database for all manufacturers. This database is currently widely used. All reference databases are separated by gender and provide the BMD mean and SD at each age; however, the lumbar spine database is manufacturer specific.

To compare a patient's BMD with the reference population BMD, two standardized scores have been developed, called the *Z-score* and *T-score* (see Fig. 19.10). In older adults, the Z-score is greater than the T-score.

The Z-score indicates the number of SDs the patient's BMD is from the average BMD for the patient's respective age and sex group. The Z-score is used to determine if the measured BMD is reasonable, and if an evaluation for secondary osteoporosis is warranted.

The T-score indicates the number of SDs the patient's BMD is from the average BMD of young, normal, sex-matched individuals with peak bone mass. The T-score is used to assess fracture risk, diagnose osteoporosis, and low bone mass *(osteopenia)*, when determining if therapy is recommended.

The Z-score, T-score, or both may be adjusted for ethnicity, weight, or both. It is incorrect to assume that because ethnicity and weight have been entered into the scan biographic information, the standardized scores have been adjusted. Some manufacturers allow an ethnicity to be entered for which there is no reference database; these patients are compared with whites. Some manufacturers adjust for weight and ethnicity on the Z-score but not the T-score. To determine what adjustments have been made, first carefully check the information on the scan printout, including footnotes. If a question remains, call the manufacturer's customer service line and ask.

The ISCD recommends the use of a uniform white (non–race adjusted) female and male normative database for women and men of all ethnic groups. All manufacturers' defaults may not be adjusted to this recommendation. The technologist needs to be familiar with the defaults of the specific equipment and know how to make adjustments.

Bone mass is normally distributed (i.e., has a bell-shaped curve) in the population, and no one exact cut point exists below which a person has osteoporosis. However, with the widespread availability of DXA and T-scores, there was pressure to declare such a cut point. The World Health Organization (WHO) recommended that the classifications presented in Table 19.4 be used in DXA studies of postmenopausal Caucasian women.

Discordance occurs when there exist different T-scores at anatomic sites within a patient, within populations, and between modalities. It makes the diagnosis of osteoporosis more complicated than simply applying T-score criteria, and the problems are being researched to find more standardized diagnostic criteria. A patient may be found to have a low T-score at the hip but not at the spine, and a QCT scan of the spine is likely to produce a lower T score than is a DXA scan of the spine in the same patient.

Applying the T-score criteria designed for DXA to other modalities (e.g., quantitative ultrasound [QUS], QCT) has proven problematic. The best practice is to apply the T-score criteria only to DXA. The T-score is one important risk factor for osteoporosis, but the patient's medical history, lifestyle, medications, and other risk factors must also be considered in a complete clinical evaluation. Physicians who interpret bone density scans need to be educated in the complexities of the task.

Large epidemiologic studies have investigated the clinical value of BMD in elderly women and have yielded information on the relationship of BMD and T-scores to fracture risk. A gradient of risk has been observed between BMD and fracture incidence, with lower BMD or T-score conferring increased risk of fracture. For each 1 SD decrease in T-score, the risk for fracture increases 1.5-fold to 2.5-fold. A woman with a T-score of −2 has approximately twice the risk of fracture compared with a woman with a T-score of −1, all other factors being equal. This information helps clinicians to explain the meaning of a bone density test to patients. Patients can then make informed decisions about the level of fracture risk they are willing to accept and whether to begin or continue therapy.

Dual Energy X-Ray Absorptiometry Scanning

RADIATION PROTECTION

Radiologic technologists receive extensive instruction in radiation physics, biology, and protection during their professional education. Practicing proper radiation protection and achieving the goal of *ALARA* (as low as reasonably achievable) is relatively simple for DXA. The effective radiation dose in micro*sieverts* (μSv) for DXA scans is low compared with conventional radiography doses and similar to natural background radiation (Table 19.5). If the positioning or acquisition parameters of a scan are questionable, the scan should be repeated because the risk from the additional radiation dose is negligible compared with the risk of an incorrect medical diagnosis.

Time, distance, and shielding relate to DXA in the following ways:

1. The manufacturer sets the time for the scan based on the array or scan mode appropriate for the thickness of the body part being scanned.
2. The manufacturer sets the distance from the x-ray tube to the patient. This is a fixed distance.
3. Distance is the best form of protection for the technologist. The technologist's console should be at least 3 ft (1 m) from the x-ray source (x-ray tube) scanner for pencil-beam scanners and up to 9 ft (3 m) from heavily used array-beam scanners (array-beam produces higher dose than pencil-beam). If these distances cannot be accommodated, a mobile radiation shield can be used.

Shielding is built into the scanner via collimation. Additional lead shielding should not be used on DXA patients.

Other important radiation safety points include the following:

- The technologist should wear an individual dosimetry device (radiation badge, thermoluminescent dosimeter, or optically stimulated luminescence device) at the collar on the side adjacent to the scanner. Another monitor can be placed outside the scan room. A staff member should be charged with understanding and monitoring the dosimetry records and performing any necessary follow-up. A radiation warning sign should be posted and highly visible.
- The technologist should always remain in the room during the scan and monitor the acquisition image, allowing the scan to be aborted as soon as the need for repositioning and rescanning is obvious.
- The technologist should have adequate education and be clinically competent with DXA experience in order to minimize repositioning and repeated scans. It is important to know how to prepare the patient to eliminate artifacts. Any questionable scan should be repeated.
- The technologist should follow proper procedures to avoid scanning a pregnant patient and place documentation in the permanent record. If a woman of childbearing age will not sign that she is not pregnant, the "10-day rule" allows scanning during the first 10 days after the first day of her last menstrual period.
- Patients should be screened at scheduling for problems that require postponement of scanning, such as pregnancy and recent barium, contrast, or nuclear medicine examinations.

The most effective radiation safety practice is a knowledgeable, well-educated, clinically competent, and conscientious DXA technologist. It is essential for DXA technologists to receive instructions from the manufacturer of a specific model of scanner. This might consist of reviewing digital information and reviewing performed scans with a field application specialist. When experience is obtained, a technologist can become certified by the ISCD. Another certification is available through the American Registry of Radiologic Technologists (ARRT). Both of these credentials can be obtained by technologists who are educationally prepared and clinically competent. Technologists must obtain continuing education in bone densitometry to meet the qualifications of maintaining current practice status for both ISCD and ARRT.

TABLE 19.4

World Health Organization classifications of bone density by T-score

Classification	Criteria
Normal	BMD or BMC T-score of ≥−1
Low bone mass (osteopenia)	BMD or BMC T-score between −1 and −2.5
Osteoporosis	BMD or BMC T-score of ≤2.5
Severe osteoporosis	BMD or BMC T-score of ≤2.5 and ≥1 fragility fractures

Data from Kanis JA. World Health Organization (WHO) Study Group: assessment of fracture risk and its application to screening for postmenopausal osteoporosis: a synopsis of the WHO report. *Osteoporos Int.* 1994;4:358.

TABLE 19.5

Bone densitometry radiation doses compared with other commonly acquired doses

Type of radiation exposure	Effective dose (mSv)
Daily natural background radiation	5–8
Round-trip air flight across the United States	60
Lateral lumbar spine radiograph	700
PA chest radiograph	50
QCT with localizer scan (from scanner offering low kV and mAs; may be 10 times higher for other scanners)	60
DXA scan (range allows for different anatomic sites; Lunar EXPERT-XL may be higher)	1–5
SXA scan	≤1
QUS	0

Data from Kalender WA. Effective dose values in bone mineral measurements by photon absorptiometry and computed tomography. *Osteoporos Int.* 1992;2:82.

PATIENT CARE AND EDUCATION

Typical DXA patients are ambulatory outpatients; however, many are frail and at increased risk for fragility fractures. Patient care and safety require attention to the following points of courtesy and common sense:

- All areas of the laboratory, including the front entrance, waiting room, and scan room, should be monitored daily and modified for patient safety. The location of floor-level cables in the scan room should be checked.
- The technologist should maintain professionalism at all times by introducing himself or herself and other staff members to the patient and explaining the procedure. Ethical conduct and professionalism in the workplace are requirements of all health care professionals. The technologist should adhere to the Code of Ethics for Radiologic Technologists (Chapter 1) and the American Society of Radiologic Technologists (ASRT) Bone Density Practice Standards.
- The technologist needs to remove all external artifacts. Some DXA laboratories have all patients gowned for consistency. However, it is possible to scan a patient who is wearing loose cotton clothing with no buttons, snaps, or zippers (i.e., "sweats"). If clothing is not removed, the bra must be undone, and all hooks and underwires must be removed from the scan field. Considering that shoes must be removed for proper height measurement, a long-handled shoehorn would be a practical aid.
- The technologist should provide a simple explanation of the expected action of the scan-arm, the proximity of the scan-arm to the patient's face and head, the noise of the motor, and the length of time for the scan. This information may reduce the patient's anxiety.

- The technologist must listen to any concerns the patient may have about the procedure and be ready to answer questions about radiation exposure, the length of the examination, and the reporting protocol used by the laboratory.
- Although the scan tables are not more than 3 ft (approximately 1 m) in height, a steady footstool with a long handle is recommended. All patients should be assisted on and off the table.
- On completion of the examination, the technologist should ensure the scan-arm has returned to the home position, clearing the patient's head. The patient should sit upright for several seconds to regain stability before descending from the scanner.

In some institutions, it is the responsibility of the DXA technologist to provide education to the patient and the family. Topics may include osteoporosis prevention, proper nutrition, calcium and vitamin D supplementation, weight-bearing exercise, and creating a hazard-free living environment. Many technologists give community educational programs, in-service staff seminars, and participate in health fairs.

PATIENT HISTORY

Each bone density laboratory should develop a patient questionnaire customized for the types of patients who are referred to undergo the exam. Before scanning is performed, any information that could postpone or cancel the scan should be identified. The questionnaire should be directed at obtaining information in four basic categories. Sample questions include the following:

1. Scanning criteria:
   - Is there a possibility of pregnancy?
   - Is it impossible for you to lie flat on your back for several minutes?

- Have you had a nuclear medicine, barium, or contrast x-ray examination performed in the last week?
- Have you had any previous fractures or surgeries in the hip, spine, abdomen, or forearm areas?
- Do you have any other medical conditions affecting the bones, such as osteoporosis, curvature of the spine, or arthritis?

2. *Patient information*: This includes identifying information, referring physician, current standing height without shoes along with current weight, and medical history including medications.

3. *Insurance information*: Because DXA scans are not universally covered by insurance, it is important to obtain information on the insurance carrier, the need for prior approval, and the information necessary for insurance coding. In 1998, the US Congress passed the Bone Mass Measurement Act (BMMA) dealing with reimbursement for Medicare patients. Central and peripheral technologies are covered. Medicare does not cover screening, so a qualified individual must meet at least one of the following requirements:
   - Estrogen-deficient woman at clinical risk of osteoporosis
   - Individuals with hyperparathyroidism
   - Individuals receiving long-term glucocorticoid (steroid) therapy
   - Individuals with vertebral abnormalities by radiograph
   - Individuals being monitored on osteoporosis therapy and have been approved by the US Food and Drug Administration (FDA)

4. *Reporting information*: The type and scope of the report that is provided determine how much information is necessary about the patient's risk factors for, and history of, low bone mass, fragility fractures, and bone diseases.

REPORTING, CONFIDENTIALITY, RECORD KEEPING, AND SCAN STORAGE

When the scan has been completed, the following guidelines should be observed:

- The technologist should end the examination by telling the patient when the scan results will be available to the referring physician. If a patient asks for immediate results, the technologist should explain that it is the ordering physician's responsibility to give the results to the patient after the scan has been interpreted by an educationally prepared and clinically competent DXA clinician.
- DXA scan results are confidential medical records and should be handled according to the institution's rules for such records. Results should not be discussed with other staff members or patients, and digital results should be shielded from inappropriate viewing. As of April 2005 the guidelines of the American Health Insurance Portability and Accountability Act of 1996 (HIPAA) must be integrated into the DXA laboratory. Manufacturers use privacy tools or HIPAA-secure tools to ensure patient confidentiality.
- Complete records must be kept for each patient. If a patient returns for *follow-up* scans, the positioning, acquisition parameters, and placement of the ROI must be reproduced as closely as possible to the original scans. The technologist must keep electronic records with the patient's identifying information and date, the file name, and the archive location of each scan. The electronic record should also identify any special information about why particular scans were or were not performed (e.g., the right hip was scanned because the left hip was fractured, or the forearm was not scanned because of the patient's severe arthritis) and any special procedures done for positioning (e.g., the femur was not fully rotated because of pain) or scan analysis (e.g., the bone edge was manually placed for the radial ultradistal region). The patient questionnaire, log sheet, and complete scan information must also be kept electronically.
- The general consensus is that DXA scan results should continually be kept electronically because all serial studies are compared with the baseline.

COMPUTER COMPETENCY

DXA scan acquisition, analysis, and archiving is controlled with a personal computer (PC). DXA technologists must be familiar with the basic PC components and how they work. Digital networking allows a scan to be performed at one location and be sent electronically to a remote location for reading or review by an interpreting or referring physician. A technologist must be able to back up, archive, locate, and restore patient scan files. Daily backup and archival are recommended to preserve patient scan files and data. A third copy of data should be stored offsite to ensure retrieval of patient data and to be able to rebuild databases if there is a computer failure, fire, flood, or theft. Most facilities have access to *picture archiving communications systems (PACS)* where all scans are stored electronically and can be retrieved when needed.

Manufacturers frequently upgrade software versions, and the technologist is responsible for performing this task. Records of upgrades and software installation should be maintained. Current software media should be accessible to service engineers at the time of preventive maintenance and repairs.

Computers consist of software and hardware. Software consists of programs written in code that instruct the computer how to perform tasks. The DXA manufacturer's software controls many aspects of DXA scanning from starting the scan to calculating and reporting the results. Hardware comprises the physical components for central processing, input, output, and storage.

Fig. 19.17 Plot of spine phantom BMD and time (in months). Two *arrows* show abrupt shifts in BMD. *Straight line* shows a slow drift downward in BMD. These indicate changes in scanner calibration.

GE Healthcare
Lunar DXA
Madison, WI 53717

QA Phantom Report
08/07/2006
8:56:22 AM

Lunar iDXA
ME+00001
(10.50)

QA Phantom

BMD Calibration	Composition Calibration

BMD Calibration (g/cm²): 1.543, 1.499, 1.453, 1.043, 0.999, 0.953, 0.540, 0.495, 0.450

Dates: 09/19/2005 01/05/2006 04/23/2006 09/09/2006 — Date

Composition Calibration (% Fat): 65.5, 61.0, 56.5, 41.0, 36.5, 32.0, 12.5, 9.0, 3.5

Dates: 09/19/2005 01/05/2006 04/23/2006 09/09/2006 — Date

QA Phantom

BMD	0.994 g/cm²	Pass
BMC	24.93 g	Pass
Area	25.09 cm²	Pass

QC Tests

X-ray and Detector Status	Pass
Mechanical Tests	Pass
Calibration Status	Pass

Precision

BMD CV	0.00%

System Status: Pass

GE Healthcare

Lunar iDXA
ME+00001
(10.50)

Fig. 19.18 GE Lunar quality assurance results printout. The technologist must perform and review the data before performing clinical patient scans.

(Courtesy GE Lunar, Madison, WI.)

DUAL ENERGY X-RAY ABSORPTIOMETRY SCANNER LONGITUDINAL QUALITY CONTROL

Longitudinal quality control procedures are performed in accordance with the manufacturer's recommendations. Manufacturers' instructions in operator manuals must be followed exactly. These procedures have the common goal of ensuring that patients are scanned on properly functioning equipment with stable calibration. Unstable calibration can take the form of abrupt shifts or slow drifts in BMD, as seen on plots of phantom scan results (Fig. 19.17). These problems make the patient's BMD values too high or too low and prohibit a valid comparison between baseline and follow-up scans. Calibration "shift" may occur if there has been a relocation, maintenance, or change of x-ray tube or detector on the scanner. Calibration "drift" may occur if there is a change in room conditions (temperature, humidity) or change in power supply or with aging of the x-ray tube or detector. It is important to monitor the plots regularly.

The procedures use either external or internal instruments to track the calibration of the DXA scanner over time. GE Lunar and Norland Swissray systems necessitate scanning an external calibration block to perform a calibration check. The technologist must observe the procedure; he or she should review the report and note whether the system passed all tests of internal parameters (Fig. 19.18). Hologic systems perform an automatic internal calibration check when the system is turned on.

Manufacturers also provide semianthropomorphic and aluminum phantoms for tracking calibration over time. Hologic systems require that daily QC be performed before patient scanning (Fig. 19.19).

When not recommended by the manufacturer, the ISCD advises the following procedures: Periodic (at least once per week) phantom scans should be performed for any DXA system as an independent assessment of system calibration. The BMD is plotted, monitored, and checked with statistical and quality control rules. The quality control rule used to check DXA scanners is modified from Shewhart Control Chart rules. Shewhart rules are a classic method of checking that a quality parameter is stable and within acceptable limits of 3 SDs. For DXA, the value of the control limits is modified to *1.5%* of the mean to provide more uniformity across scanners.

483

The mean and SD are calculated from the first 25 measurements of the parameter. A graph is created displaying the mean and the control limits 1.5 SDs above and below the mean. The parameter measurements are plotted over time and checked for violation of rules, such as one measurement more than 1.5 SDs from the mean. DXA control charts display the mean as the center line with control limits (1.5% of the mean) above and below. The Hologic software produces this graph automatically (see Fig. 19.15). For other manufacturers, the graph and plotting must be done by hand. The technologist must verify the phantom BMD after any service is performed on the scanner. When the phantom BMD value falls outside the control limits, the scan should be repeated once; if it fails, service should be called and patient scans should be canceled. If the BMD remains outside the control limits, the manufacturer must be contacted. No patients should be scanned until the equipment has been repaired and is operating within the known values.

Ten phantom scans should be performed and plotted before and after scanner preventive maintenance, repair, relocation, and software or hardware upgrades. This practice is to ensure that the calibration has not been altered and proper adjustments can be made. These phantoms and values should be reviewed before the service engineer leaves the DXA laboratory. Recalibration adjustments should be made before scanning any patients. The technologist is required to oversee this operation.

Inconsistent phantom scanning, analysis, or interpretation of the results may lead to false precision and patient outcomes. The DXA technologist must understand the quality control procedures and follow them consistently. DXA laboratories should have written standard operating procedures (SOPs) and documented instructions to ensure consistency among technologists. The technologist is required to maintain service logs and compliance with government inspections, radiation surveys, and regulatory requirements.

Fig. 19.19 Hologic phantom.

Fig. 19.20 Examples of incorrect and correct follow-up scan positioning. Note difference in BMD between the scans. (A) Baseline hip scan. (B) Incorrectly positioned follow-up scan. Size and shape of lesser trochanter and angle of femoral body do not match baseline. (C) Correctly positioned follow-up scan.

ANATOMY, POSITIONING, AND ANALYSIS

Radiologic technologists receive extensive instruction in anatomy during their radiology training. DXA scanning requires knowledge of DXA-specific anatomy. This anatomy relates to positioning the patient properly for scan acquisition. The points presented in this section generally apply to all DXA scanners; however, instruction from the specific manufacturer is required before operating the scanner.

Similar to all technologies, DXA has operating limits. Accuracy and precision may be impaired if the bone mass is low, the patient is too thick or thin, the anatomy is abnormal, or there have been significant changes in soft tissue between serial scans. The added value of an experienced DXA technologist is recognition and adaptation to abnormal situations. Any anomaly or protocol variation that may compromise the scan results must be noted by the technologist and taken into consideration by the interpreting physician.

DXA calculations are based on soft tissue and bone. Adequate amounts of soft tissue are essential for valid results.

Serial scans

DXA is a qualitative instrument used to monitor BMD change over time. True comparison of BMD results requires that serial scans be performed on the same scanner that was used for the baseline scans.

Scan results are more precise with less intervention from the technologist and the DXA equipment, reflecting a true biologic change. It is imperative that the patient positioning be exactly the same for baseline and serial scans. The same scan settings (e.g., field size, mode, or speed and current) and ROI should be placed identically on the images. These steps ensure that scan results are comparable over time. The software's *compare feature or copy* should be used. The baseline scans should be available at the time of the patient's appointment. Documentation of any procedures out of the range of the laboratory's SOP needs to be available when performing serial scans. ISCD recommends comparing any serial scan to the baseline scan. If the baseline scan has been previously analyzed incorrectly, always reanalyze correctly and then compare. Note this information for the interpreting clinician.

Fig. 19.20 shows the comparison of a patient's baseline hip scan (see Fig. 19.20A) and a follow-up scan done 6 years later. It is an example to demonstrate why follow-up positioning must match baseline if the BMD measurements are to be compared. The first follow-up scan (see Fig. 19.20B) did not reproduce the baseline positioning. The rotation of the femoral neck was different, as indicated by the larger lesser trochanter and the femoral shaft being more abducted, and resulted in the midline being placed differently by the software and a different angle for the neck ROI. The scan was repeated (see Fig. 19.20C) to reproduce the baseline positioning correctly. The difference in total hip BMD between scans *A* and *B* is −13% compared with a difference of −10% between scans *A* and *C*.

PA lumbar spine

Spine scans are most appropriate for predicting vertebral fracture risk. It is noted that vertebral fractures are the most common osteoporotic fracture. Underestimation of fracture risk occurs in patients older than 65 years who present with degenerative changes that can artificially elevate spinal BMD. The following points can help with positioning patients for PA lumbar spine DXA scans, analyzing the scan results, and evaluating the validity of the scans:

1. Degenerative changes in the spine, such as *osteophytosis*, overlying calcification, compression fractures (Fig. 19.21), or scoliosis greater than 15 degrees (Fig. 19.22), can falsely elevate the BMD. Artifacts in the vertebral bodies or very dense artifacts in the soft tissue may also affect the BMD, depending on the model of the scanner and version of the software. The interpreting clinician should develop policies and protocols for the technologist in these circumstances (e.g., do not include the spine but include another site, such as forearm). These are considered SOPs and should be followed by all technologists for consistency.

2. The lumbar spine is centered in the scan field. In a patient with scoliosis, L5 may need to be off center so that adequate and relatively equal amounts of soft tissue are on either side of the spine throughout the scan.

3. Some visualization of iliac crests should be acquired in the scan region. This ensures the inclusion of all of L4. The iliac crest is an excellent landmark for consistent placement of the intervertebral markers at baseline and follow-up scanning.

Region	Area(cm²)	BMC(g)	BMD(g/cm²)
L1	13.56	10.07	0.743
L2	13.75	11.63	0.846
L3	14.56	11.83	0.812
L4	16.44	14.34	0.872
TOTAL	58.31	47.87	0.821

A

Region	Area(cm²)	BMC(g)	BMD(g/cm²)
L1	11.45	10.88	0.951
L2	12.97	11.72	0.903
L3	14.95	11.80	0.789
L4	16.50	14.35	0.870
TOTAL	55.87	48.75	0.873

B

Fig. 19.21 Use of Hologic compare feature indicates that L1 bone map and ROI from baseline scan (A) no longer fit the follow-up scan (B) because of a compression fracture of L1. Both scans should be analyzed to exclude L1 before comparing total BMD. Note differences in BMD and area measurements.

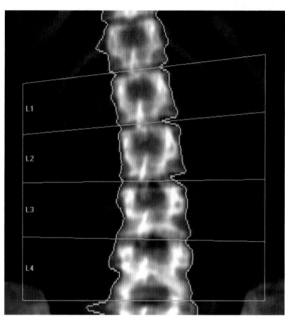

Fig. 19.22 DXA PA spine scan with scoliosis and scoliosis analysis technique.

Fig. 19.23 Characteristic shapes of L1-5 and their relationship to the iliac crests as seen on DXA PA spine scan.

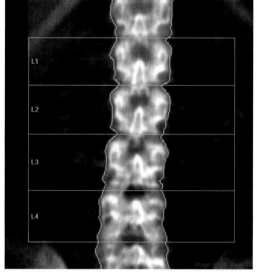

Fig. 19.24 Six lumbar vertebrae. Vertebral labeling is done from the bottom to the top according to the shape of the vertebrae.

4. The PA spine scan image displays the posterior vertebral elements, which have unique characteristic shapes, in contrast to a general lumbar radiograph. These shapes can be used to differentiate placement of the intervertebral markers. When degenerative disease has obscured the intervertebral spaces, these shapes can aid in determining proper labeling of the vertebral levels. L1, L2, and L3 have a U shape; L4 has an H or X shape and appears to have "feet," and L5 looks like a sideways I or "dog bone" (Fig. 19.23). Another aid is that L3 typically has the widest transverse processes. L1, L2, and L3 are approximately the same height. L4 is a bit taller than the others, whereas L5 is the shortest in height. The iliac crest usually lies at the level of L4-5 intervertebral space.

5. A small percentage of patients appear to have four or six lumbar vertebrae rather than five, which is most commonly seen. The vertebrae can be labeled by locating L5 and L4 on the basis of their characteristic shapes and then counting upward (Fig. 19.24). The procedure of counting from the bottom greatly biases toward a higher BMD and avoids including T12 without a rib, which significantly lowers the BMD. This procedure ensures a conservative diagnosis of low BMD. If necessary, the technologist can adjust the scan parameters manually to accommodate the six lumbar vertebrae.

6. Do not adjust the bone edges or angle or move the intervertebral markers unless absolutely necessary. These techniques should be performed in a fashion that is easy to reproduce for serial scans. Variations to protocol should be documented.

7. Check that the patient is lying straight by observing from the head or foot end of the table. If a patient is lying straight on the table, but the spine is not straight on the scan, do not attempt to twist the patient to get the image straight. This unusual positioning would not be reproducible at follow-up. Make a note in the record that the patient was positioned straight on the table.

8. The purpose of the leg-positioning block is to reduce the lordotic curve, open up the intervertebral spaces, and reduce the part-image distance. Consistency in using the same height of the leg-positioning block when a patient returns for serial scans is important. Document the block height.

9. A checklist for a good PA spine scan (see Fig. 19.21A) includes the following:
   • The spine is straight and centered in the scan field. Patients with scoliosis should have equal amounts of soft tissue on either side of the spine if possible.
   • The scan contains a portion of the iliac crest and half of T12; the last set of ribs is shown, when applicable.
   • The entire scan field is free of external artifacts.
   • The intervertebral markers are properly placed.
   • The vertebral levels are properly labeled.
   • The bone edges are correct.

Proximal femur

The hip scan is perhaps the most important because it is the best predictor of future hip fracture, which is the most devastating of fragility fractures. Compared with the spine scan, the hip scan is more difficult to perform properly and precisely because of variations in anatomy and the small ROI. The following points can help in positioning patients for hip DXA scans, analyzing the results, and evaluating the validity of the scans:

1. With the patient in a supine position, rotate the entire leg 15 to 25 degrees internally to place the femoral neck parallel with the tabletop and perpendicular to the x-ray beam. Successful rotation is achieved when the lesser trochanter is diminished in size and only slightly visible (or not visible). A large, pointed lesser trochanter may indicate a low degree of rotation (see Fig. 19.20B and C). However, patient anatomy is not always as shown in textbooks. Patients can have a prominent lesser trochanter, and proper rotation is achieved when the femoral neck region is free of overlapping ischium, and appropriate pelvis separation is visualized. This positioning allows proper placement of the femoral neck ROI. All scanners come with positioning aids that should be used according to the manufacturer's instructions.

2. The shaft of the femur must be straight and parallel to the long axis of the table.

3. A few patients have little or no space between the ischium and femoral neck. In some cases, part of the ischium lies under the femoral neck, elevating the BMC and falsely elevating the femoral neck BMD (Fig. 19.25). This could be caused by the rotation of the ischium (pelvis). The patient should be removed from the table and repositioned. If the problem persists, slightly adjust the leg until the ischium and neck are separated. Variations in positioning should be noted and reproduced at the time of the serial scan.

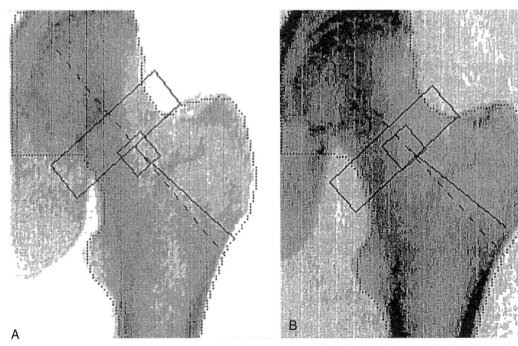

A   B

Fig. 19.25 (A) Despite use of the software tool to "cut out the ischium," bone from the ischium underlies the femoral neck ROI. The BMC is increased, increasing the BMD. (B) The same patient was positioned for a follow-up scan 1 year later. The pelvis is no longer rotated, as indicated by the narrower width of the ischium. Adequate space exists between the neck and ischium, and there is no ischium beneath the neck ROI. This is an example of poor pelvis positioning in A; the patient must be lying flat on the pelvis as in B. These two scans *cannot* be compared for rate of bone loss. The scan in B should be considered a new baseline and compared with a properly performed follow-up scan in the future.

4. To compare proximal femur BMD over time, the positioning must be exactly reproduced and the angle of the neck box ROI must be the same (see Fig. 19.20). Check these points on the baseline and serial scan images:
   - The lesser trochanter must be of same size and shape. If not, change the hip rotation. More rotation would make the lesser trochanter appear smaller.
   - The femoral shaft must be abducted the same amount. Adjust the abduction or adduction accordingly.
   - The neck box ROI is automatically placed perpendicular to the midline, so the midline must be at the same angle in each scan. If it is not, reposition as required. If positioning is not the problem, proper software adjustments must be made according to the manufacturer's guidelines.
5. A fractured hip with orthopedic hardware should not be scanned. If arthritis is present in the scan, it can cause an increase in the density of the medial hip with shortening of the femoral neck (Fig. 19.26). The less affected hip should, therefore, be scanned for an accurate diagnosis. The DXA diagnosis should always be based on the lowest BMD value. The limits of the technology are taxed by patients who are very thin or thick or have very low bone mass. These problems are revealed by poor bone edge detection, a mottled appearance of the image, or both. Some images show the bone edges, and it is obvious when the proper edge cannot be detected. For images that do not show the bone edges, the area values must be checked and compared. The operator's manual may not adequately cover these problems. The technologist is responsible for recognizing problems and querying the manufacturer's application department about the best ways to handle such difficulties. If a patient is deemed unsuitable for a DXA hip scan, another site, such as a forearm, may prove to be valuable.
6. A basic checklist for a good DXA hip scan (see Fig. 19.20A) includes the following:
   - The lesser trochanter is small or barely visible.
   - The midline of the femoral shaft is parallel to the lateral edge of the scan.
   - Adequate space is present between the ischium and femoral neck.
   - The midline through the femoral neck is reasonably placed, resulting in a reasonable angle for the femoral neck box.
   - The proximal, distal, and lateral edges of the scan field are properly located.
   - No air is present in the scan field on GE Lunar scans.

Fig. 19.26 Hip arthritis. Note increased density in medial hip and foreshortened femoral neck. The technologist may be required to intervene in this situation. Notation of difficulty with positioning and known arthritis should be mentioned on the patient's history form.

Forearm

Two important ROIs are present on the DXA forearm scan: the ultradistal region, which is the site of the common Colles fracture, and the one-third (33%) region, which measures an area that is primarily cortical bone near the mid-forearm (see Table 19.1). Although the ulna is used for forearm length measurement and available for analysis, only the one-third (33%) region of the radius is reported. The following guidelines can aid in positioning, acquisition, and analysis of forearm DXA scans and evaluating the validity of the scans:

1. The nondominant forearm is scanned because it is expected to have slightly lower BMD than the dominant arm. A forearm should not be scanned in patients with a history of wrist fracture, internal hardware, or severe deformity resulting from arthritis. An indication for scanning the forearm would be documented hyperparathyroidism.

2. The same chair should be used for all patients to ensure consistency over time. The chair should have a back but no wheels or arms.

3. At the time of the baseline scan, the forearm should be measured according to the manufacturer's instructions. The ulna is measured from the ulnar styloid to the olecranon process. The distal one-third of this measurement is used to place the one-third, or 33%, ROI. A manufacturer estimates the forearm length based on the height. The directions for determining the starting and ending locations of the scan must be followed exactly (Fig. 19.27A).

4. The forearm must be straight and centered in the scan field (see Fig. 19.27A).

Correct use of the appropriate positioning aids must be applied. For Hologic models, the forearm scan requires adequate amounts of air in the scan field. Soft tissue must surround the ulna and radius, and several lines of air must be present on the ulnar side. If the forearm is wide, the scan must be manually set for a wider scan region so that adequate air is included.

5. Motion is a common problem in forearm scan acquisition (see Fig. 19.27A). The patient should be in a comfortable position so that the arm does not move during the scan. The hand and proximal forearm can be secured with straps or tapes placed outside the scan field. Avoid unnecessary conversation during the scan to minimize movements.

Fig. 19.27 DXA forearm scans. (A) DXA forearm scan shows several positioning and acquisition mistakes: The forearm is not straight or centered in the scan field, and motion has occurred in the radius and ulna. (B) Scan shows good patient positioning, scan acquisition, and scan analysis.

6. The placement of the ultradistal ROI should be just below the radial end plate. This placement is easy to reproduce on serial scans. The ultradistal ROI is subject to low BMD, which could create bone edge detection problems. The bone edge should be adjusted if necessary. Baseline and serial scan bone edges must match for proper analysis, comparison, and report of percent change over time.

7. A basic checklist for a good DXA forearm scan (see Fig. 19.27B) includes the following:
   - The forearm is straight and centered in the scan field.
   - Adequate amounts of soft tissue and air are included.
   - No motion is present.
   - The proximal and distal ends of the scan field are properly placed.
   - Bone edges are properly and consistently placed.
   - No artifacts or clothing are present in the scan field.

Other Bone Densitometry Techniques

CENTRAL (OR AXIAL) SKELETAL MEASUREMENTS

QCT is an established method using cross-sectional CT images from commercial scanners equipped with QCT software and a bone mineral reference standard. QCT has the unique ability to provide separate BMD measurements of trabecular and cortical bone and true volumetric density measurements in grams per cubic centimeter (g/cm^3). QCT of the spine is used to measure the trabecular bone within the vertebral bodies to estimate vertebral fracture risk and age-related bone loss; it is also used for follow-up of osteoporosis and other metabolic bone diseases and their therapies (Fig. 19.28). Other current uses of QCT involve measuring BMD at the hip and producing high-resolution three-dimensional images to analyze trabecular bone architecture.

Lateral lumbar spine DXA scans can be performed with the patient in the decubitus lateral position using fan-beam technology. Decubitus lateral scans are obtained with fixed-arm scanners. Lateral spine DXA allows partial removal of the outer cortical bone and gives a truer measurement of the inner trabecular bone, which experiences earlier bone loss and is more responsive to therapy (see Fig. 19.10). However, lateral spine DXA is often confounded by superimposition of the ribs and iliac crest with the vertebral bodies and has poorer precision than does PA spine DXA. Lateral DXA is more widely used in clinical practice for early detection of vertebral fractures and abdominal aortic calcifications.

The term *vertebral fracture assessment (VFA)* encompasses looking at the spine "morphometrically" in the lateral projection, which means visualizing the shapes of the vertebral bodies of the lumbar and thoracic spine to determine if there has been some deformity with resultant

Fig. 19.28 Examples of various elements of QCT examination. *Upper left,* Lateral scout image of lumbar spine. *Upper right,* Localizer lines for midvertebral slices through L1 and L2. *Lower left,* CT slice showing calibration phantom below the patient. *Lower right,* Elliptic ROI positioned in the trabecular bone of the vertebral body.

compression of the vertebral bodies. Dual energy vertebral assessment (DVA), lateral vertebral assessment (LVA), instant vertebral analysis (IVA), and radiologic vertebral assessment (RVA) are synonymous for this process. The manufacturers of bone densitometers have devised their own way of either enhancing the image or improving the scan acquisition and analysis. Images are obtained in dual energy acquisition and the single energy method. Both methods are comparable. VFA is used for the sole purpose of detecting vertebral fractures.

In contrast to traditional lateral spine x-rays, VFA has the capability of visualizing the lumbar and the thoracic spine as one continuous image. This capability aids the interpreting physician in identifying the vertebral level where abnormalities

are present. PA views can also be incorporated into a VFA study. For an accurate representation of the vertebral bodies, the patient's spine must be as straight as possible.

The PA view can help identify artifacts and deformities, such as scoliosis. Scoliosis is a condition that can cause the greatest challenge in VFA and could possibly make a study "unreadable." VFA also exposes the patient to approximately $\frac{1}{100}$ the radiation dose of just a single lateral x-ray image. VFA is an adjunct to DXA scanning in cases where a patient might not have been x-rayed for vertebral fracture beforehand. General spine x-ray is still the "gold standard" for visualizing abnormalities in the spine.

VFA uses single energy x-ray absorptiometry (for image only) or DXA (for

image and BMD) lateral scans of the thoracic and lumbar spines from the level of approximately T4 to L5 (Fig. 19.29). The images are used to determine abnormalities in vertebral shape that may indicate vertebral fragility fractures, which are a strong risk factor for future vertebral fractures. The upper right corner of Fig. 19.29 shows the Genant grading system. The three columns on the right show the types of fracture, and the rows show the grades of severity. Seeing a severe fracture is easy, and seeing a moderate fracture is relatively easy, but it is difficult to determine if a mild deformity is normal for the patient or the beginning of a problem. VFA should be interpreted by a trained physician who is viewing the images on the scan monitor (Fig. 19.30).

Fig. 19.29 Morphometric x-ray absorptiometry scan to detect vertebral shape abnormalities. Genant grading system is in the *upper right corner.*

(Courtesy Hologic, Inc, Bedford, MA.)

Fig. 19.30 Dual VFA.

Total body and body composition

Whole-body DXA measures bone mass (i.e., area, BMC, BMD) and *body composition* for the total body and subregions of the body (e.g., arms, legs, trunk). Body composition can be measured as fat and fat-free mass (with or without BMC) in grams or percent body fat (Fig. 19.31). Careful positioning is required to separate the bones of the forearm and lower leg. Obese patients present a problem when not all of the body fits in the scan field. The ROI must be carefully placed according to the manufacturer's instructions. Having internal or external artifacts that cannot be removed is not unusual; the effect of such artifacts depends on size, density, and location. Hip joint replacement hardware would have more effect than a woman's thin wedding band. Each DXA laboratory should have written SOPs so that all patients are scanned and analyzed consistently. All deviations from normal and artifacts should be noted for the interpreting physician. Whole-body DXA data are useful for studying energy expenditure, energy stores, protein mass, skeletal mineral status, and relative hydration. These measurements have been used in research studies and clinical trials of osteoporosis therapies, obesity, and weight change, fat and lean distribution, and diabetes. Clinically, whole-body scans are used routinely in pediatrics and body fat analysis in athletes and patients with underweight disorders (e.g., anorexia nervosa).

Total Body Bone Density

COMMENTS: D:\data\desktop.dfb

A

Region	BMD¹ (g/cm²)	Young-Adult² T-Score	Age-Matched³ Z-Score
Head	2.467	-	-
Arms	1.115	-	-
Legs	1.341	-	-
Trunk	1.012	-	-
Ribs	0.748	-	-
Pelvis	1.277	-	-
Spine	1.186	-	-
Total	1.278	1.9	2.1

Trend: Total

Measured Date	Age (years)	BMD¹ (g/cm²)	Change vs Baseline (%)	Change vs Baseline (%/yr)
05.14.02	35.1	1.278	0.0	0.0
06.22.00	33.2	1.278	baseline	baseline

Total Body Tissue Quantitation

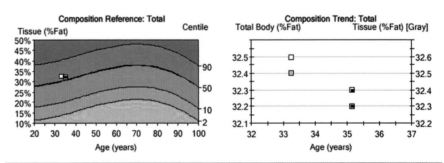

Trend: Total

Measured Date	Age (years)	Tissue (%Fat)	Centile²,³	T.Mass (kg)	Region (%Fat)	Tissue (g)	Fat (g)	Lean (g)	BMC (g)	Fat Free (g)
05.14.02	35.1	32.3	58	62.9	30.8	59,950	19,346	40,603	2,956	43,559
06.22.00	33.2	32.5	61	63.2	31.0	60,256	19,560	40,697	2,922	43,618

Trend: Fat Distribution

Measured Date	Age (years)	Android (%Fat)	Gynoid (%Fat)	A/G Ratio	Total Body (%Fat)
05.14.02	35.1	24.7	44.5	0.55	32.3
06.22.00	33.2	26.3	45.0	0.58	32.5

B

Fig. 19.31 (A) Hologic DXA whole-body scan with printout of total body composition results. (B) Percent body fat (*% Fat*) is reported. *YA,* Young adult.

SKELETAL HEALTH ASSESSMENT IN CHILDREN FROM INFANCY TO ADOLESCENCE

Fracture prediction and definition of osteoporosis

- Evaluation of bone health should identify children and adolescents who may benefit from interventions to decrease their elevated risk of a clinically significant fracture.
- The finding of one or more vertebral compression (crush) fractures is indicative of osteoporosis in the absence of local disease or high-energy trauma. In such children and adolescents, measuring BMD adds to the overall assessment of bone health.
- The diagnosis of osteoporosis in children and adolescents should not be made on the basis of densitometric criteria alone.
- In the absence of vertebral compression (crush) fractures, the diagnosis of osteoporosis is indicated by the presence of both a clinically significant history of fracture and BMD Z-score less than or equal to −2.0. A clinically significant fracture history is one or more of the following: (1) two or more long bone fractures by age 10 years; (2) three or more long bone fractures at any age up to 19 years of age. A BMC/BMD Z-score greater than −2.0 does not preclude the possibility of skeletal fragility and increased fracture risk.

DXA assessment in children and adolescents with disease that may affect the skeleton

- DXA measurement is part of a comprehensive skeletal health assessment in patients with increased risk of fracture.
- In patients with primary bone disease or at risk for a secondary bone disease, a DXA should be performed when the patient may benefit from interventions to decrease their elevated risk of a clinically significant fracture, and the DXA results will influence that management.
- DXA should not be performed if safe and appropriate positioning of the child cannot be ensured.

QCT in children and adolescents

There is no preferred method for QCT for clinical application in children and adolescents. QCT, pQCT peripheral quantitative computed tomography (pQCT), and high-resolution-peripheral quantitative computed tomography (HR-pQCT) are primarily research techniques used to characterize bone deficits in children. They can be used clinically in children when appropriate reference data and expertise are available. It is imperative that QCT protocols in children using general CT scanners implement appropriate exposure factors, calibration phantoms, and software to optimize results and minimize radiation exposure.

Densitometry in infants and young children

DXA is an appropriate method for clinical densitometry of infants and young children. DXA lumbar spine measurements are feasible and can provide reproducible measures of BMC and areal bone mineral density (aBMD) for infants and young children 0 to 5 years of age. DXA whole-body measurements are feasible and can provide reproducible measures of BMC and aBMD for children 3 years or older. DXA whole-body BMC measurements for children younger than 3 years are of limited clinical utility due to feasibility and lack of normative data. Areal BMD should not be used routinely due to difficulty in appropriate positioning. Forearm and femur measurements are technically feasible in infants and young children, but there is insufficient information regarding methodology, reproducibility, and reference data for these measurement sites to be clinically useful at this time. In infants and children younger than 5 years, the impact of growth delay on the interpretation of the DXA results should be considered, but it is not currently quantifiable (Fig. 19.32) (ISCD 2019 Position Statements).

DXA interpretation and reporting in children and adolescents

- DXA is the preferred method for assessing BMC and areal BMD.
- The PA spine and total body less head (TBLH) are the preferred skeletal sites for performing BMC and areal BMD measurements in most pediatric subjects. Soft tissue measures in conjunction with whole-body scans may be helpful in evaluating patients with chronic conditions associated with malnutrition or with muscular and skeletal deficits.
- The hip is not a preferred measurement site in growing children due to variability in skeletal development.
- If a follow-up DXA scan is indicated, the minimum interval between scans is 6 to 12 months.
- In children with short stature or growth delay, spine and TBLH BMC and areal BMD results should be adjusted. For the spine, adjustment should be done using either bone mineral apparent density (BMAD) or the height Z-score. For TBLH, adjust using the height Z-score.
- An appropriate reference data set must include a sample of healthy representatives of the general population sufficiently large to capture variability in bone measures that takes into consideration gender, age, and race/ethnicity.
- When upgrading densitometer instrumentation or software, it is essential to use reference data valid for the hardware and software technologic updates.

Fig. 19.32 Pediatric BMD and soft tissue assessment.

- Baseline DXA reports should contain the following information:
  - DXA manufacturer, model, and software version
  - Referring physician
  - Patient age, gender, race-ethnicity, weight, and height
  - Relevant medical history including previous fractures
  - Indication for study
  - Tanner stage or bone age results, if available
  - Technical quality
  - BMC and areal BMD
  - BMC and/or areal BMD Z-score
  - Source of reference data for Z-score calculation
  - Adjustments made for growth and interpretation
  - Recommendations for the necessity and timing of the next DXA study are optional
- Serial DXA reports should include the same information as for baseline testing. In addition, indications for follow-up scan, technical comparability of studies, changes in height and weight, and changes in BMC and areal BMD Z-scores should be reported.
- Terminology
  - T-scores should not appear in pediatric DXA reports.
  - The term "osteopenia" should not appear in pediatric DXA reports.
  - The term "osteoporosis" should not appear in pediatric DXA reports without a clinically significant fracture history.
  - "Low bone mineral mass or BMD" is the preferred term for pediatric DXA reports when BMC or areal BMD Z-scores are less than or equal to −2.0 SD. (ISCD 2019 Position Statements)

PERIPHERAL SKELETAL MEASUREMENTS

Peripheral bone density measurements include scans of the hand, forearm, heel, and tibia. The scanners are smaller (some are portable), making the scans more available to the public and less expensive than conventional DXA. Peripheral measurements can predict *overall risk of fragility fracture* to the same degree as measurements at central skeletal sites but are not generally accepted for following skeletal response to therapy.

Radiographic absorptiometry is a modern adaptation of the early bone density technique. Digital radiographic absorptiometry uses a hand radiograph that is scanned (digitized) into a computer (Fig. 19.33A). ROI is placed on the digital image of the metacarpals, and estimated BMD is reported (see Fig. 19.33B).

Single energy x-ray absorptiometry, peripheral DXA, and peripheral QCT are adaptations of DXA or QCT for measuring the thinner, easier to penetrate, peripheral skeletal sites. Most scanners measure the wrist (Fig. 19.34) or the heel.

With *QUS* of the heel, ultrasound waves are transmitted laterally through the calcaneus using water, gel, or alcohol (dry system) as a coupling medium (Fig. 19.35). Attenuation increases as the velocity of the ultrasound waves increases, and normal bone attenuates more than osteoporotic bone. These properties of bone and ultrasound signals permit the assessment of the QUS parameters of broadband ultrasound attenuation (BUA) and speed of sound (SOS). BUA, SOS, and proprietary combinations of the two (e.g., stiffness) characterize the mechanical properties of bone relating to elasticity, strength, and consequently fracture risk.

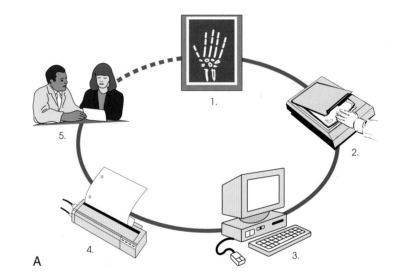

Selected Measurement

Date of recording	1/28/01
Est. BMD	0.480 g/cm²
T-Score	-2.18
Z-Score	-2.51
T-Score (% of H.Y.A)	82
Z-Score (%)	81
Porosity (1-19)	8.2

B

Fig. 19.33 Pronosco X-posure System for digital BMD estimates. (A) Five steps of acquiring and digitizing a standard hand x-ray, keying in patient data, receiving a printout, and discussing results with the patient. (B) Partial report showing automatically placed ROI on the metacarpals, estimated BMD, T-score and Z-score, and a unique porosity measurement.

(Courtesy Pronosco A/S, Vedbaek, Denmark.)

Fig. 19.34 Norland model peripheral DXA performs peripheral DXA bone mineral analysis of the wrist.

(Courtesy Norland/Swissray, Ft. Atkinson, WI.)

Fig. 19.35 QUS of the heel uses either water as a coupling mechanism *(top)* or a dry system using a gel on the transducers *(bottom).*

(Courtesy GE Lunar, Madison, WI.)

FRACTURE RISK MODELS

The University of Sheffield, UK has developed the *FRAX* tool to evaluate the fracture risk of patients. It is based on individual patient models that integrate the risks associated with clinical risk factors and BMD at the femoral neck. It uses clinical risk factors with the femoral BMD to estimate the 10-year probability risk of a major osteoporotic fracture. FRAX is intended to assess fracture risk only and assist the physician in treatment decisions for patients between the ages of 40 and 90 years. It cannot be used if the patient is on pharmacologic treatment for osteoporosis. The FRAX tool and other fracture risk models may assist physicians in making decisions about who to treat, especially patients with low bone mass. Fracture prediction models should be used judiciously in managing individual patients and are not meant to replace clinical judgment (http://www.shef.ac.uk/FRAX).

Trabecular bone score

Trabecular bone score (TBS) is an analytic tool developed in 2008 that performs measurements on lumbar spine DXA images that capture information relating to trabecular microarchitecture. TBS is not a direct measurement of bone microarchitecture but is related to three-dimensional bone characteristics. These include the trabecular number, the trabecular separation, and the connectivity density. ISCD 2019 Position Statements state that TBS is associated with vertebral, hip, and major osteoporotic fracture risk in postmenopausal women and in postmenopausal women with type II diabetes. However, it is associated only with hip and major osteoporotic fracture risk in men over the age of 50 years. TBS is not useful for monitoring bisphosphonate treatment in postmenopausal women with osteoporosis and should not be used alone to determine treatment recommendations in clinical practice. ISCD also states that TBS can be used in association with FRAX and BMD to adjust FRAX probability of fracture in postmenopausal women and older men.

Best Practices for Dual-Energy X-Ray Absorptiometry (DXA)

DXA is a technology used worldwide to diagnose osteoporosis, monitor changes in BMD, and assess fracture risk. The clinical results of the DXA scan are highly dependent on the quality of the scan acquisition, analysis and interpretation. The following best practices describe quality standards for BMD testing that have been derived from the International Society for Clinical Densitometry (ISCD.org). These practices will aid patients, health care providers, and payers in facilitating recognition of high-quality DXA services.

1. *Qualifications:* All bone densitometry technologists should be educated and competent in the areas of anatomy, radiation protection, patient care, history taking, basic computer operation, scanner quality control, patient positioning, scan acquisition and analysis, and proper record keeping and documentation. At least one practicing DXA technologist and preferably all technologists practicing in the DXA department should have a valid certification in bone densitometry. This includes keeping up to date on continuing education. Each DXA technologist should have performed an in vivo precision assessment according to standard methods and calculation of the facility's LSC. Precision Assessment should be standard clinical practice and completed by all technologists. Adherence to state and local safety regulations is necessary.

2. *Radiation safety:* The DXA facility must comply with all applicable radiation safety requirements for both the patient and the technologist. A DXA scan should not be performed unless there is a net benefit to the patient. Radiation exposure should be as low as reasonably achievable (ALARA). Pregnant patients should never be scanned and, if in doubt, follow the "10 day" rule. The technologist should wear an individual dosimetry device to monitor any radiation that might be received. Adhere to all safety regulations that are required by the facility, city, state, and country to minimize radiation exposure.

3. *Standard operating procedures:* Each DXA facility should have a detailed SOP for DXA procedures that is updated routinely and available for all personnel to follow. Examples of three different categories of SOPs include pre-testing, testing, and post-testing. *Pre-testing* consists of patient scheduling, patient preparation, patient education, instrument calibration, and maintenance. *Testing* should include the selection of accurate skeletal sites, scan mode, acquisition, and patient positioning. *Post-testing* should be accurate analysis, interpretation, and reporting. Individuals who are involved in all aspects of bone density should participate in the development of the document. This will help reduce errors, improve patient and technologist safety, and produce consistent quality scans. Failure to follow SOPs may result in invalid data, which can lead to potentially harmful patient care.

4. *Professionalism:* Ethical conduct and professionalism in the workplace is a requirement of all health care professionals. The technologist should adhere to the Code of Ethics for Radiologic Technologists (Chapter 1) and the ASRT Bone Density Practice Standards. The HIPAA of 1996 must also be followed to ensure the privacy of the patient's health information.

5. *Scan acquisition and analysis:* There are important manufacturer-specific differences in DXA hardware, software, instrument operation, and requirements for patient positioning, acquisition, and analysis. Each technologist must be knowledgeable in their specific DXA manufacturer as it is the primary source for quality control standards, instrument maintenance, patient scanning, and data analysis. Deviation from the recommended procedures may adversely affect the validity of the BMD measurements. The accuracy and precision of BMD measurements by DXA can be directly affected by changes in instrument performance that may occur as a calibration "shift" or "drift." Phantom scanning on a regular basis can determine when a DXA system is out of calibration and requires service. If the phantom falls outside acceptable ranges, then patient scanning should be postponed until machine service occurs.

6. *Interpretation and reporting:* It is recommended that at least one practicing DXA interpreter/clinician, and preferably all interpreters, have a valid certification in bone densitometry. This includes keeping up to date on continuing education. DXA reports must provide correct and meaningful information for the referring health care provider to provide quality bone health care. By passing an examination and receiving a certification in Bone Densitometry, an interpreter provides evidence that this skill set has been met.

Conclusion

The main purpose of bone densitometry is to assist the diagnosis of osteoporosis by detecting low bone mass before fractures occur. Osteoporosis is a preventable and treatable disease. Patients concerned about their risk of this disease should consult their physicians for a complete evaluation.

DXA scans of the hip and spine are the most widely performed techniques and considered the gold standard, but simpler, less expensive peripheral scans of the extremities are also available for screening purposes. Radiographers using bone densitometry equipment must be properly trained in scanner quality control, anatomy, patient scan positioning, acquisition, and analysis. This training ensures accurate and precise bone density results.

Knowledge of current treatments and expected changes is important for complete technical evaluation of the scan results. History taking and data input are valuable tools for completion of this examination. Technologists are frontline educators to patients, and knowledge in the field is ever changing. The technologist must keep informed about the treatment options and their effects on bone density.

Quality assurance is a key factor in accurate and precise DXA acquisition and analysis. Technology changes frequently, so it is important for the technologist to understand the changes within the industry. The technologist must be able to oversee these applications to maintain and update equipment properly.

Definition of Terms

ALARA (as low as reasonably achievable): Principle of reducing patient radiation exposure and dose to lowest reasonable amounts.

anthropomorphic: Simulating human form.

areal technique: See *projectional technique.*

array-beam collimation: Dual-energy x-ray absorptiometry system that uses a narrow "slit" x-ray collimator and a multielement detector. The motion is in one direction only, which greatly reduces scan time and permits supine lateral spine scans. It introduces a slight geometric distortion at the outer edges, which necessitates careful centering of the object of interest.

biochemical markers: Laboratory tests on blood and urine to detect levels of bone formation or resorption.

body composition: Results from whole-body scans obtained by dual energy x-ray absorptiometry; reported as lean mass in grams, percent body fat, and bone mineral density of the total body and selected regions of interest.

bone densitometry: Art and science of measuring bone mineral content and density of specific anatomic sites or the whole body.

bone mass: General term for amount of mineral in a bone.

bone mineral content (BMC): Measure of bone mineral in the total area of a region of interest.

bone mineral density (BMD): Measure of bone mineral per unit area of a region of interest.

bone remodeling: Process of bone resorption by osteoclasts, followed by bone formation by osteoblasts. The relative rates of resorption and formation determine whether bone mass increases, remains stable, or decreases.

celiac disease: Disease characterized by hypersensitivity to gluten (wheat protein).

compare feature: Software feature of dual energy x-ray absorptiometry that replicates the size and placement of regions of interest from the reference scan to the follow-up scan.

cortical bone: Dense, compact outer shell of all bones and the shafts of the long bones; supports weight, resists bending and twisting, and accounts for approximately 80% of the skeletal mass.

cross-calibration: Cross-calibration of numbers is needed to calculate the average BMD relationship and least significant change between the initial machine and new machine of a DXA facility. It is not possible to quantitatively compare BMD or to calculate LSC between facilities without cross-calibration.

discordance: Patient may have T-score indicating osteoporosis at one anatomic site but not at another site or by one modality but not by another.

dual energy x-ray absorptiometry (DXA): Bone density measurement technique using an x-ray source separated into two energies. It has good accuracy and precision and can scan essentially any anatomic site, making it the most versatile of the bone density techniques.

dual photon absorptiometry (DPA): Obsolete method of measuring bone density at the hip or spine using a radio-isotope source that produces two sources of photons; replaced by dual energy x-ray absorptiometry.

fragility fractures: Nontraumatic fractures resulting from low bone mass, usually at the hip, spinal vertebrae, wrist, proximal humerus, or ribs.

FRAX: Fracture risk assessment tool developed by the World Health Organization.

HIPAA: The American Health Insurance Portability and Accountability Act of 1996 (HIPAA) is a set of rules to be followed by health plans, physicians, hospitals, and other health care providers. HIPAA took effect on April 14, 2003. In the health care and medical profession, the great challenge that HIPAA has created is the assurance that all patient account handling, billing, and medical records are HIPAA compliant.

hyperparathyroidism: Disease caused by excessive secretion of parathyroid hormone (PTH) from one or more parathyroid glands, resulting in excessive calcium in the blood; affects cortical bone more than trabecular bone.

kyphosis: Exaggerated outward curvature of the thoracic spine, also called *dowager's hump.*

least significant change (LSC): Amount of change in bone density needed to be statistically confident that a real change has occurred.

longitudinal quality control: Manufacturer-defined procedures performed on a regular basis to ensure that patients are scanned on properly functioning equipment with stable calibration. Scanning must be postponed until identified problems are corrected.

mean: Statistic commonly called the average; sum of the data values divided by the number of data values.

morphometric x-ray absorptiometry (MXA): Lateral scans of the thoracic and lumbar spine using single energy or dual energy x-ray absorptiometry to determine vertebral abnormalities or fractures from the shapes of the vertebrae.

osteoblasts: Bone-building cells that fill the pits left by resorption with new bone.

osteoclasts: Bone-destroying cells that break down and remove old bone, leaving pits.

osteomalacia: Bone disorder characterized by variable amounts of uncalcified osteoid matrix.

osteopenia/low bone mass: Reduction in bone mass, putting a person at increased risk of developing osteoporosis. By World Health Organization criteria, it is a bone mineral density or bone mineral content T-score between −1 and −2.5. *Low bone mass* or *low bone density* is the preferred term.

osteophytosis: Form of degenerative joint disease resulting from mechanical stress that increases measured spinal bone mineral density.

osteoporosis: Systemic skeletal disease characterized by low bone mass and deterioration of bone structure, resulting in decreased mechanical competence of bone and an increase in susceptibility to fracture. By World Health Organization criteria, it is a bone mineral density or bone mineral content T-score of less than −2.5.

overall risk of fragility fracture: Risk of sustaining an unspecified fragility fracture. The risk for hip fracture specifically is best measured at the hip.

peak bone mass: Maximum bone mass, usually achieved between 20 and 30 years of age. Population mean peak bone mass is used as a reference point for the T-score.

pencil-beam collimation: Dual energy x-ray absorptiometry system using a circular pinhole x-ray collimator that produces a narrow x-ray stream, which is received by a single detector. Its motion is serpentine (or raster) across or along the length of the body. Modern systems have improved scan time and image quality. Off-centering of the object does not cause geometric distortion.

percent coefficient of variation (%CV): Statistic used to compare standard deviations from different data sets, which may have different means; also a measure of precision; calculated as SD ÷ mean × 100. A smaller %CV indicates better precision.

peripheral dual energy x-ray absorptiometry (pDXA): Dual energy x-ray absorptiometry system designed to scan only the peripheral skeleton; smaller and simpler to operate than DXA scanners.

peripheral quantitative computed tomography (pQCT): Dedicated QCT system designed to measure bone density on the peripheral skeleton, usually the forearm.

picture archiving communication system (PACS): Medical imaging technology that provides economical storage and convenient access to images from multiple modalities.

primary osteoporosis: Osteoporosis not caused by an underlying disease, classified as type I or type II.

projectional (or areal) technique: Two-dimensional representation of a three-dimensional object.

quantitative computed tomography (QCT): System for quantitative CT measurements of bone density, allowing true measurement of volume and separation of trabecular and cortical bone; usually measured at the spine or forearm, sometimes at the hip.

quantitative ultrasound (QUS): Quantitative measurement of bone properties related to mechanical competence using ultrasound. The results are reported in terms of broadband ultrasound attenuation (BUA); speed of sound (SOS); and a non-standardized proprietary mathematic combination of the two, called the *stiffness* or *quantitative ultrasound index* (QUI). It predicts overall or spine fracture risk without using ionizing radiation and is usually measured at the calcaneus.

radiogrammetry: Older method of measuring bone loss by comparing the outer diameter and inner medullary diameter of small tubular bones, usually the finger phalanges, or metacarpals.

radiographic absorptiometry (RA): Visual comparison of hand x-ray density with a known standard in the exposure field.

reference population: Large, sex-matched, community-based population used to determine the average bone mineral density and standard deviation at each age; used as reference base for T-scores and Z-scores; may also be matched on ethnicity and weight.

regions of interest (ROI): Defined portion of bone density scans where the bone mineral density is calculated; may be placed manually or automatically by computer software.

scintillation counter: Counter using a photomultiplier tube for detection of radiation.

secondary osteoporosis: Osteoporosis caused by an underlying disease.

serial scans: Sequential scans, usually performed 12, 18, or 24 months apart, to measure changes in bone density. Scans are best done on the same scanner or on a new scanner cross-calibrated to the original scanner.

Shewhart Control Chart rules: Classic quality control rules based on comparing a data value with the mean and standard deviation of a set of similar values.

sieverts (Sv): Measurement of effective radiation dose to a patient. Bone density doses are measured in microsieverts (µSv), which are one millionth of 1 sievert.

single energy x-ray absorptiometry (SXA): Bone density technique for the peripheral skeleton, making use of a single energy x-ray source and an external medium, such as water, to correct for the effects of soft tissue attenuation. Scanners are smaller and simpler to operate than dual energy x-ray absorptiometry scanners.

single photon absorptiometry (SPA): Obsolete method of measuring bone density at the forearm using a single radioisotope source; replaced by single energy x-ray absorptiometry.

standard deviation (SD): Measure of the variability of data values around the mean value.

subtraction technique: Removal of the density attributable to soft tissue so that the remaining density belongs to bone only

total body less head (TBLH): Total body scanning less head analysis.

trabecular bone: Delicate, latticework structure within bones that adds strength without excessive weight; supports compressive loading at the spine, hip, and calcaneus and is found in the ends of long bones, such as the distal radius.

trabecular bone score (TBS): Analytic tool that performs measurements on lumbar spine DXA images to capture information relating to trabecular microarchitecture.

T-score: Number of standard deviations an individual's bone mineral density (BMD) is from the average BMD for sex-matched, young normal peak bone masses.

type I osteoporosis: Primary osteoporosis related to postmenopausal status.

type II osteoporosis: Primary osteoporosis related to aging.

vertebral fracture assessment (VFA): Encompasses looking at the spine "morphometrically" in the lateral projection. Common synonymous terms are *dual energy vertebral assessment (DVA), lateral vertebral assessment (LVA), instant vertebral assessment (IVA),* and *radiologic vertebral assessment (RVA).*

volumetric density: Bone mineral density calculated by dividing by the true three-dimensional volume.

Ward triangle: Region on proximal femur lying on the border of the femoral neck and greater trochanter; has low bone mineral density. Cannot be used in diagnosis.

Z-score: Number of standard deviations the individual's bone mineral density (BMD) is from the average BMD for a sex-matched and age-matched reference group.

Resources for information and instruction

American College of Radiology: ACR standard for the performance of adult dual or single x-ray absorptiometry (DXA/pDXA/SXA). Contact the Standards & Accreditation Department, Preston White Drive, Reston, VA, 1891, American College of Radiology. 22091.

American Registry of Radiologic Technologists: Provides a postprimary examination leading to a certificate of added qualifications in bone densitometry. For details, see the Examinee handbook for bone densitometry. Contact the American Registry of Radiologic Technologists, 1255 Northland Drive, St Paul, MN 55120-1155. Web site: www.arrt.org.

American Society of Radiologic Technologists: Approved elective curriculum in bone densitometry for radiography programs. Contact the American Society of Radiologic Technologists, 15000 Central Avenue SE, Albuquerque, NM 87123. Web site: www.asrt.org.

Best Practices for Dual-Energy X-ray Absorptiometry Measurement and Reporting: International Society for Clinical Densitometry Guidance. Journal of Clinical Densitometry Assessment & Management of Musculoskeletal Health.

Contact International Society for Clinical Densitometry 955 South Main St. Building C Middletown, CT 06457. Web site: www.iscd.org.

International Society for Clinical Densitometry: Certification courses, annual and regional meetings, continuing education, newsletter, Journal of Clinical Densitometry, and web site with links to Official Positions and Pediatric Official Positions. Contact International Society for Clinical Densitometry 955 South Main St. Building C Middletown, CT 06457. Web site: www.iscd.org.

National Osteoporosis Foundation: Excellent source of osteoporosis information and educational materials for technologists, physicians, and patients. Contact the National Osteoporosis Foundation, 1232 22nd Street NW, Washington, DC 20037-1292. Web site: www.nof.org.

Scanner manufacturers: source for technologist instruction and answers to scanner-specific application questions. Refer to the operator's manual for contact information.

StrongerBones.org

Surgeon General's Report. Web site: www.surgeongeneral.gov.

References

1. Gowin W, Felsenberg D. Acronyms in osteodensitometry. *J Clin Densitomet.* 1998;1:137.

2. National Institutes of Health Consensus Development Panel on Osteoporosis Prevention. Diagnosis, and Therapy: Osteoporosis prevention, diagnosis, and therapy. *JAMA.* 2001;285:785–795.

Selected bibliography

American Society of Radiologic Technologist (ASRT). Available at: https://www.asrt.org/main/standards-and-regulations/professional-practice/practice-standards. (Accessed August 17, 2020.)

Blunt BA, et al. Good clinical practice and audits for dual x-ray absorptiometry and x-ray imaging laboratories and quality assurance centers involved in clinical drug trials, private practice, and research. *J Clin Densitomet.* 1998;1:323.

Bone Health and Osteoporosis. Available at: https://www.bones.nih.gov/health-info/bone/SGR/surgeon-generals-report. (Accessed August 17, 2020.)

FRAX. WHO Fracture Risk Assessment tool. Available at: http://www.shef.ac.uk/FRAX. (Accessed August 15, 2020.)

Genant HK. Development of formulas for standardized DXA measurements. *J Bone Miner Res.* 1995;9:997.

Genant HK, et al. Universal standardization for dual x-ray absorptiometry: patient and phantom cross-calibration results. *J Bone Miner Res.* 1994;9:1503.

Harvey NC, Glüer CC, Binkley N, et al. Trabecular bone score (TBS) as a new complementary approach for osteoporosis evaluation in clinical practice. *Bone.* 2015;78:216–224.

International Osteoporosis Foundation. Facts and Statistics (website). Available at: www.iofbonehealth.org. (Accessed August 17, 2020.)

International Society for Clinical Densitometry. Official positions. Available at: http://www.iscd.org/Visitors/positions/OfficialPositionsPowerPoint.cfm ISCD.org. (Accessed August 15, 2020.)

Mayo Clinic. Available at: https://www.mayoclinic.org/diseases-conditions/osteoporosis/diagnosis-treatment/drc-20351974. (Accessed August 17, 2020.)

National Institutes of Health Consensus Development Panel on Osteoporosis Prevention, Diagnosis, and Therapy. Osteoporosis prevention, diagnosis, and therapy. *JAMA.* 2001;285:785.

National Osteoporosis Foundation. Available at: www.nof.org. (Accessed August 17, 2020.)

National Osteoporosis Foundation physician's guide. Washington, DC: National Osteoporosis Foundation; 1998.

National Osteoporosis Foundation. Available at: https://www.nof.org/2014/06/02/54-million-americans-affected-by-osteoporosis-and-low-bone-mass/. (Accessed August 17, 2020.)

ADDENDUM B
SUMMARY OF ABBREVIATIONS, VOLUME TWO

ACR	American College of Radiology	EU	excretory urogram	MVTA	motor vehicle traffic accident
AML	acanthiomeatal line	GFR	glomerular filtration rate	NPO	nil per os (nothing by mouth)
AP	anteroposterior	GML	glabellomeatal line	OID	object–to–image receptor (IR)
ASRT	American Society of Radiologic	GSW	gunshot wound		distance
	Technologists	HSG	hysterosalpingography	OML	orbitomeatal line
BE	barium enema	IAM	internal acoustic meatus	PA	posteroanterior
BPH	benign prostatic hyperplasia	IOML	infraorbitomeatal line	PTC	percutaneous transhepatic
BUN	blood urea nitrogen	IPL	interpupillary line		cholangiography
CDC	Centers for Disease Control and	IR	image receptor	RUQ	right upper quadrant
	Prevention	IUD	intrauterine device	SID	source–to–image receptor (IR)
CNS	central nervous system	IV	intravenous		distance
CPR	cardiopulmonary resuscitation	IVP	intravenous pyelogram	SMV	submentovertical
CR	central ray	IVU	intravenous urography	TEA	top of ear attachment
CSF	cerebrospinal fluid	KUB	kidneys, ureters, and bladder	TMJ	temporomandibular joint
CT	computed tomography	LES	lower esophageal sphincter	UES	upper esophageal sphincter
CTC	CT colonography	MBSS	modified barium swallow study	UGI	upper gastrointestinal
CVA	cerebrovascular accident	MCP	midcoronal plane	UPJ	ureteropelvic junction
EAM	external acoustic meatus	MML	mentomeatal line	UVJ	ureterovesical junction
ED	emergency department	MPR	multiplanar reconstruction	VC	virtual colonoscopy
ERCP	endoscopic retrograde	MRI	magnetic resonance imaging	VCUG	voiding cystourethrogram
	cholangiopancreatography	MSP	midsagittal plane	VFSS	videofluoroscopic swallow study

INDEX

Page numbers followed by *f*, *t*, or *b* indicate figures, tables, or boxes, respectively. **Boldface** numbers indicate the volume.

Index

Index

Index

Index

Index

Egas Moniz
(1874-1955)

Schüller
(1874-1957)

Lysholm
(1891-1947)

Albers-Schönberg
(1865-1921)

Béclère, H.
(1880-1937)

Fuchs
(1895-1962)

Waters
(1888-1961)